Computational Cytology

Pranab Dey

Computational Cytology

Advancements and Applications with Artificial Intelligence

Springer

Pranab Dey
Professor of Oncopathology, Homi Bhabha
Cancer Hospital and Research Centre
(Tata Memorial Center), New Chandigarh
Homi Bhabha Cancer Hospital and Research Centre
(Homi Bhabha National Institute), New Chandigarh
Chandigarh, Chandigarh, India

ISBN 978-981-95-3271-1 ISBN 978-981-95-3272-8 (eBook)
https://doi.org/10.1007/978-981-95-3272-8

This Springer imprint is published by the registered company Springer Nature Singapore Pte Ltd.
The registered company address is: 152 Beach Road, #21-01/04 Gateway East, Singapore 189721, Singapore

Dedicated to

Shree Shree Satyananda Giri,

Shree Shree Paramahansa Yogananda,

Rini, and Madhumanti

Preface

Currently we are in an age of digital technology and machine learning. Artificial intelligence is now considered as an emerging technology with high potential. In the field of cytology, the amalgamation of digital cytology and artificial intelligence has given birth to a completely new branch entitled "Computational Cytology". The book discusses the various aspects of computational cytology. Special emphasis has been given to artificial intelligence and its subset deep learning. The book is equipped with multiple boxes, tables and figures to make the chapters updated and simplified. In addition, practical guidelines are given to make the neural network model. I strongly believe that this book will help pathologists and researchers to understand artificial intelligence and also to apply it in the respective field.

Chandigarh
July 2025

Pranab Dey

Acknowledgements

I am thankful to Vandana Joshi, Associate Editor of Springer Nature, who suggested the topic of the book and offered me the opportunity to write this book. I express my sincere thanks to Jayanthi Adilingam, production editor.

My heartiest thanks to my wife, Rini, and my daughter, Madhumanti, for their continuous cooperation and patience towards me.

I express my gratitude to God Almighty, without His grace nothing is possible. He is the ultimate intelligence in this comic world.

Chandigarh
July 2025

Pranab Dey

Contents

Abbreviations

AdaIN	Adaptive Instance Normalization
ADC	Adenocarcinoma
AUC	Area Under Curve
AI	Artificial Intelligence
ANN	Artificial Neural Network
AUS	Atypia of Undetermined Cases
AE	Autoencoder
BGD	Batch Gradient Descent
BERT	Bidirectional Encoder Representations from Transformers
BigGAN	Big Generative Adversarial Network
BIF	Big Image File
BQP	Bounded-Error Quantum Polynomial Time
CCE	Categorical Cross-Entropy
cfDNA	Cell Free DNA
ctDNA	Circulating Tumour DNA
cPTC	Classic Papillary Thyroid Carcinoma
CDS	Clinical Decision Support
CAP	College of American Pathologists
CRC	Colorectal Cancers
CMOS	Complementary Metal-Oxide-Semiconductor
Ccyt	Computational cytology
cGAN	Conditional GAN
CNN	Convolutional Neural Network
CNV	Copy Number Variant
CycleGAN	Cycle-Consistent Generative Adversarial Network
DCCA	Deep Canonical Correlation Analysis
DCNN	Deep Convolutional Neural Network
DL	Deep Learning
DLS	Deep Learning System
DICOM	Digital Imaging and Communications in Medicine
D	Discriminator Network
DCIS	Ductal Carcinoma In Situ
HER	Electronic Health Record
EPIC-seq	Epigenetic Expression Inference from Cell Free DNA-Sequencing

ER	Estrogen Receptor
FN	False Negative
FP	False Positive
FNN	Feed Forward Neural Network
FNAC	Fine Needle Aspiration Cytology
FISH	Fluorescence In Situ Hybridization
FPGS	FocalPoint GS Imaging System
FLUS	Follicular Lesions Of Undetermined Significance
FDA	Food and Drug Association
GRU	Gated Recurrent Unit
GRU	Gated Recurrent Units
GEO	Gene Expression Omnibus
GAN	Generative Adversarial Networks
G	Generative Network
GPT	Generative Pre-Trained Transformer
GATK	Genome Analysis Toolkit
GCS	Google Cloud Space
GBM	Gradient Boosting Machine
GD	Gradient Descent
GCN	Graph Convolutional Network
GPU	Graphics Processing Unit
H&E	Haematoxylin and Eosin
HEIF	High Efficiency Image Format
HSIL	High Grade Squamous Intraepithelial Lesions
MSI-H	High microsatellite instability
HASHI	High-throughput Adaptive Sampling for whole-slide Histopathology Image analysis
HIS	Hospital Information Service
HDFF	Hybrid Deep Feature Fusion
Tanh	Hyperbolic Tangent
ICC	Immunocytochemistry
IHC	Immunohistochemistry
INDEL	Insertion or Deletion of Nucleotides
ICGA	International Cancer Genome Consortium
JPEG	Joint Photographic Expert Group
LIS	Laboratory Information Systems
LCNE	Large Cell Neuroendocrine Carcinomas
LMMF	Large Multimodal Foundation Models
LED	Light Emitting Diode
LBC	Liquid-Based Cytology
LSTM	Long Short-Term Memory
LSIL	Low Grade Squamous Intraepithelial Lesions
MSH-L	Low Microsatellite Instability
ML	Machine Learning
MAE	Mean Absolute Error

MSE	Mean Squared Error
MSI	Microsatellite Instability
miRNA-Seq	miRNA Sequencing
MMR	Mismatch Repair
MMF	Multimodal Foundation Models
NER	Named Entity Recognition
NLP	Natural Language Processing
NST	Neural Style Transfer
NGS	Next-Generation Sequencing
NILM	No Intraepithelial Lesion and Malignancy
NSCLC	Non-Squamous Cell Lung Carcinoma
NIFTP	Noninvasive Follicular Thyroid Neoplasm with Papillary-like nuclear features
OpenCV	Open Source Computer Vision Library
OD	Optical Density
OUTRIDER	Outlier in RNA-Seq Finder
ONT	Oxford Nanopore Technologies
PTC	Papillary Thyroid Carcinoma
PQC	Parametrized Quantum Circuits
PSO	Particle Swarm Optimization
PCR	Polymerase Chain Reaction
PNG	Portable Network Graphics
PR	Progesterone Receptor
PDL-1	Programmed Cell Death Ligand-1
PPI	Protein-Protein Interaction
QADA	Quantum Adversarial Domain Adaptation
QNN	Quantum Artificial Neural Network
QCNN	Quantum Convolutional Neural Network
QFT	Quantum Fourier Transform
QKM	Quantum Kernel Method
QML	Quantum Machine Learning
RF	Random Forests
ROC	Receiver Operating Characteristic
ReLU	Rectified Linear Units
RNN	Recurrent Neural Network
RGB	Red Green Blue
ROI	Region of Interest
RL	Reinforcement Learning
RAG	Retrieval-Augmented Generation
SSL	Self-Supervised Learning
SMILES	Simplified Molecular Input Line Entry System
SNP	Single Nucleotide Polymorphism
SNV	Single Nucleotide Variants
SVD	Singular Value Decomposition
SCC	Small Cell Carcinoma

SCCE	Sparse Categorical Cross-Entropy
SQC	Squamous Cell Carcinoma
SGD	Stochastic Gradient Descent
StyleGAN	Style-Based Generative Adversarial Network
SVM	Support Vector Machine
TIFF	Tagged Image File Format
TFN	Tensor Fusion Networks
TBSRTC	The Bethesda System Reporting for Thyroid Cytopathology
TCGA	The Cancer Genome Atlas
TCIA	The Cancer Imaging Archive
TF	Transcription Factor
TLS	Transfer Learning
TN	True Negative
TP	True Positive
TIL	Tumour Infiltrating Lymphocytes
TME	Tumour Microenvironment
TMB	Tumour Mutation Burden
TPS	Tumour Proportion Score
TSR	Tumour-Stromal Ratio
VQA	Variational Quantum Algorithm
VQA	Visual Question Answering
WGAN	Wasserstein GAN
WSI	Whole Slide Imaging

Part I

Computational Integration in Cytology

Introduction to Computational Cytology 1

Abstract

Recently, there have been significant progress in digital cytology, whole-slide imaging, and Artificial Intelligence (AI). Artificial intelligence (AI) can help to make a mathematical model that can extract actionable clinical information regarding disease identification, stratification and management. The "computational cytology" is an emerging field that encompasses the digital cytology, patient's metadata and artificial intelligence. By definition, it refers to the incorporation of digital imaging data from the cytology smear, patient metadata and molecular data into a mathematical model using a computer to obtain clinically useful information. In the present chapter, the development of computational cytology and its potential applications in cytology are discussed.

Keywords

Computational cytology · Artificial intelligence · Digital cytology · Whole slide imaging

1.1 Introduction

In the last few decades, significant developments have occurred in the medical field. The rapid progress of high-throughput laboratory and information technologies has brought a revolution in pathology. The digitization of the whole slide by whole slide imaging (WSI) helps to analyse the cellular pattern and individual cell morphology. There is also a huge accumulation of data from the molecular and proteomics profiles. It is becoming more difficult to handle such huge data in a systematic and actionable way. The rapid progress of computational power and artificial intelligence has brought a revolution in the medical field. The patient's raw data including imaging of the slide, molecular data and clinical data can be analysed in a

P. Dey, *Computational Cytology*, https://doi.org/10.1007/978-981-95-3272-8_1

mathematical model. AI can help to make a mathematical model that can extract actionable clinical information regarding disease identification, stratification, management, etc. By definition, "computational cytology" means the incorporation of digital imaging data of the cytology smear, patient metadata and molecular data in a mathematical model by a computer to obtain clinically useful information [1, 2].

Computational cytology is a newly developed and emerging branch of pathology. In the world of rapid outburst of data technology, computational cytology will help us to reach a clinically useful data extraction.

1.2 Evolution of Cytology: From Microscope to Machine Learning

The history of evolution of computational cytology is depicted in Fig. 1.1. There are certain revolutions in the field of pathology. The first revolution is immunohistochemistry/immunocytochemistry in the late 1980s. The second revolution occurred when molecular biology was introduced in clinical pathology in the year 2005. The third revolution is the digital pathology and artificial intelligence [3] (2017).

Light Microscope The introduction of the light microscope in 1850 started the new age of microscopy-based diagnosis in pathology. The cytologists are habituated to reporting by observing cellular patterns and individual cell morphology on the smear. A simple microscopic examination was enough to gather information from the smear and to draw inferences [4]. The simple microscopic examination of the cytology smear is easy and effective. However, traditional microscopy is manual, subjective and labour-intensive and may affect diagnostic consistency and accuracy. Moreover, cytopathologists should have years of experience to diagnose difficult cases by simple microscopic examination (Box 1.1). In comparison, the digital microscopy provides images easy to read, transferable and easy to store with objective estimation of the cellular morphometric features (Fig. 1.2).

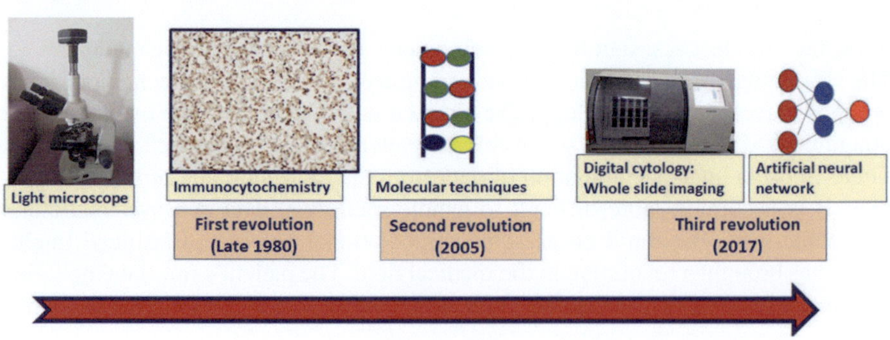

Fig. 1.1 Historical evolution of computational cytology

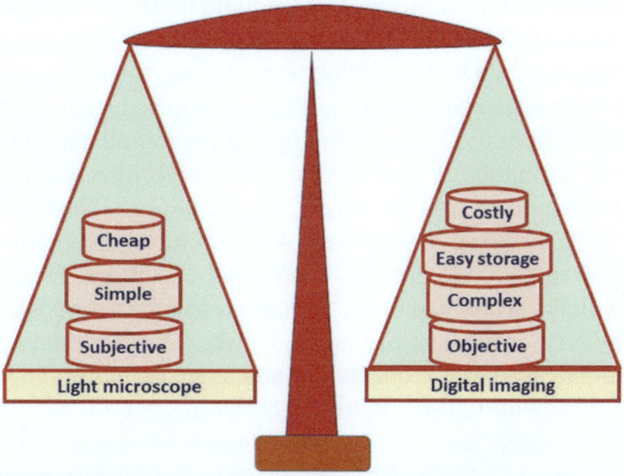

Fig. 1.2 The comparison of light microscopy versus digital imaging

Box 1.1: Limitations of Light Microscope

- Subjective interpretation
- Variable diagnostic accuracy
- Expert and experienced pathologist needed
- Occasionally, it may be difficult to correlate the image data with immunocytochemistry and molecular data

Immunocytochemistry (ICC) In the late 1980s and early part of 1990, immunohistochemistry (IHC) was introduced in the laboratories [5].

The application of IHC and ICC on histopathology and cytology samples can be considered the first revolution in pathology/cytology. With the help of ICC, the character of the cells can be identified. ICC is widely useful in the diagnosis of undifferentiated malignancy, source of primary sites, prognostic assessment and management [6]. Anyone in the laboratory can do the ICC. It is a relatively cheap and easy-to-do technique (Box 1.2). The ICC involves visual interpretation and also to some extent subjective.

Box 1.2: Pros and Cons of Immunocytochemistry

Advantages

- Easy to perform
- Relatively cheap
- Provides essential information to diagnose problematic cases

Limitations

- Needs strict validation
- Interpretation is subjective

Molecular Technique DNA double helix was discovered in the year 1950. In the years 1960 to 1980, DNA was extracted and gel electrophoresis was done. Southern blotting for DNA and Northern blotting for RNA were done with labelled probe. Polymerase chain reaction (PCR) was introduced in the year 1983. It revolutionized the field of molecular pathology as the minute amount of DNA can be analysed by this technique. Fluorescence in Situ Hybridization (FISH) helped to visualize the DNA mutation in the tissue. Post 2000 era, Next-Generation Sequencing (NGS) was introduced in pathology which allowed comprehensive analysis of the genome and epigenomic changes with rapid speed and excellent accuracy [7]. NGS was widely used in pathology laboratories in the year 2010 onwards. The data generated by NGS is huge and complex. Unlike ICC, the interpretation of the molecular techniques does not require the knowledge of morphology. The molecular techniques are difficult to do in routine laboratories and the technique is complex and difficult to interpret (Box 1.3). The applications of molecular techniques in cytology/pathology can be considered as the second revolution in pathology.

Box 1.3: Next-Generation Sequencing

Advantages

- Provides thorough knowledge of the gene sequence and mutational changes.
- Gives comprehensive analysis of the genome, transcriptome and epigenetics.

Limitations

- Costly
- Needs special skills to do
- NGS provides huge and complex data that often needs AI to interpret

Digitalization and AI The introduction of the whole slide scanner along with the application of AI has brought revolutionary changes in cytology [8]. Previously, only a part of the cytology smear was analysed. The whole slide imaging (WSI) uploads the entire smear in the computer. The digital images are easy to transport from one place to another. Several whole slide scanners are available commercially. Each of the scanners has its own merit and demerits. In April 2017, Food and Drug Association (FDA) approved Philips IntelliSite digital scanner for the reporting of Pathology slides [9]. Later on, Aperio AT2 DX Digital Pathology System of Leica Biosystems was also approved by FDA [10].

Previously, WSI was used mainly for research and educational purposes. However, now WSI are used in diagnostic and prognostic purposes. AI is a rapidly developing science. It can analyse the complex data efficiently and meaningfully. Deep learning is a part of AI that can extract the features from the images without any external intervention [11, 12].

The comparison of different techniques in cytology is highlighted in Table 1.1.

Table 1.1 The comparison of different techniques in cytology

Feature	Light microscope	Immuno-cytochemistry	Molecular techniques	Computational cytology
Accessibility	Easy	Relatively easy	Difficult	Difficult
Cost	Cheap	Relatively cheap	Costly	Costly
Technical complexity	Simple	Relatively simple	Complex	Complex
Interpretation	Easy	Relatively easy	Difficult	Difficult
Visualization	Possible and dependent on morphology	Morphology dependent	Independent of morphology	Comprehensive and morphology included

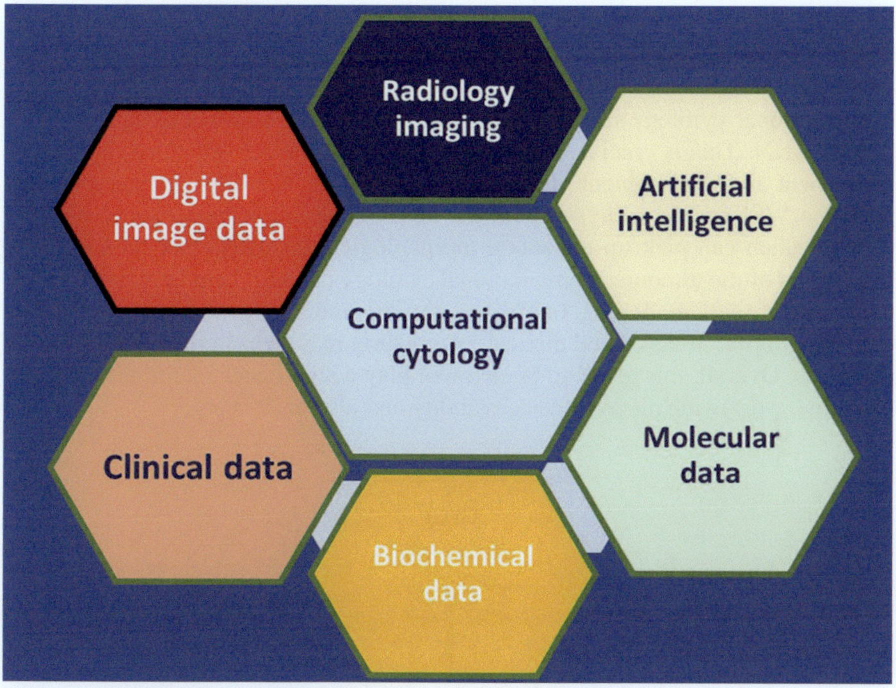

Fig. 1.3 Computational cytology at a glance

1.3 Computational Cytology: A Journey in the Unknown Path

Currently, the cytologist deals with a vast amount of data that include clinical information, biochemical investigation, radiological imaging data, digital image data and molecular data (Fig. 1.3). It is a great challenge to extract the actionable information from these huge data. Moreover, the molecular data is often complex, particularly the data from NGS (Box 1.4). Computational cytology can integrate different dimensional data and apply the information in diagnosis, sub-classification, prognostic assessment and management of disease. Moreover, it is immensely useful in personalized medicine.

Box 1.4: Importance of Computational Cytology
- To handle a vast amount of data
- To handle complex data
- The integration of different datasets
- Model development to solve specific problems
- Development of personalized medicine

1.4 Conclusions

Computational cytology revolutionized the analysis of multimodal data with the help of ANN. This is crucial for the early diagnosis, cancer screening, prognostic assessment and management of the patient (Fig. 1.4). The digital image obtained from the WSI can be analysed with the help of a convolutional neural network (CNN) which can pick up the subtle morphological changes associated with the behaviours of the tumours. Computational cytology can also help in biomarker discovery and disease modelling. In addition, the integration of genomic and proteomic data with digital imaging and clinical information may help in the comprehensive diagnosis. Overall, this growing branch will play a significant role in personalized medicine, worldwide diagnostic accessibility and also basic research.

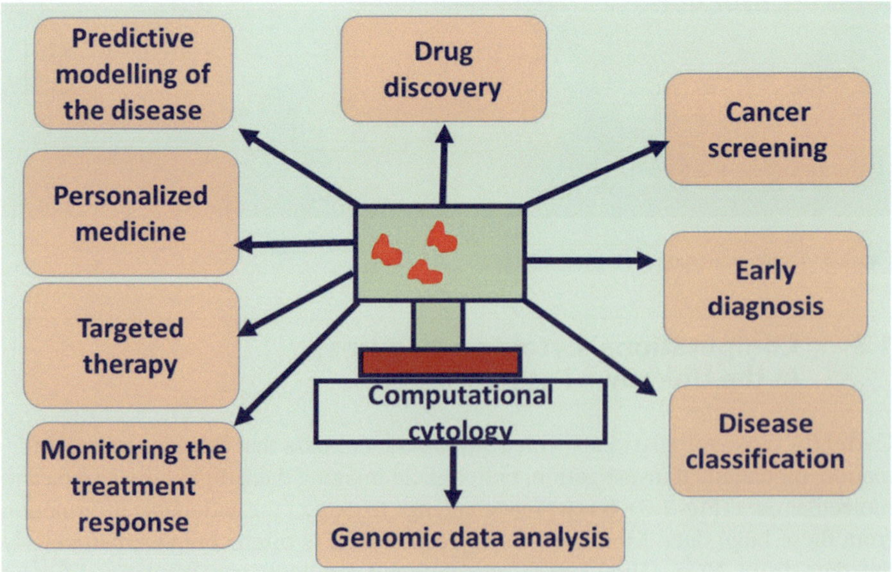

Fig. 1.4 Future potentials of computational cytology

References

1. Dey P, Bansal B, Saini T. An emerging era of computational cytology. Diagn Cytopathol. 2023;51(4):270–5.
2. Dey P. In: Dey P, editor. Chapter 10: 'computational pathology: an emerging discipline with vast potential' in recent advances in pathology-1. New Delhi: Jaypee Brothers Medical Publishers; 2025.
3. Salto-Tellez M, Maxwell P, Hamilton P. Artificial intelligence-the third revolution in pathology. Histopathology. 2019;74(3):372–6.
4. Ball CS. The early history of the compound microscope. Bios. 1966;37:51–60.
5. Soilleux E, Gatter KC. The antibody revolution: how 'immuno' changed pathology. In: Hall P, Wright NA, editors. Understanding disease: a centenary celebration of the Pathological Society. Chichester: John Wiley & Sons Ltd; 2006. p. 174–84.
6. Dey P. Immunocytochemistry in diagnostic cytology. New Delhi: Jaypee Brothers Medical Publishers; 2021.
7. Dey P. Chapter 23: Sanger sequencing and next generation gene sequencing: basic principles and applications in pathology. In: Basic advanced technology in histopathology and cytology. 2nd ed. Springer nature; 2023.
8. Saini T, Bansal B, Dey P. Digital cytology: current status and future prospects. Diagn Cytopathol. 2023;51(3):211–8.
9. US Food and Drug Administration. FDA news release: FDA allows marketting of first whole slide imaging system for digital pathology. 2017. Available at https://www.fda.gov/news-events/press-announcements/fda-allows-marketing-first-whole-slide-imaging-system-digital-pathology.
10. https://www.accessdata.fda.gov/cdrh_docs/reviews/K190332.pdf.
11. Dey P. The emerging role of deep learning in cytology. Cytopathology. 2021;32(2):154–60. https://doi.org/10.1111/cyt.12942. Epub 2020 Dec 17.
12. Sanyal P, Dey P. Using a deep learning neural network for the identification of malignant cells in effusion cytology material. Cytopathology. 2023;34(5):466–71. https://doi.org/10.1111/cyt.13260. Epub 2023 Jun 23.

Digital Cytology: The Cornerstone of Computational Cytology

2

Abstract

Digital cytology means the digital conversion of a microscopic image of a cytology smear along with the acquisition of the clinical data and the patient's metadata. The introduction of whole slide imaging (WSI) has given a new dimension to the digitization of images. WSI helps to view the slides at any magnification without losing the image features. WSI image is known as a digital slide which can be stored in cloud space and can be transferred and retrieved any time. In the current chapter, the various aspects of WSI are discussed such as the hardware, software, scanning techniques and various challenges to implement WSI. In addition, the guidelines for diagnostic use of WSI cases have been discussed.

Keywords

Digital cytology · Whole slide imaging · WSI · Digital slide · Scanning

2.1 Introduction

Weinstein in 1986 for first time introduced the term "digital pathology" [1]. Digital cytology is a part of digital pathology which deals with cytology image. The digital cytology means the digital conversion of a microscopic image of a cytology smear along with the acquisition of the clinical data and the patient's metadata. The microscope attached with a digital camera can acquire a static image of the glass slide. In comparison, the whole slide scanning deals with the entire microscopic image of the glass slide. The cytopathologist can view the whole slide imaging (WSI) from the viewer area at any magnification. Ferreira et al. [2] for first time published their work on whole slide imaging in the year 1996. They designed the software system for WSI in a robotic microscope. Multiple static images are captured and then stitched to make the complete image. The process was very slow and each image

P. Dey, *Computational Cytology*, https://doi.org/10.1007/978-981-95-3272-8_2

took a lot of space.in the computer. Over the years, the WSI technology has been improved significantly with significantly high speed and better resolution of the images. Currently, WSI is one of the leading technologies to implement computational cytology as it is best suited for artificial neural networks [3].

2.2 Essential Components of WSI

Each WSI system has two essential parts: Hardware and software system (Fig. 2.1).

The whole slide imaging is a composite structure and most of the WSI system is a closed one.

2.2.1 Hardware System

The hardware system consists of the following parts (Fig. 2.2) (Box 2.1):

1. *Robotics and Slide Loader*: The main function of the robotics is to load the slides, maintain the proper alignment, move the slides into the x and y axes and unload the slides. Robotics helps in the high-throughput and precision scanning. The slide loader loads a single slide to few hundred slides, depending on the need of the individual laboratories.

Components of Robotic Systems

- Robotic Arms: Robotics picks up the glass slide and places it properly with accurate alignment to the scanner.
- Conveyor system: The conveyor system transports the slides from one station to another station and takes the major part of loading and unloading the glass slides.

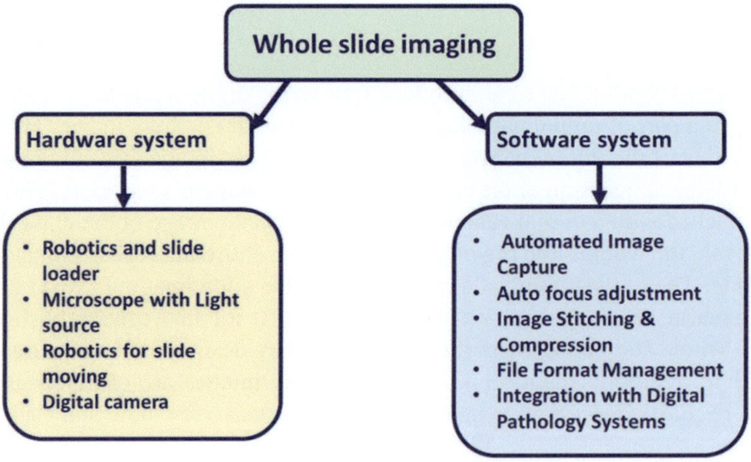

Fig. 2.1 The components of whole slide imaging

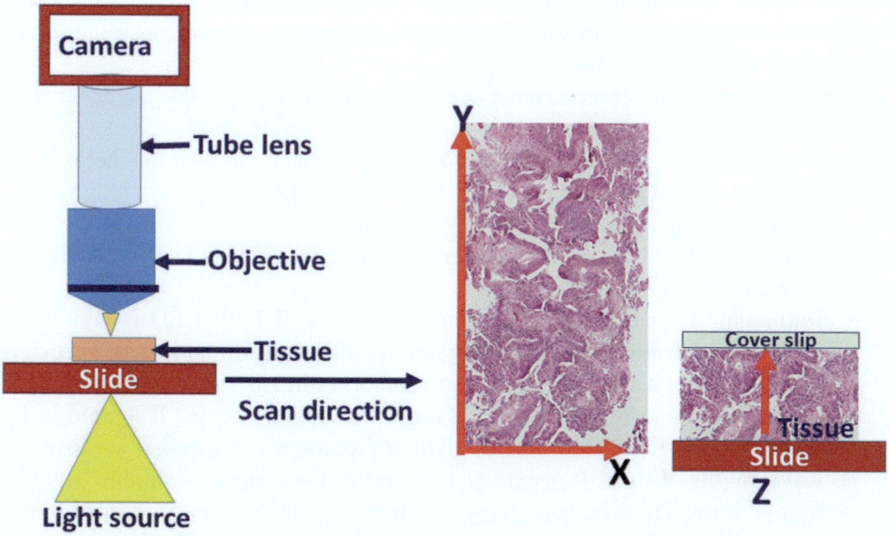

Fig. 2.2 Schematic diagram of the hardware system of whole slide imaging

- Slide holder and racks: They store and organize the slides before and after scanning.
- Sensors and vision system: They help in the alignment of the slide, reading the barcode label and avoid any potential errors.

Slide Loaders in Whole Slide Imaging

Slide loader is the specialized part of the WSI that helps to upload the slides into the scanner.

The types of slide loading are:

Batch loader: Here, the whole bulk of the slide is loaded as a batch and the individual slides are loaded sequentially.

Continuous loaders: In the case of the continuous loader, the slides can be loaded in between the process without any interruption of the scanning.

Single slide loading: It is used for the scanning of a single slide.

Steps of Slide Loading

- Slide placement: Slide is taken from the rack to the scanning stage.
- Barcode scanning: The barcode of the slide is scanned.
- Alignment: The slide is aligned properly by the robotic arm.
- Scanning: The slide is moved under the objective of the lens for digital acquisition of the data.
- Unloading: After the end of the scanning, the slides are picked up from the stage and returned to the tray.

Technological Advancements in Robotics and Slide Loaders

- *Optical Sensors*: The optical sensor helps to detect the exact positioning and alignment of the glass slides.
- *Laser Scanners*: The laser scanner scans the barcode and verifies the accuracy.

2. *Microscope*: The microscope is the main component of the WSI that helps in the digitization of the cytology slide with high precision.

   The microscope has the following components:
   - Objective lenses: The objective are of 4×, 10×, 20× and 40×. Occasional scanners may have 100×.
   - Illumination system: (A) Light Emitting Diode (LED): LED is commonly used in the current WSI system. It gives stable, uniform and energy-efficient illumination. There is minimal heat generation in LED and so the chance of sample degradation is least. (B) Halogen or Xenon Lamps: It is used in the older WSI system. This type of light source provides a broad spectrum of wavelengths of light. It generates heat and so the chance of sample degradation is more. The frequent change of the light source may be needed in this type of illumination. (C) Laser Light Sources: It is used in high-end fluorescence microscopy. It provides high-intensity and narrow bandwidth light which is perfect for a fluorescence WSI system.
3. *Robotics for slide moving*: Automating slide movement by robotics is essential for the quick and thorough scanning without manual intervention. *X-Y Stage Movement*: It moves the slide in the X and Y axes and helps in complete scanning of the whole slide.

   Z-axis autofocus: It helps in adjusting the autofocus in the Z-axis.

   Piezoelectric Stages: It gives ultra-precise movement of the stage to capture the high-resolution images.
4. *Digital Cameras*: Mainly, there are two types of digital cameras:
   A. *Charge-Coupled Device (CCD) Cameras*: CCD cameras are highly sensitive and produce low noise. It produces good-quality images. It is less suitable for high-throughput system as the readout of the LED is slow.
   B. *Complementary Metal-Oxide-Semiconductor (CMOS) Cameras*: CMOS is less expensive than LED cameras and so commonly used in modern WSI. It rapidly and efficiently acquires images.

Box 2.1: Hardware System of Whole Slide Imaging

- *Robotics and slide loader*:
  - Components of Robotic Systems:
    Robotic Arms
    Conveyor system
    Slide holder and racks
    Sensors and vision system

(continued)

Box 2.1 (continued)

- *Robotics for slide moving*:
  - *X-Y Stage Movement*: It moves the slide in the X and Y axes and helps in complete scanning of the whole slide.
  - *Z-axis autofocus*: It helps in adjusting the autofocus in the Z-axis.
  - *Piezoelectric Stages*: It gives ultra-precise movement of the stage to capture the high-resolution images.
- *Digital camera*

  A. *Charge-Coupled Device (CCD) Cameras*: CCD cameras are highly sensitive and produce low noise.

  B. *Complementary Metal-Oxide-Semiconductor (CMOS) Cameras*: CMOS is less expensive than LED cameras and so commonly used in modern WSI.
- *Microscope*:
  - *Objective lenses*: The objectives are of 4×, 10×, 20× and 40×. Occasional scanners may have 100×.
  - *Illumination system*:

    A. Light Emitting Diode (LED): It gives stable, uniform and energy-efficient illumination. Commonly used in WSI.

    B. Halogen or Xenon Lamps: It is used in the older WSI system

    C. Laser Light Sources: It is used in high-end fluorescence microscopy.

2.2.2 Software System

The software system of WSI mainly works on scanning and image acquisition, image viewing, image management and image analysis.

The key functions of this software are (Box 2.2):

- *Automated Image Capture*: It involves the systematic movement of the stage of the scanner and camera to acquire the image of the whole slide. The images are acquired either by tile-based scanning or by line-based scanning.
- A*uto focus adjustment*: The software dynamically maintains the focal plane so that the image is acquired with proper focus and high clarity.
- *Image Stitching and Compression*: The software stitches the tiles of the small parts of the image to make a single complete image. It also compresses the image to store it without losing its quality.
- *File Format Management*: The software saves the image in a digital format so that the image can be readable in different formats. The images are finally viewed by the pathologists in the viewer's station. The software also helps to analyse the image.
- *Integration with Digital Pathology Systems*: The software helps to integrate the digital image into the Laboratory Information Systems (LIS).

Box 2.2: Software System

- *Automated Image Capture*: Acquire the image of the whole slide.
- A*uto focus adjustment*: Properly focuses the image with high clarity.
- *Image Stitching and Compression*: The software makes a single complete image.
- *File Format Management*: The software saves the image in a suitable digital format.
- *Integration with Digital Pathology Systems*: The software integrates the digital image into the Laboratory Information Systems.

2.3 Challenges in WSI Software

The software of WSI faces several challenges (Fig. 2.3):

- *Storage Capacity*: The digital slide of WSI takes huge storage space and so there is a need for advanced storage solutions and optimum compression techniques of the images.
- *Standardization of the Digital Format*: The digital format of different vendors of WSI are different and there is a need of compatible format across the platform.
- *Processing Speed*: Acquisition of images in high resolution needs high-speed processing algorithms and good computational power.
- *Integration of Artificial Intelligence*: The artificial neural network software should be included in the WSI software. It will help in the automated image analysis and diagnosis.
- *Cloud-Based Solutions*: Currently, data are stored and remotely accessed in the cloud. The software should be compatible with cloud storage and analysis.

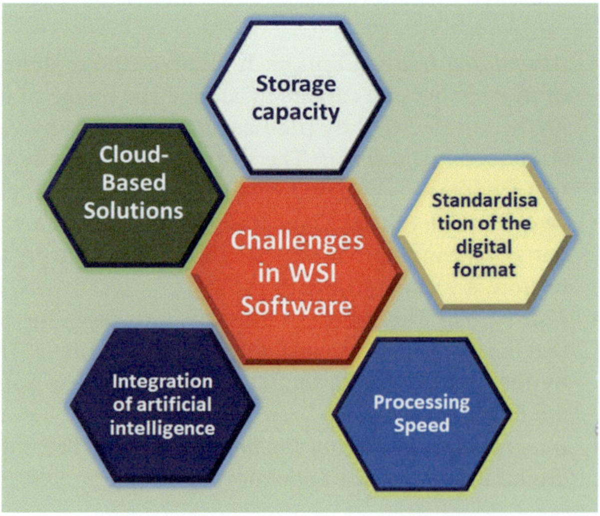

Fig. 2.3 Challenges and limitations of the software system of whole slide imaging

2.4 Scanning Techniques by WSI

The different scanning techniques are used by different WSI (Fig. 2.4) (Box 2.3).

A. *Tile-Based Scanning*

Work pattern: In tile-based scanning, the machine captures a large number of tiles of the entire glass slide in high resolution. These tiles are stitched together to get a composite image.

Advantages:

(a) It is suitable for acquiring images in higher magnification.

(b) The focus is adaptable in various parts of the glass slide.

Limitations:

(a) Relatively slower than the line scanning technique.

(b) Stitching artefact may appear in the composite image.

B. *Line-Based Scanning*

Work pattern: In the line-based scanning, the sensor moves longitudinally and narrow linear strips of the images are captured. These longitudinal strips are stitched together to get a composite image.

Advantages:

(a) Faster than tile-based scanning.

(b) Consistent in resolution and focus.

Limitations:

(a) It needs accurate slide movement and proper alignment.

(b) Stitching artefact may occur in case of malalignment.

C. *Z-Stack Scanning*

Work pattern: Here, the images are captured in different focal planes and then are combined to get a better-focused image.

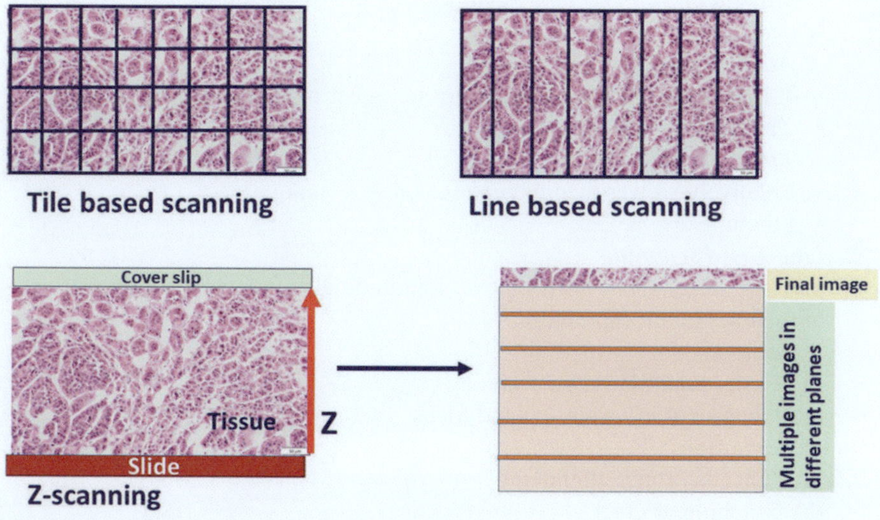

Fig. 2.4 Scanning processes in whole slide imaging

Advantages:

(a) Z-stacking is very helpful in cytology, where the cells are often clustered and the smears are thick.
(b) Three-dimensional structures can be assessed as the images are sharp.

Limitations:

(a) Time-consuming
(b) The images need a lot of space
(c) Additional computation work is needed

D. *Continuous Scanning*

Work pattern: Here, the slide moves continuously under the line-scan camera.

Advantages:

(a) Fast scanning reduces mechanical wear.

Limitations:

(a) The hardware should be highly precise.
(b) Motion blurring may occur.

E. *Hybrid Scanning*

Work pattern: Multiple techniques are combined together to get accurate image rapidly.

Advantages:

(a) High speed with good resolution.

Limitations:

(a) High cost.
(b) Complex system.

Box 2.3: Scanning Techniques

1. *Tile-based scanning*

Work pattern: The large number of tiles of the entire glass slide is scanned.

Advantages:

- It is suitable for acquiring images in higher magnification.
- The focus is adaptable.

Limitations:

- Relatively slower than the line scanning technique.
- Stitching artefact.

2. *Line-based scanning*

Work pattern: The sensor moves longitudinally and marrow linear strips of the images are captured.

Advantages:

(a) Faster than tile-based scanning
(b) Consistent in resolution and focus

Limitations:

(a) It needs proper alignment
(b) Stitching artefact

(continued)

Box 2.3 (continued)

3. *Z-Stack Scanning*

   Work pattern: Here, the images are captured in different focal planes

   Advantages:

   (a) Z-stacking is very helpful in cytology, where the cells are often clustered and the smears are thick.

   (b) Three-dimensional structures can be assessed.

   Limitations:

   (a) Time-consuming

   (b) Additional computation work is needed

4. *Continuous scanning*

   Work pattern: The slide moves continuously under the line-scan camera.

   Advantages:

   (a) Fast scanning

   Limitations:

   (a) The hardware should be highly precise.

   (b) Motion blurring may occur

5. *Hybrid scanning*

   Work pattern: Multiple techniques are combined to get an accurate image rapidly

   Advantages:

   (a) High speed with good resolution

   Limitations:

   (a) High cost

   (b) Complex system

2.5 File Format in WSI

The WSI in pathology images are usually huge and the file size ranges from several hundred megabytes to a few gigabytes. This is particularly true for the cytological images where Z-scan is done. Many vendors use the proprietary file format that are vendor-specific. In these situations, the viewing of the slides need that particular software used by the vendor.

The vendor-specific image file extensions are:

Philips: Philips IntelliSite Pathology solutions use TIFF-based proprietary file format. However, it is not a standard TIFF and the proprietary software is needed to open the file. The file stores the images as pyramid multiresolution level for rapid zooming.

Aperio: Leica Biosystems uses a proprietary SVS format which is a variant of TIFF. It also uses pyramid multiresolution for rapid zooming. The software utilizes JPEG, JPEG 2000 for efficient compression to store the images.

Table 2.1 Comparison of different whole slide imaging systems

Company	Key models	Scanning Speed	Slide capacity	Z-stacking	Artificial intelligence (AI) integration
Philips	IntelliSite Ultra-Fast Scanner (UFS)	1 min/slide (15 × 15 mm)	Up to 300 slides	No	Possible by Deep learning plugins, Philips AI Manager
Aperio (Leica)	AT2, GT 450, CS2	50 s/side (15 × 15 mm)	GT450: 450 slides	Yes (AT2 supports)	Advanced (HALO AI compatible)
Hamamatsu	NanoZoomer S360, XR, RS	60 s/slide in 20× (S360)	S360: 360 slides	Yes	AI through third-party
Roche Ventana	iScan HT, iScan Coreo	80 s/slide	HT: 360 slides	Yes	Excellent
3DHISTECH	Panoramic 1000, MIDI II, SCAN II	1 min/slide	P1000: 1000 slides	Yes (advanced)	Advanced (many AI modules available)

Hamamatsu: Hamamatsu scanner uses a modified TIFF format called NDPI. This is a proprietary file format. It uses JPEG or JPEG2000 for the compression and storing the image. The scanner uses multi multi-resolution pyramidal storage system for rapid zooming.

Roche Ventana: Roche Ventana uses a proprietary Big Image File (BIF) format. The BIF supports a large image size. It uses JPEG 2000 for the compression and storage of the image.

3DHistech: It uses a proprietary MRXS file format. It is a modified Tagged Image File Format (TIFF)-based file format. The file can handle large images with high resolution. JPEG or JPEG2000 is used for file compression and storage.

Table 2.1 compares the different whole slide imaging systems.

2.6 Digital Slides Versus Glass Slides

The traditional cytologists are still habituated to report on the glass slides. The glass slide is easy to report by simple light microscopic examination. The slides are easy to handle and do not need any special skill. However, the interpretation of the slides can be observer-dependent. The accurate objective quantitation of the different components such as mitotic count, expression of immunological markers may often be difficult on a light microscope. In contrast, the digital slides are easy to circulate, and the objective quantification of different components can be done with great accuracy. The digital slides maintain all the information of the original slides and one can see them in different magnifications. In addition, artificial neural networks can be applied to digital slides. There are several advantages of the digital slides over the glass slides.

Table 2.2 Digital versus glass slides

Features	Digital slides	Glass slides
High resolution	Yes	Yes
Transportation	Easy and rapid	Slow
Multiple view	Possible by a large number of viewers	Not possible
Physical storage	Not needed	Needed
Retrieval	Rapid	Slow
ANN	Best suited	Can be studied for ANN

2.7 Advantages of the Digital Slides

1. Easy transport: The digital slides are easy to transport from one place to another in this planet.
2. Multiple viewing: The DS can be seen by multiple observers at a time.
3. Good image quality: High-resolution good quality images are seen in the digital slides.
4. Easy storage: The digital slides are easy to store and no physical space is needed.
5. Easy retrieval: It is easy to retrieve the digital slides.
6. Artificial neural network (ANN): The digital slides are best suited for the ANN.

The comparison of the digital slides and the glass slides is shown in Table 2.2.

2.8 Limitations of Digital Slides

- *Cost*: The initial cost of the WSI system and the software is high. So the digital slides are costly.
- *Storage of the digital slides*: The digital slides are usually of higher resolution and so they need a huge storage capacity of the computer.
- *Slow processing time*: The digital slides take huge storage space and so the loading of the slides on the viewing port may take a long time. Viewing of the slides in higher magnification may often take a longer time.
- *Software compatibility to view slides*: Most of the WSI companies use the proprietary software to view the digital slides. There may be problem to view the digital slides on other computers with different software platforms.
- *Training*: Initial training is needed to report directly on the digital slides. Most of the pathologists are not habituated to reporting on the digital slides.
- *Impaired image quality*: The compression of the digital image at the time of storage may affect the quality of the image, particularly fine details in higher magnification.

- *Internet dependency*: The digital slides often need internet access to download and view the images from distant places. The internet service should be fast and stable for the good performance of the WSI system.
- *Legal issues*: The reporting of the digital slides in the clinical setting across the nations may need the approval of the concerned authority. Moreover, the patient's data needs protection from misuse by commercial people.
- *Resistance to report on digital slides*: Unfortunately, the pathologists are overall reluctant to report on the digital slides and they prefer to report on light microscopic examination for routine reporting.

2.9 Guidelines for Using Digital Slides in Diagnostic Purposes

In the year 2021, the College of American Pathologists (CAP) released the updated guidelines for diagnostic use of WSI cases [4].

They passed three strong recommendations and nine statements for good practice for reporting digital slides for the diagnosis. Each laboratory should have internal validation before the introduction of WSI-based reporting. The strong recommendations are:

(1) The validation set should include the entire spectrum of specimen types routinely used in the laboratory. In each category, at least 60 cases should be taken.
(2) The diagnostic concordance between the digital and glass slides of the same observer should be established and the concordance should be more than 95%.
(3) At least a 14-day washout period is needed between the viewing of the digital slides and glass slides.

Table 2.3 mentions the good practice statements regarding the validation of the WSI.

In a meta-analysis study, Antonini et al. [5] showed that out of 25 series, only 4 studies followed strong recommendations and one study followed complete guidelines issued by CAP. The authors concluded that the various validation studies should be well-designed and rigorous to maintain the criteria of CAP.

Table 2.3 The brief notes of the validation for the primary diagnosis on whole slide imaging

Strong recommendations	Good practice statements
The validation set should include the entire spectrum of specimen types routinely used in the laboratory and each category should have at least 60 cases.	GPS1: Before the implementation of WSI for diagnostic purpose, each laboratory should have its own validation study.
	GPS2: The validation process should be designed according to clinical use.
The diagnostic concordance between the digital and glass slides by same observer should be more than 95%.	GPS3: The validation system should be according to the real-world clinical environment
	GPS4: The validation study should include the entire WSI system (both software and hardware).
At least a two-week gap is needed between the viewing of the digital slides and glass slides.	GPS 5: The laboratories should have procedures to mention the changes in WSI system.
	GPS 6: Only WSI competent pathologists should join in the validation process.
	GPS 7: All the contents of the glass slide should be scanned in the digital slides.
	GPS 8: There should be proper documentation of the methods, measurements and final report of the validation
	GPS 9: The pathologists should review the slides randomly both the digital and glass slides

2.10 Conclusions

A whole slide scanner provides WSI of the glass slide. WSI maintains all the information on the original glass slides. There are several whole slide scanners available in the market. The cytology slides need Z-axis scanning due to cellular aggregations. The WSI of the cytology slides is one of the prerequisites to go for computational cytology. The digital images can be uploaded in the system and can be further analysed by an artificial neural network.

References

1. Weinstein RS. Prospects for telepathology. Hum Pathol. 1986;17:433–4.
2. Ferreira R, Moon B, Humphries J, Sussman A, Saltz J, Miller R, Demarzo A. The virtual microscope. Proc AMIA Annu Fall Symp. 1997:449–53.
3. Saini T, Bansal B, Dey P. Digital cytology: current status and future prospects. Diagn Cytopathol. 2023;51(3):211–8.
4. https://documents.cap.org/documents/wsi-teaching-presentation.pdf.
5. Antonini P, Santonicco N, Pantanowitz L, Girolami I, Rizzo PC, Brunelli M, Bellevicine C, Vigliar E, Negri G, Troncone G, Fadda G, Parwani A, Marletta S, Eccher A. Relevance of the College of American Pathologists guideline for validating whole slide imaging for diagnostic purposes to cytopathology. Cytopathology. 2023;34(1):5–14.

Digital Workflow in Cytology

3

Abstract

The digital workflow in computational cytology means the acquisition of data from the cytology samples along with metadata, viewing the digitized images and interpreting the cytology-related data by artificial intelligence. The digital workflow is the cornerstone of computational cytology. It integrates digital cytology and advanced computational techniques such as artificial neural networks. The current chapter discusses the various steps of the digital workflow including sample collection and preparation, digitalization of the slide, image storage and management, image pre-processing and storage.

Keywords

Workflow · Cytology · Sample collection · Image storage

3.1 Introduction

The digital workflow in computational cytology means the acquisition of data from the cytology samples along with metadata, viewing the digitized images and interpreting the cytology-related data by artificial intelligence [1, 2]. The digital workflow is the cornerstone of computational cytology. It integrates digital cytology and advanced computational techniques such as artificial neural networks.

3.2 The Steps of Digital Workflow

The steps of Digital Workflow are shown in Fig. 3.1.

P. Dey, *Computational Cytology*, https://doi.org/10.1007/978-981-95-3272-8_3

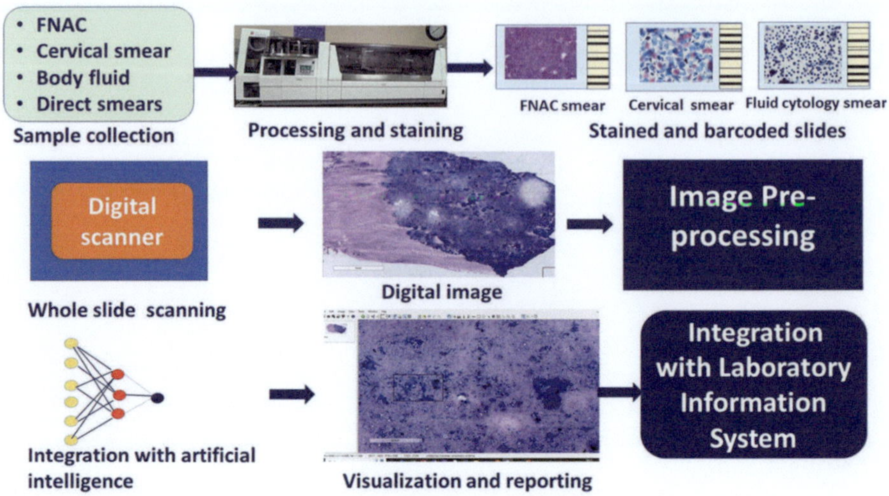

Fig. 3.1 Steps of digital workflow

A. *Sample Collection and Preparation*

Types of Specimen: The cytology samples consist of fine needle aspiration cytology (FNAC), body fluid samples and cervical smears or materials in liquid.

Sample Preparation: FNAC material can be spread directly on the smear or can be put in the liquid-based cytology fixative for the smear preparation. Body fluids are processed by centrifugation or by liquid-based preparation. CSF is processed by cyto-centrifugation. Cell block preparation is often used in cytology samples and the sections are cut for haematoxylin and eosin staining.

B. *Digitalization of the Slide:* The well-stained slides are digitized by a whole slide imagining (WSI) scanner. A high-throughput scanner rapidly scans multiple images in high resolution. This type of scanner is needed in a busy laboratory. The file is stored in a suitable format, e.g. JPEG, TIFF and DICOM (Digital Imaging and Communications in Medicine).

C. *Image Storage and Management*

Storage Platform: The digital slides are stored in a cloud-based system. The images are accessed by laboratory information systems (LIS).

Data Security: The data security means the protection of the digital images from any unauthorized access. It prevents the tampering of the image or theft of the original image.

File Format: The file is stored in a suitable format. The compression algorithms help to reduce the storage space and transmission costs without losing the quality of the digital image.

There are two types of compression algorithms:

1. *Lossless Compression*: In lossless compression, there is no loss in image quality. However, the compression ratio is low. The original image is well-maintained in lossless compression. This type of compression is ideal for medical images.

2. *Lossy Compression:* In lossy compression, the file size is reduced by discarding some amount of unnecessary data while maintaining the diagnostic quality.

Table 3.1 shows different compression algorithms.

D. *Image Pre-processing*: Image pre-processing includes the improvement of the quality of the images, normalization and correction of the colour. The details of data pre-processing are mentioned in the previous chapter (Chap. 2).
E. *Integration with Artificial Intelligence*: The machine learning/artificial intelligence software is integrated with WSI. The AI software will help to perform specific tasks such as screening for malignancy, mitosis counting, tumour grading, prognostic assessment and management.
F. *Visualization and Reporting:* Images are visualized by the pathologist and are reported. The report is generated automatically or semi-automatically.
G. *Integration with Laboratory Information Systems (LIS):* The report of the cytology samples is connected with the laboratory information system (LIS). This helps in the rapid retrieval of the patient report for management and also in research purposes.
H. *Collaboration and Communication*: The WSI can be circulated to colleagues or experts for confirmation or an alternate opinion.
I. *Archiving and Compliance:* Image is finally archived in a hard disc or cloud storage. The data of patients can be restored whenever required.

Table 3.1 Comparison of different compression algorithms

Algorithm	Compression type	Ratio of compression	Advantages	Disadvantages	Best use
JPEG2000 (Joint Photographic Experts Group)	Lossless	2:1 to 3:1	DICOM support, good-quality image	Slow	Medical images
LZW (TIFF TIFF, Tagged Image File Format)	Lossless	1.5:1 to 2:1	Widely supported and simple	Large file size	Archival storage
FLIF (Free Lossless Image Format)	Lossless	2:1 to 3:1	Better compression than TIFF, highly efficient	Limited software support	Web-based viewers
HEIF (High Efficiency Image Format)	Lossy	20:1 to 50:1	High compression efficiency	Limited adoption in medical imaging	Histopathology
PNG (Portable Network Graphics)	Lossless	1.5:1 to 2:1	Widely supported	Takes more storage space	Smaller pathology data set

J. *Quality Control & Validation:* The training of an AI model gives feedback which helps to increase the diagnostic accuracy. The standard protocol of the digital workflow helps to maintain consistency in different laboratories.

3.3 Benefits of Digital Cytology Workflow

The key benefits of implementing the digital cytology workflow in the laboratory include improving diagnostic accuracy, storage, data management, and extending research capabilities (Fig. 3.2). These benefits are described below:

A. *Improved Diagnostic Accuracy*
   1. *High Resolution*: Digital cytology acquires the image in high resolution and allows the cytopathologists to view these images in full detail.
   2. *AI Assistance:* The application of AI in digital cytology can help to identify subtle abnormalities and detect malignancy more accurately.
   3. *Standardization:* Automated digital workflow reduces the variation of diagnosis from person to person as the image quality is consistently maintained.
B. *Increased Efficiency*
   1. *Rapid Turnaround Time:* Automated digital workflow enhances rapid turnaround time because it accelerates the task of scanning slides, organization of data, and curtails the manual effort.
   2. *Regularized workflow:* Digital workflow provides a continuous flow of image acquisition, data integration, analysis and reporting of the slides. This makes the diagnosis faster and more efficient.

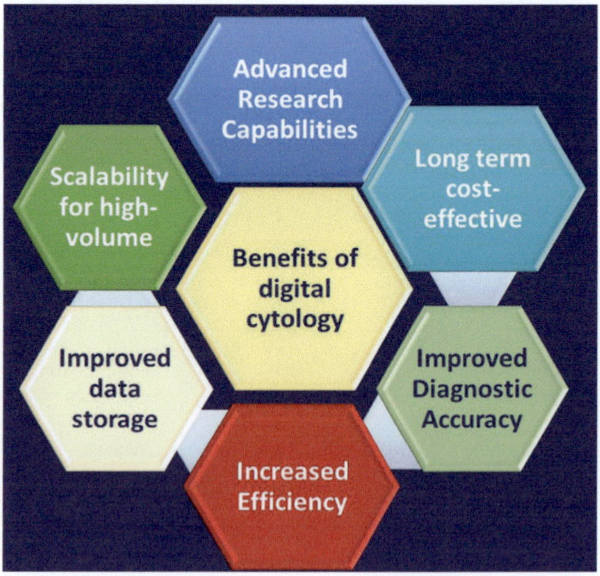

Fig. 3.2 Benefits of digital cytology

3. *Batch Processing:* A high-throughput system allows the batch processing of scanning and analysis of multiple samples simultaneously.

C. *Improved Data Storage and Management*

The successful implementation of the digital workflow will help in the storage and integration of the cytological digital images and other metadata systematically. This may help in the rapid retrieval of archival data for clinical and research purposes.

D. *Scalability for High-Volume*

The digital workflow can handle large volumes of data without affecting the work performance. The scalability of high volume is achieved by an automated screening process that can screen a large volume of digital slides. The implementation of advanced infrastructures may also help in the scalability of handling large volumes.

E. *Advanced Research Capabilities*

The successful digital cytology workflow helps in the storage of huge data to train the artificial neural network model for the research analysis. In addition, data fusion such as a combination of digital image data, clinical data, genomics, proteomics and molecular data will have immense effect in personalized medicine.

F. *Patient-Centric Benefits*

Rapid Diagnosis: Implementation of the digital workflow will give rise to faster diagnosis.

Personalized medicine: Digital cytology provides high diagnostic accuracy and personalized treatment facility.

G. *Long-Term Cost-Effectiveness:*

Digital cytology is cheaper in the long term as it eliminates the physical storage problem and lowers the manual cost of labour.

3.4 Challenges in Digital Workflow to Implement in Cytology

The implementation of the digital workflow in the cytology laboratory encounters several challenges (Fig. 3.3):

- High cost: The initial cost of a WSI scanner is very high, and making the complete infrastructure for digital workflow is expensive.
- Regulatory hurdles: There is no universal standard for digital cytology and so there may be wide variation in image acquisition, processing, storage and management from laboratory to laboratory.
- Training: The cytologists need adequate training to work with digital cytology.
- Storage of data: WSI of high-resolution cytology smears takes large volumes of storage space. Therefore, the system needs a high storage capacity.

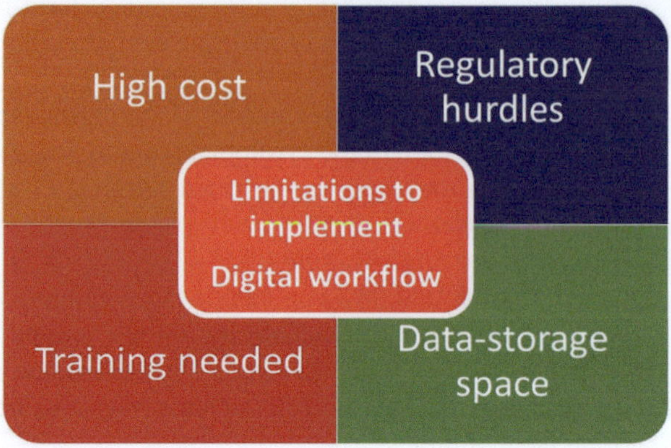

Fig. 3.3 Limitations of digital workflow to implement in Cytology

3.5 Conclusions

Digitalization of the laboratory system is an essential step towards computational cytology. The steps of digitalization starts from the sample collection and barcoding to the visualization and reporting of the digital slides. The advantages of digitalization include increased diagnostic efficiency, rapid turnaround time, improved data storage and management and enhanced research capabilities. However, there are several challenges and limitations of digitalization such as high cost, training of the staff and limitation of data storage space. It is expected that in course of time, these hurdles will be overcome.

References

1. Saini T, Bansal B, Dey P. Digital cytology: current status and future prospects. Diagn Cytopathol. 2023;51(3):211–8.
2. Dey P. In: Dey P, editor. Chapter 10: ‘Computational pathology: an emerging discipline with vast potential’ in recent advances in pathology-1. New Delhi: Jaypee Brothers Medical Publishers; 2025.

Automation in Cytology Laboratory

4

Abstract

The automation in the cytology laboratory plays an important role in standardization of the processing, staining, digitization and reporting of slides. Liquid-based cytology (LBC) prepares the smear and stains it automatically. The automated stainer stains different stains automatically. Whole slide scanning (WSI) helps to digitize the cytology smears which can be interpreted by multiple cytologists from multiple locations. Artificial intelligence (AI) also has a major role in automation by automated capturing of images, extracting the features and diagnosing the diseases. The present chapter discusses the various aspects of automation in the Cytology laboratory.

Keywords

Automation · Cytology · Laboratory · Artificial intelligence · Liquid-based cytology · Autostainer

4.1 Introduction

In recent years, there has been significant technological progress in cytology. This includes automated preparation, staining, scanning and interpretation of the cytology samples. The automation in cytology laboratory helps in standardization of the processing and staining. Moreover, the introduction of WSI and artificial intelligence (AI) has a significant impact on Cytology [1]. WSI scans the cytology smears which can be interpreted by multiple cytologists from multiple locations. The digital slides are best suited for AI. AI makes a paradigm shift by automated image capturing, feature extraction and diagnosis [2]. In the present chapter, the various aspects of automation have been discussed.

P. Dey, *Computational Cytology*, https://doi.org/10.1007/978-981-95-3272-8_4

4.2 Rationality to Go for Automation (Box 4.1)

- *Standardization*: Automation provides high-quality standardization processing of the samples.
- *Reducing Workload*: Automation greatly reduces the manual workload.
- *Efficient*: Automated screening shortens the time of screening by the cytotechnologists.
- *Enhanced Accuracy*: By applying an artificial neural network (ANN), the reports are more consistent and accurate.
- *Scalability*: The ANN model can screen many thousands of slides in a short period of time. So it is fit for any National screening program.

Box 4.1 Rationality for Automation

- *Standardization*: High-quality standardised processing of the samples.
- *Reducing workload*: It greatly reduces the manual workload.
- *Efficient*: It shortens the time of screening.
- *Enhanced accuracy*: It is consistent and accurate.
- *Scalability*: Large number of cases in a short period of time.

4.3 Scopes of Automation in Cytology Laboratory

The automation in the cytology laboratory starts from receiving the sample to final reporting (Fig. 4.1).

Barcoding Barcoding each sample is the first step of automation. Barcoding gives a unique number to the sample. It helps to trace the sample at any time.

4.3.1 Processing

Samples

1. The fine needle aspiration cytology (FNAC): FNAC samples may come as direct air-dried smear or alcohol-fixed smears. It may also be sent as liquid-based cytology (LBC) preparation.

   Processing: Air-dried and alcohol fixed smears are processed by an autostainer. Samples collected in LBC fixatives are processed in the LBC instrument.
2. Body fluid: Body fluid may come with anticoagulants or in LBC fluid.

   Processing: It may be processed in the LBC instrument.
3. Cervical cytology: The samples are collected in LBC fixative.

   Processing: It can be processed in the LBC instrument.
4. Other samples as smear such as crushed smear or imprint smear can be stained directly by an autostainer.

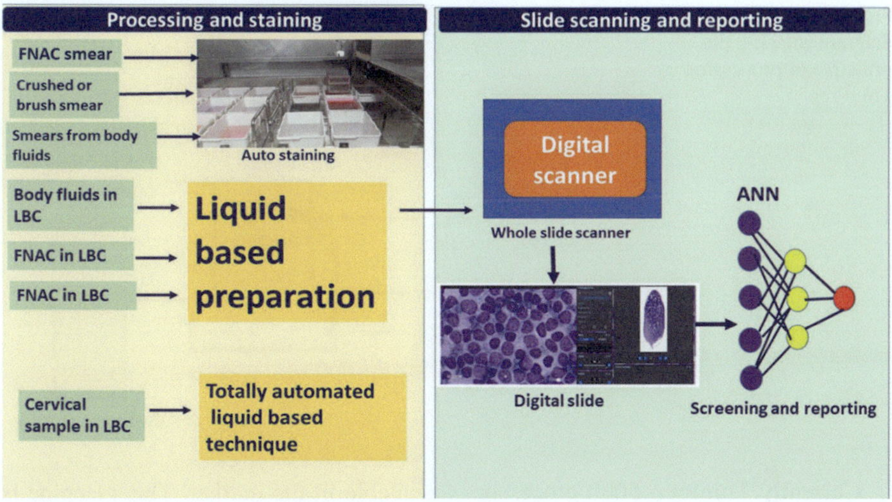

Fig. 4.1 Automation in a cytology laboratory

4.3.2 Staining

FNAC slides: These slides are stained directly by the autostainer.

Cervical cytology: Slides are stained by LBC machines.

Body fluid: Body fluids processed by LBC are stained directly by LBC machines. Only Papanicolaou's staining is done by the LBC machine.

Liquid-based cytology (LBC) is an important part of automation in cytology samples. LBC can process the cytology samples collected in LBC fixatives and can also stain the slides. There are two commercially available FDA-approved LBC machines in the market: ThinPrep and SurePath [3]. The cervical samples are collected by a cervix-brush supplied by the company. The body fluids and FNAC samples can be directly put into the LBC fixatives supplied by the companies.

ThinPrep In the ThinPrep technique, the sample is collected in PreservCyt solution supplied by the company (Box 4.2). A cylindrical hollow tube with an attached filter in one end is rotated rapidly within the vial containing the sample to disperse the cells (Fig. 4.2). The negative suction is applied to the cylindrical tube so that the fluid in the vial is sucked and the cells are attached to the filter. The trapped cells on the outer surface of the filter are transferred to the glass slide. The smear is immediately dipped in the fixative to avoid air drying.

So basically, ThinPrep works as:

- Cell dispersion: By the rotation of the cylinder with a filter
- Cell collection: Continuous negative suction in the cylinder
- Cell transfer: Impressing the filter on the glass slide helps to transfer the cells

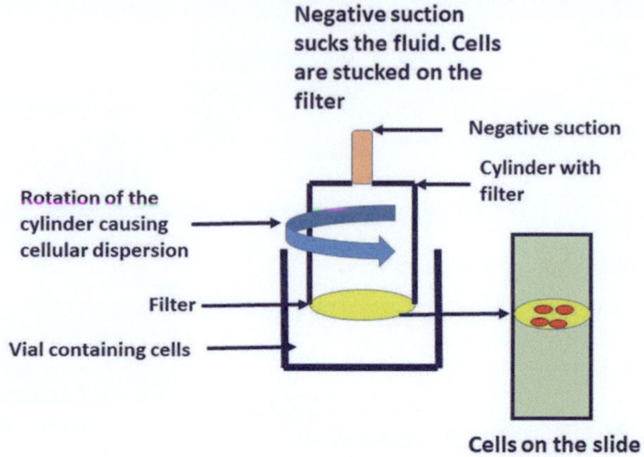

Fig. 4.2 Schematic diagram showing the principle of processing by ThinPrep

Currently ThinPrep 5000 processor is available in the market. This machine is fully automated and can process 20 vials or slides at a time. The processed slides can be sent for staining directly. The machine can read barcoded vials and therefore reduces any chance of mismatching.

Box 4.2 Thin Prep

FDA-approved liquid-based cytology machine

Basic principles

- Cell dispersion: By the rotation of the cylinder with filter
- Cell collection: Continuous negative suction in the cylinder
- Cell transfer: Impressing the filter on the glass slide.

Main advantages

- Monolayer preparation
- Automated processing
- Clean background
- The residual fluid is fit for HPV testing

Disadvantages

- Comparatively less cell enrichment

4.3.3 SurePath

SurePath is also an effective technique for LBC (Box 4.3).

The basic working principles of SurePath are (Fig. 4.3):

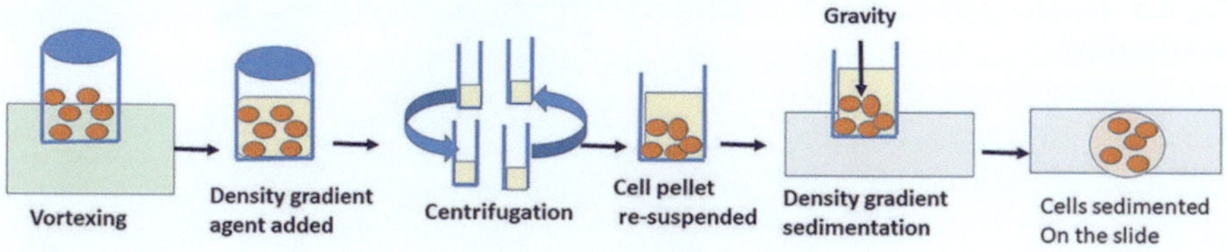

Fig. 4.3 Schematic diagram showing the basic principles of SurePath

- *Vortexing*: To disperse the cells mechanically
- *Cell enrichment*: The cells are enriched by mixing the sample with PREPSTAIN® Density Reagent, followed by centrifugation. The unwanted debris and mucus are removed. A pellet is formed by centrifugation.
- *Resuspension*: The concentrated cells in the cell pellet are re-suspended for staining.
- *Density Gradient Sedimentation*: In the PREPSTAIN® Settling chamber, the cells are sedimented on a pre-coated slide by simply gravity (Fig. 4.4).

Currently, BD totalys ™ multiprocessor is available in the market which is a fully automated machine. This present machine process 96 vials in a batch at a time.

Box 4.3 SurePath
FDA-approved liquid-based cytology machine

Basic principles
- *Vortexing*: The cells are mechanically dispersed by vortexing.
- *Cell enrichment*: The cells are enriched by buffy coat preparation adding PREPSTAIN® Density Reagent and centrifuging the sample.
- *Density gradient Sedimentation and staining*: The cells are sedimented on a pre-coated slide by gravitational force followed by staining.

Advantages
- Good enrichment of cells
- The residual fluid is fit for HPV testing

Disadvantages
- Multiple layered cells

Automated screening Automated screening procedure should be designed in such a way that (1) no dysplastic or malignant cells should be passed as normal or negative and (2) it should not label the normal cell as malignant cells. In addition, the automated screening technique should be economically cost-effective and it should shorten the period of screening. Therefore, the two main goals of automated screening are to increase the accuracy and productivity of cervical screening.

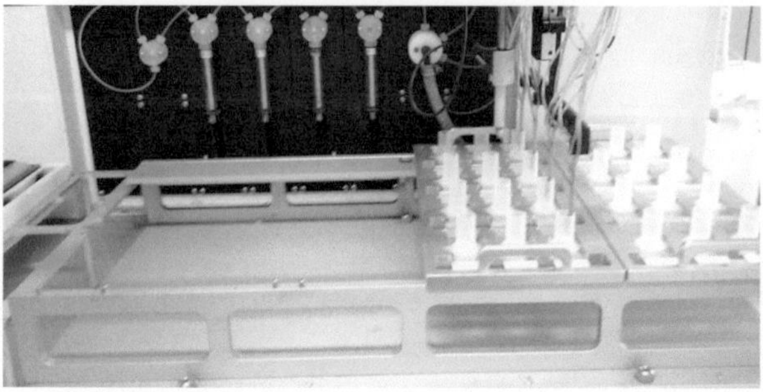

Fig. 4.4 Density gradient sedimentation

4.4 Automated Screening

To date, there is no fully automated screening device in the market. Semi-automated screening devices are available in the market: (1) BD FocalPoint GS Imaging System and (2) HOLOGIC ThinPrep Imaging System [4].

BD FocalPoint GS Imaging System (FPGS) The device is FDA-approved and can be used for the screening of both SurePath and conventional smear.

There are two major parts of FPGS:

1. *BD FocalPoint* ™ *Slide Profiler*: The slides are screened at lower and higher magnifications. Based on several cytological features, the slide is given a "device score" that indicates the probability of abnormality. Each slide is categorized as "no review" and "review". The data is transferred to the review station.
2. *BD FocalPoint GS Review Station*: The slides for "review" is manually screened in the review station by cytotechnologists. Abnormal smear is further reviewed by the cytopathologists.

HOLOGIC ThinPrep Imaging System The system includes (1) ThinPrep imaging system and (2) ThinPrep review system.

1. *ThinPrep image processor*: The system scans for abnormal cells and records the potential abnormal cells It records the locations of 22 microscopic fields and transfer the data to the review scope.
2. *Review scope*: In the review scope, the cytologists review the 22 microscopic fields. The presence of any abnormal cells are screened carefully and confirmed.

Whole Slide Scanning and Artificial Neural Network (ANN) The digital slides generated by WSI are perfectly suitable for ANN. In fact, automation is the first step to implement ANN. WSI provides complete images of the cytology slides and eliminates the bias of selecting areas Moreover, deep learning, particularly convolutional neural network (CNN), is able to extract the features without any manual intervention [5]. However, ANN from WSI faces several challenges:

- *Large image size*: The huge size of WSI is difficult to handle by AI.
- *Smaller cell size*: Relative to the large size of WSI, the cells are too small.
- *Huge data*: Each WSI of cytology smear contains huge data which is difficult to handle by AI.

Solutions Subgraph-based approach: Uniformly partitioning the WSI into subgraphs may be easy to annotate and detect the abnormal cells.

4.5 Challenges of Implementing Automation

There are several challenges to implement automation in the cytology laboratory.

1. *Cost*: Automated screening devices are costly and difficult to afford by the developing countries.
2. *Technical*: The technical staff needs proper training.
3. *Integration*: The automated system should be properly integrated in the existing laboratory system.
4. *Medico-legal*: In primary screening, the error in the system may have primary screening issues.

4.6 Conclusions

Automation brings a paradigm shift in cytology laboratory. It provides high efficiency, reproducibility and is focussed on precise diagnosis. Automation provides standardized approach with high consistency. The application of the AI on WSI images gives a more comprehensive approach in cytology. AI will open various newer avenues by the integration of clinical and molecular data along with the analysis of WSI.

References

1. Saini T, Bansal B, Dey P. Digital cytology: current status and future prospects. Diagn Cytopathol. 2023;51(3):211–8.
2. Dey P. Chapter 19: Automation and liquid based cytology in cytology sample. In: Basic and advanced laboratory techniques in histopathology and cytology. Springer nature; 2023.
3. Dey P. Chapter 21: Automation and liquid-based cytology. In: Diagnostic cytology. Jaypee brothers medical publishers Pvt. Ltd; 2024.
4. Dey P. Chapter 2: Sample collection, liquid based cytology and automated screening. In: Handbook on cervical cytology: special emphasis on liquid based cytology. 2nd ed. Jaypee brothers medical publishers Pvt. Ltd; 2023.
5. Dey P. The emerging role of deep learning in cytology. Cytopathology. 2021;32(2):154–60. https://doi.org/10.1111/cyt.12942. Epub 2020 Dec 17. PMID: 33222315.

Part II

Major Components of Computational Cytology

Data Acquisition and Preparation in Computational Cytology

5

Abstract

Data and its acquisition are the prime components of computational cytology. The data can be classified as Internal and external databases. The internal database is generated from the local hospital or laboratory data. The main components of the internal database are microscopic images, clinical, biochemical, radiological and molecular genetics. The external database is acquired from the medical journals, clinical trials or other databases from the various sources. The complete utilization of both databases can help to make an effective neural network model. The present chapter discusses the various components of the databases.

Keywords

Data · Internal database · External database · Clinical data · Molecular data · Data pre-processing

5.1 Introduction

Data and its acquisition are the prime components of computational cytology (CCyt). The data are acquired from various sources. The main components of the data are microscopic images, clinical, biochemical, radiological and molecular genetics [1]. The pre-processing of data is needed to train the artificial intelligence (AI) model.

P. Dey, *Computational Cytology*, https://doi.org/10.1007/978-981-95-3272-8_5

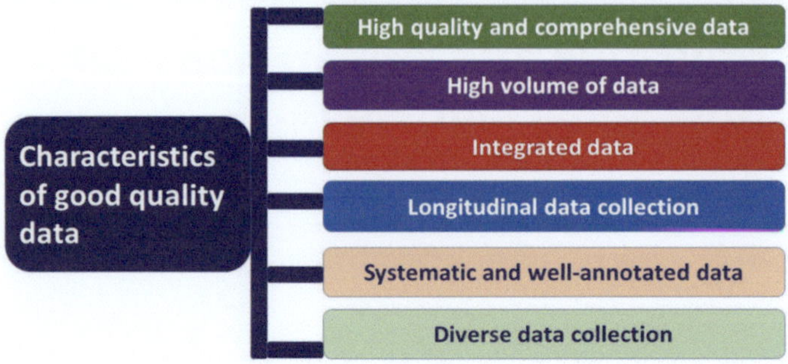

Fig. 5.1 Characteristics of high-quality data collection

5.2 Data Collection: What are the Characteristics of Good Quality Data?

The salient features of data collections are described below [2, 3] (Fig. 5.1):

1. *Good-quality comprehensive data*: The high-quality and complete data is required to have a robust model.
2. *Quantity*: The data should be in a huge volume to generate a robust AI model.
3. *Integration*: The multimodal data fusion gives a holistic approach to the tumour.
4. *Longitudinal data series*: The longitudinal data collection gives the overview of the disease and helps in prognostic prediction and management of the disease.
5. *Annotated and organized data*: Annotated and organized data is essential.
6. *Wide range of data collection*: A wide range of data collection from various areas helps to eliminate bias.

5.3 Types of Data

The types of data can be classified as Internal and external databases.

5.3.1 Internal Database

It is generated from the local hospital or laboratory data.

5.3.1.1 Clinical Data (Box 5.1)

It includes the clinical details of the patient such as chief complaints, medical history, treatment history and other demographic data.

Characteristics

The characteristics of the clinical data are:

- It is well-oriented.
- The clinical data is in the form of text data. So to make an AI model, we have to convert the text data into digital data.
- Clinical data along with microscopic image (WSI) and molecular data help to predict the prognosis.

Applications
- Building the prognostic model in CCyt.
- The multimodal fusion of clinical data with image data helps to make a successful AI model.

Challenges
- This data is usually extensively variable from laboratory to laboratory.
- To keep the privacy of the individuals.

Box 5.1 Clinical Data

Contents
- Chief complaints
- Past medical history
- Therapy history
- Other essential data

Characteristics
- Structured data
- The text data needs to be converted into digital data

Applications
- Building the prognostic model in CCyt
- The multimodal fusion of clinical data with WSI

Challenges
- Data secrecy

5.3.1.2 Whole Slide Imaging (WSI)

The WSI provides image data (Box 5.2). It digitally records the entire slide and can be visualized in different magnifications. WSI images are easy to transfer in distant places.

Main Characteristics
- The WSI images occupy a vast amount of storage space (several thousand megapixels).
- The WSI provides the distinct cellular details.
- A whole slide scanner is essential to have WSI slides.

Applications

- Digitized image may help in the identification, sub-classification and grading of tumour.
- The architectural pattern of the tumour cells is discernible.
- The WSIs are used to train an AI model.

Challenges

- The huge data in WSI.
- Expert pathologists are needed for annotation of the image.

Box 5.2 Digital Imaging by Whole Slide Imaging (WSI)

- WSI is the source of digital slide
- Cytology images need additional Z-axis scan

Main Characteristics

- The WSI images occupies vast amount of storage space

Applications

- To identify the morphological pattern of the tumour cells from WSI
- WSI is the source of training data for AI model

Challenges

- Massive data in WSI
- Annotation is a cumbersome process

5.3.1.3 Molecular Genetics (Box 5.3)

The sources of molecular genetics are: genomic, epigenetic, proteomic, structural and molecular interaction data.

Characteristics

- It shows mutation, gene expression profile and epigenetic changes.
- The data is expressed as sequencing files.

Applications

- Molecular genetics along with WSI may find new biomarkers.
- In precision medicine.
- Multimodal model generation.

Challenges

- Molecular genetics is expensive.
- It is complex.
- Integration of the molecular data with other data is a major challenge.

Box 5.3 Molecular Genetics

Main sources: Genomic data, epigenetic data, proteomic data, structural data and molecular interaction data

Characteristics

- Molecular data is viewed as specific digital file formats (sequential file).

Applications

- Helpful to detect the newer biomarkers.
- It is the building block of personalised medicine.
- It helps to make the multimodal model.

Challenges

- Costly to generate
- Complex data
- Multimodal data fusion of molecular data with WSI, clinical data is a challenging task.

5.3.1.4 Biomarker Data

The biomarker data helps to diagnose and predict the therapeutic response of the disease (Box 5.4).

Characteristics

- Multimodal data fusion is possible with the biomarker data and WSI and clinical data.
- The biomarkers help in the assessment of the pathological process.
- Biomarkers are often the targets of therapy.

Applications

- To diagnose and predict prognosis.
- To assess the patient's response to treatment.

Challenges

- The biomarker measurement needs standardization.

Box 5.4 Biomarker Data

Characteristics

- Integration of the biomarker data with clinical data, imaging data and molecular data provides an effective model
- The biomarkers are the therapeutic targets.

Applications

- Diagnostic and prognostic markers of the disease.
- The common predictors of therapeutic response.

Challenges

- Standardization is needed.

5.3.1.5 Radiology Imaging

It includes simple radiographic image, computerized tomographic scan, magnetic resonance image and positron emission tomographic scan (Box 5.5).

Characteristics

- Radiological imaging is useful in determining the exact location, local extension and distant metastasis of the lesion.

Applications

- The multimodal data fusion of the radiology and WSI images may provide a more accurate diagnosis.

Challenges

- To do fusion of the radiological and cytological data is a challenge.

Box 5.5 Radiology Imaging Data

Contents

- Simple radiographic image.
- Computerised tomographic scan.
- Magnetic resonance image.
- Positron emission tomographic scan.

Characteristics

- To locate the lesion.
- To notice invasion and distant metastasis.

Applications

- The multimodal data fusion of the radiology and WSI images may provide a more accurate diagnosis.

5.3.1.6 Environmental and Lifestyle Data

These include the patient's environmental settings, behaviours and personal habits that can influence their health.

Characteristics

- The data is collected directly from the list of questions asked to patients.
- The data may be unreliable.

Applications

- To determine the role of environmental factors in the pathogenesis of the disease.
- To make a predictive model.

Challenges

- Limited obtainability and reliability of data.

5.3.2 External Database

External database is acquired from the medical journals, clinical trials or other databases (Fig. 5.2). It is accessible to all the medical personnel.

Examples of External Databases

1. *The Cancer Genome Atlas (TCGA)*: TCGA contains the data of the molecular genetics along with histopathology, cytology of several cancers.
2. *The Cancer Imaging Archive (TCIA)*: TCIA contains the WSI of pathology and radiology images of the different tumours.
3. *Gene Expression Omnibus (GEO)*: GEO includes the genomic and transcriptomic data in different diseases.

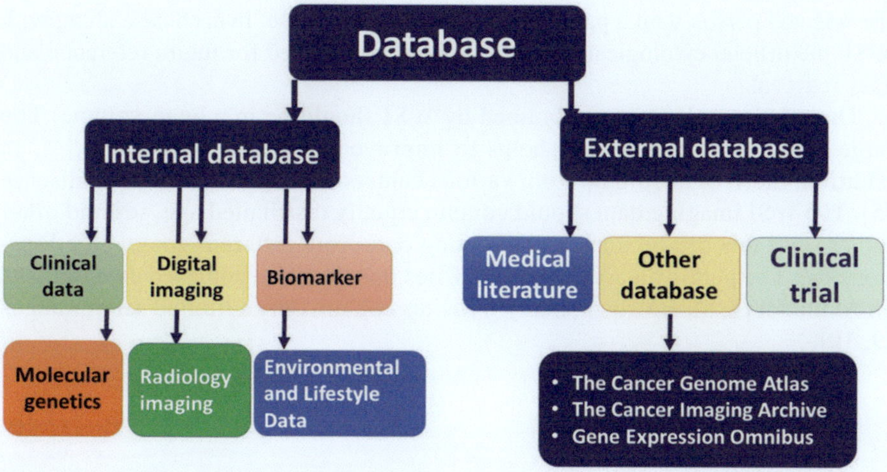

Fig. 5.2 Internal and external databases

5.3.2.1 Characteristics of an External Database

- *Publicly available*: It is open to all. Occasionally, the data may be password-protected.
- *Centralized data*: The data is centralized and can be downloaded by multiple institutions and studies.
- *Annotated dataset*: Many external databases are annotated.
- Examples:
  1. *NuInsSeg*: NuInsSeg contains images of a huge number of segmented nuclei extracted from the WSI.
  2. *Lizard*: The dataset is derived from the colonic tissue.
  3. *Acrobat*: It has the WSI of the Hematoxylin and eosin-stained slides histopathology section of breast cancer cases.
- *Security*: The frequent internet hacking makes the external database insecure. It should be a strong password-protected.
- *Data transfer*: The data transfer should be secured by the encryption protocol and monitored continuously.

5.4 Data Preparation

Data preparation is a multistep process that incorporates data collection, annotation, formatting and pre-processing. The different modalities of the data should be properly stored with a rapid retrieval facility.

Digital slide The whole slide imaging (WSI) of the cytology sample should be taken routinely from every cytology case. A cytopathologist should personally select the slide for scanning, as only certain slides may be representative. The slide should be well-stained, clean and free from artefact. The WSI should be properly labelled and if possible, should be attached with the hospital information service (HIS) and electronic health record (EHR). Access to the WSI should be restricted to the selected person with a password to prevent any misuse. In each case along with WSI, the official cytological diagnosis should be attached for future reference and easy retrieval.

The microscopic images obtained by WSI should be in a huge volume. The large amount of training data helps to improve the performance of AI [4]. In addition, the WSI should be from various centres and various subsets of disease [5]. The WSI imaging data should contain equally distributed age, sex and other factors and this can be done by collecting data from different geographic locations [6]. The public dataset on the websites may be more unbiased data to make an AI model [7, 8]. However, many websites contain only a limited set of images [9, 10].

5.5 Conclusions

The dataset is the main source of neural network models. The good-quality data collection is very much needed. The data is mainly of two types: internal and external databases. The internal databases are generated from the local laboratories and these are the main sources of data. The external data bases are usually collected from the medical literatures and publicly accessible webpages. The complete utilization of both the datasets can help to make an effective neural network model.

References

1. Choudhuri KBR, Mangrulkar RS. Data acquisition and preparation for artificial intelligence and machine learning applications in the book design of intelligent applications using machine learning and deep learning techniques. 1st ed. Chapman and Hall; 2023.
2. Chen L, Acun B, Ardalini N et al. Data acquisition: a new frontier in data-centric AI. https://doi.org/10.48550/arXiv.2311.13712.
3. Yang Y, Sun K, Gao Y, Wang K, Yu G. Preparing data for artificial intelligence in pathology with clinical-grade performance. Diagnostics (Basel). 2023;13(19):3115. https://doi.org/10.3390/diagnostics13193115.
4. Campanella G, Hanna MG, Geneslaw L, Miraflor A, Silva VWK, Busam KJ, Brogi E, Reuter VE, Klimstra DS, Fuchs TJ. Clinical-grade computational pathology using weakly supervised deep learning on whole slide images. Nat Med. 2019;25:1301–9.
5. Skrede OJ, De Raedt S, Kleppe A, et al. Deep learning for prediction of colorectal cancer outcome: a discovery and validation study. Lancet. 2020;395(10221):350–60. https://doi.org/10.1016/S0140-6736(19)32998-8.
6. Iizuka O, Kanavati F, Kato K, Rambeau M, Arihiro K, Tsuneki M. Deep learning models for histopathological classification of gastric and colonic epithelial tumours. Sci Rep. 2020;10:1504.
7. Cruz-Roa A, Gilmore H, Basavanhally A, Feldman M, Ganesan S, Shih NN, Tomaszewski J, González FA, Madabhushi A. Accurate and reproducible invasive breast cancer detection in whole-slide images: a deep learning approach for quantifying tumor extent. Sci Rep. 2017;7:srep46450.
8. Yu G, Sun K, Xu C, Shi X-H, Wu C, Xie T, Meng R-Q, Meng X-H, Wang K-S, Xiao H-M, et al. Accurate recognition of colorectal cancer with semi-supervised deep learning on pathological images. Nat Commun. 2021;12:6311.
9. Foucart A, Debeir O, Decaestecker C. SNOW: semi-supervised, noisy And/Or weak data for deep learning in digital pathology. In: Proceedings of the 2019 IEEE 16th International Symposium on Biomedical Imaging (ISBI 2019), Venice, Italy, 8–11 April 2019. p. 1869–72.
10. Khened M, Kori A, Rajkumar H, Krishnamurthi G, Srinivasan B. A generalized deep learning framework for whole-slide image segmentation and analysis. Sci Rep. 2021;11:11579.

Image Processing in Cytology

6

Abstract

The proper processing of the images of cytology is essential to implement computational cytology. Image processing includes image acquisition, pre-processing, segmentation and feature extraction. Noise reduction is an important part of image pre-processing. It can be done by spatial domain filtering, frequency domain filtering, wavelet-based denoising and deep learning-based approaches. Stain normalization and artefact removal are also important. The section or smear often needs annotation to highlight the region or cells of interest. In the present chapter, the various steps of image processing have been discussed.

Keywords

Image Processing · Noise · Annotation · Gaussian noise · Salt-and-Pepper Noise Poisson Noise · Speckle Noise

6.1 Introduction

The processing of the images of cytology is an important step to implement Computational cytology (CCyt). The conversion of a cytology slide into a digital slide needs careful attention. Image processing means a set of steps that consist of image acquisition, pre-processing, segmentation and feature extraction. The final stage of diagnosis is assisted by artificial intelligence (AI) in the case of CCyt. In the present chapter, the image processing technique is discussed.

P. Dey, *Computational Cytology*, https://doi.org/10.1007/978-981-95-3272-8_6

6.2 Image Acquisition

Image acquisition is the first and most important step. The cytology slides are commonly stained by Papanicolaou's stain, May Grunwald Giemsa stain and Haematoxylin and Eosin stain.

Box 6.1 Screening of Cytology Slides Before Digitization

- Select the representative slide
- Discard grossly under-stained or over-stained smears
- Avoid air bubbles
- Avoid stain deposit
- No artefact
- Clean the slides

Screening of slides for digitization The screening of slides is the first step before digitization by whole slide imaging (WSI) (Box 6.1). Archival slides often have many artefacts due to long storage. The slides with stain precipitation, bubbles under the cover slip and gross staining anomalies should be discarded. Before WSI, the cleaning of the slides is needed. Precautions should be taken not to dissolve the special coverslip (used in some WSI scanners) by xylene.

Digitization of the slides WSI scans the slide and digitises them in high resolution. The cells are often present as 3D clusters in cytology smears. So the Z-axis scanning is mandatory in cytology scanning (Box 6.2). Therefore, careful selection of a digital scanner is needed. The high-quality images with higher resolution in different magnifications are preferable for WSI. Care should be taken on proper focusing and illumination.

The details of the scanning are described in the subsequent chapters.

Box 6.2 Digitization by WSI

- Z-scanning facility
- Proper focusing
- High resolution
- Different magnifications
- Well illumination

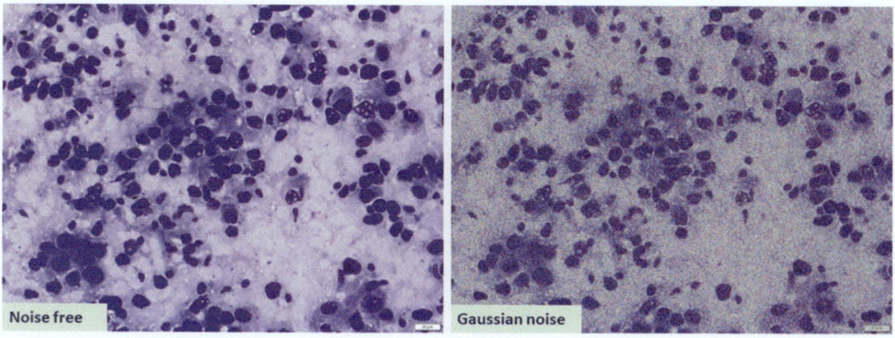

Fig. 6.1 Gaussian noise showing fine-grained variation in the entire image

6.3 Data Pre-Processing

1. *Noise and ways to reduce*: Noise in the digital image means the unwanted random variation of pixel value distorting colour or brightness (Box 6.3).

   Types of noise:

   (a) *Gaussian Noise*: It is the commonest type of noise encountered in the digital image. It is called Gaussian noise because the noise values show a Gaussian (normal) distribution. It means that the majority of the noise values are close to zero and only a few values have large deviations. Gaussian noise is caused by poor lighting. The noise appears as fine-grained or soft static variation in brightness scattered over the entire image (Fig. 6.1). The use of a Gaussian filter can avoid this noise.

Box 6.3 Noise and its Reduction in Digital Image

Noise: Unwanted random variation of pixel value resulting in variation of colour or brightness

Type of noise

- *Gaussian Noise*: Here, noise values show a Gaussian (normal) distribution
  Appearance: Fine-grained or soft static variation in brightness scattered over the entire image.
- *Salt-and-Pepper Noise*: It is due to faulty sensors or hardware of the camera or an error during analog-to-digital conversion.
  Appearance: Random black and white pixels.
- *Poisson Noise*: It is related to the quantum nature of light.
  Appearance: A grainy texture is noted in the high contrast region.
- *Speckle Noise*: It is due to interference between coherent wave fronts.
  Appearance: A grainy or textured appearance.

(continued)

Box 6.3 (continued)

Noise Reduction Techniques

- Spatial Domain Filtering
- Frequency Domain Filtering
- Wavelet-Based Denoising
- Deep learning-based approaches

(b) *Salt-and-Pepper Noise*: It is seen as random "'black and white'" pixels (Fig. 6.2). This type of noise is due to faulty sensors or a camera or an error during the analog-to-digital conversion of the image.

(c) *Poisson Noise*: Here, a grainy texture is noted in the high contrast region. Poisson noise is signal-dependent and it is related to the quantum nature of light.

(d) *Speckle Noise*: Speckle noise appears as a grainy or textured appearance. The noise is multiplicative. It is commonly seen in ultrasound or MRI images. Speckle noise arises due to interference between coherent wave fronts.

6.3.1 Noise Reduction Techniques

Different filters can be applied to reduce the noise.

(i) Spatial Domain Filtering: In this approach, the filters (mean filter, Gaussian filter, etc.) directly operate on the pixels of the image.

(ii) Frequency Domain Filtering: In this approach, at first, the image is transformed and then filtered. After reducing the noise, the image is again transformed back.

(iii) Wavelet-Based Denoising: Here, discrete wavelet transform is applied to separate the image into different frequency bands.

(iv) Deep learning-based approaches: In this approach, convolutional neural network (CNN) or Generative Adversarial Networks (GAN) is trained to generate noise-free image.

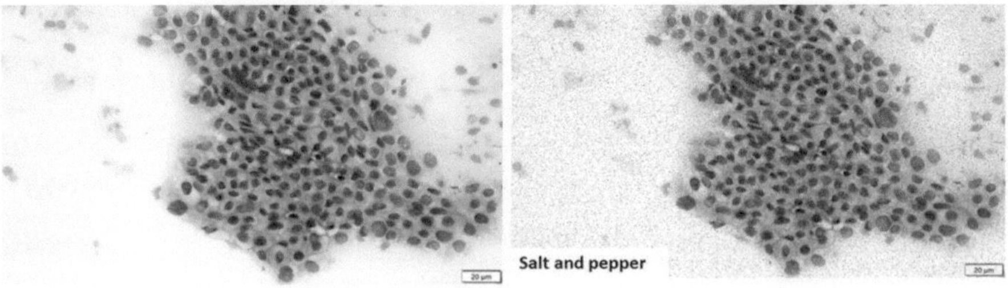

Fig. 6.2 Salt-and-pepper noise: Note the black and white specks

Table 6.1 highlights different types of noise and the reduction techniques.

2. *Stain normalization*: The inconsistency of the staining may be due to (a) the different methods of sample processing, (b) variable intensity of the stain component and (c) differences of WSI scanner setting. The techniques of stain normalization are: (i) to match the colour, (ii) normalize the colour and (iii) staining separation. The various practical methods are described below:
   A. *Histogram Matching* (Fig. 6.3): Here, the histogram of the test image is modified so that the histogram looks like that of reference image [1].

Steps (Box 6.4)

- Both test and standard images are uploaded.
- Here, we adjust the pixel intensity distribution of a source image with that of a standard image.

Advantages A simple technique.

Table 6.1 Comparison of different types of noise

Type of noise	Nature	Cause	Appearance	Removal technique
Gaussian Noise	Additive	Poor lighting	Fine-grained over the entire image	Gaussian filter
Salt-and-Pepper Noise	Impulsive	Faulty sensors or hardware of camera, or an error during analog-to-digital conversion.	Random black and white specks	Median filter, or adaptive median filter
Poisson Noise	Signal-dependent	Quantum variation in photon counting	Grainy and more in bright areas	Gaussian filter, Deep learning
Speckle Noise	Multiplicative	Coherent wave interference	Grainy, textured, depends on intensity	Kuan filters

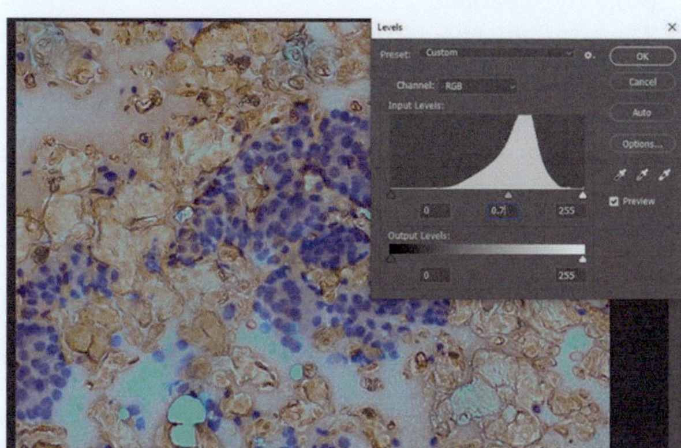

Fig. 6.3 Colour normalization by histogram

Limitations

- Due to contrast stretching forces applied here, the unnatural effect may be seen.
- The histogram technique may not solve the local colour variation.

Box 6.4 Stain Normalization by Histogram Matching

The histogram of the test image is modified so that the histogram looks like that of the reference image.

Steps

- Both test and standard images are uploaded.
- Adjust the pixel intensity distribution of a source image with that of a standard image.

Advantages: A simple technique.

Limitations

- The unnatural effect may be seen.
- It may not solve the local colour variation.

B. Stain Separation Technique

Here, individual parts of the image are normalized.

Methods

(a) *Macenko Method*: In Macenko method, the singular value decomposition (SVD) in the optical density space is applied [2] to eliminate staining variation (Fig. 6.4). The red-green-blue channel of the image is converted to optical density (OD). OD value of the image helps in normalization of the staining (Box 6.5).

Limitations

- Good-quality reference images are needed and the stain components should be properly separated.
- The accurate calculation of SVD and OD is mandatory.

Box 6.5 Macenko Method of Stain Separation Technique

Here, the singular value decomposition (SVD) in the optical density space is applied.

Steps

- Convert RGB to Optical Density (OD) Space.
- Remove Low-Intensity Pixels from Background.
- Perform Singular Value Decomposition (SVD): Apply *SVD* on the filtered OD values.

- Project OD values onto the Stain Plane.
- Select the Stain Vectors.
- Normalize Stain Concentrations.

Limitations
- Good-quality reference images are needed.
- The accurate calculation of SVD and OD are mandatory.

(b) *Reinhard Method*: The Reinhard method is simple. Here, the mean and standard deviation of the test images are matched with the standard image (Box 6.6).

Steps
- Red-green-blue image is transformed into the LAB colour space.
- The statistics are calculated in the "test" and "standard" images.
- Now, the individual channel of the test image is adjusted with that of the standard one.
- Lastly, the test image is transformed into an RGB image.

Limitations
- Both the images may not have a direct linear relation and the stain variability may be complex.
- It is inferior to the Macenko Method.

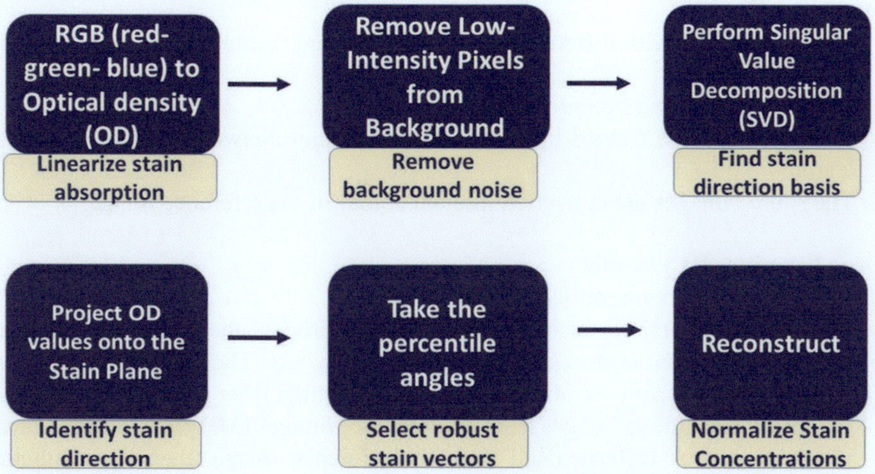

Fig. 6.4 The steps of the Macenko Method of stain separation technique

Box 6.6 Reinhard Method

Here, the mean and standard deviation of the test images are matched with the standard image.

Steps
- RGB image is transformed into the LAB colour space.
- The statistics are calculated in the "test" and "standard" images.
- The individual channel of the test image is adjusted with that of the standard one.
- The test image is transformed into the RGB image.

Limitations
- Both images may not have a direct linear relation.
- It is inferior to the Macenko Method.

C. *Deep Learning (DL) in Normalization* (Box 6.7): DL is unique to normalize the colour of the image [3].

Characteristics
- Highly adaptable.
- High scalability: Can handle a large dataset.
- Accurate: Superior to other techniques.
- Automated: No manual interference.

Steps
- Raw image data with different staining colours and resolution is acquired from different sources.
- The image is altered in a proper format.
- The image data is trained by Convolutional Neural Networks (CNNs), a deep learning model.
- The source images are converted into the colour of the reference image.

Deep learning (DL) Model
1. CNN: The most commonly used DL is CNN.
2. Generative Adversarial Networks (GANs): To process the complex data, one should use a GAN. It works with two neural networks. The generator generates artificial images from the original image. The distinguisher network tries to distinguish the synthetic images from the reference images [3]. When the generated image cannot be differentiated from the reference image, then the synthetic image is acceptable.
3. *Neural Style Transfer (NST)*: NST is applied to match the colour with the reference image [4].

Advantages of DL DL is well-suited for the complex and non-linear colour transformation of the image.

Limitations DL needs a large volume of images for training the model.

Box 6.7 Deep Learning (DL) in Normalization

Characteristics

- Highly adaptable
- High scalability
- Accurate
- Automated

Steps

- Raw image data with different staining colours and resolution is acquired.
- The image is altered in a proper format.
- The image data is trained by Convolutional Neural Networks (CNNs).
- The source images are converted into the colour of the reference image.

Deep learning (DL) model

- CNN
- Generative Adversarial Networks
- Neural Style Transfer

Tiling WSI images take huge space and so difficult to manage. It is necessary to have a subplot of the WSI image (Fig. 6.5).

Removing Artefacts The air bubbles, pen marks, stain precipitations, etc., should be removed.

Scaling and Compression The large image is compressed and stored with detailed information.

Annotation Supervised learning method of the AI model works better if the region of interest (ROI) is already demonstrated. An annotated image helps to locate *the* ROI.

Aims of annotation The main aim of annotation is to identify the objects of interest.

Types of annotation

- Manual Annotation: Here, the annotation is done manually by the pathologists.

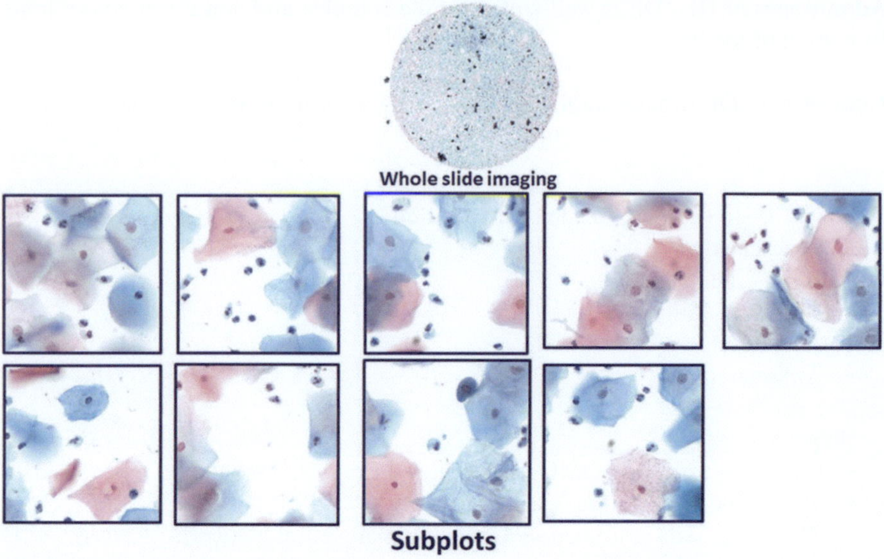

Fig. 6.5 The whole slide imaging smear is divided into several subplots

- Semi-Automated Tools: It is partly manual and a software (e.g. QuPath) platform is used for the annotation. It is less time-consuming and easy to do.
- Crowdsourcing: In crowdsourcing, a non-expert does the annotation under the supervision of a pathologist.

Selection of Different Types of Annotation

(a) *Image Classification*: It is a crude technique. The image is only labelled in a category, e.g. cat or dog.

(b) *Object Detection*: The specific objects of interest are labelled Workflow
   - *Dataset*: The images are acquired
   - Annotation
     1. Image is loaded in the proper annotation-platform
     2. The boxes are drawn around the object.
     3. Every bounding boxes are is labelled accordingly
     4. Annotation is saved (Fig. 6.6)

Export in the format

- *YOLO*: The TXT files with the normalized bounding boxes are used.
- *Pascal VOC*: XML files with the bounding box coordinates are applied.
- *COCO*: JSON files with supporting features are used.
- *TFRecord*: It is used for TensorFlow models.

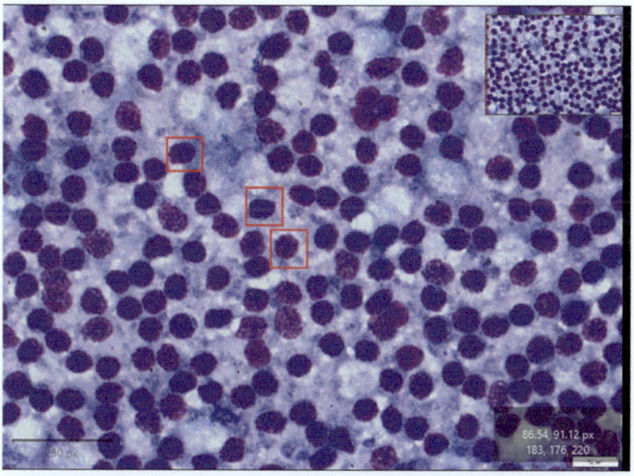

Fig. 6.6 Annotated image by bounding box and saved in jpg format

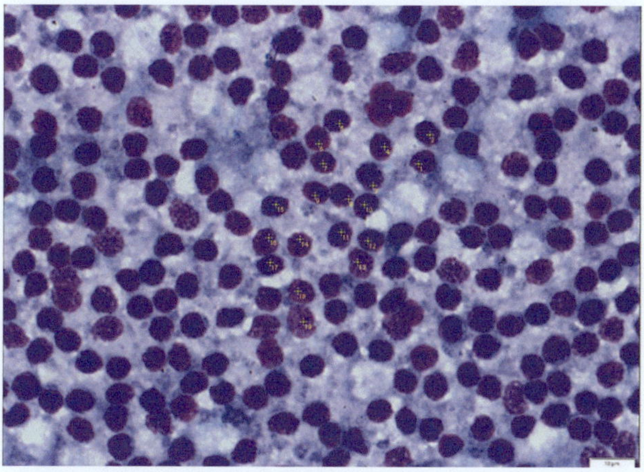

Fig. 6.7 Keypoint annotation by identifying the cells with the click

(c) *Semantic Segmentation*: Here each pixel of the image is classified into a specific category and pixel with same labels belongs to same class.
(d) *Instance Segmentation*: Instance Segmentation not only differentiate each pixel by category, but also identifies each object in the same category.
(e) *Keypoint Annotation*: The object of interest is marked (Fig. 6.7)
(f) *Line and Polygon Annotation*: The lines or polygons are drawn around the object (Fig. 6.8)
(g) *Scribble Annotation*: Rough line is drawn surrounding the object of interest (Fig. 6.9)
(h) *3D Bounding Boxes*: Three dimensional bounding boxes are applied around the object of interest

Table 6.2 shows the comparison of different types of annotations.

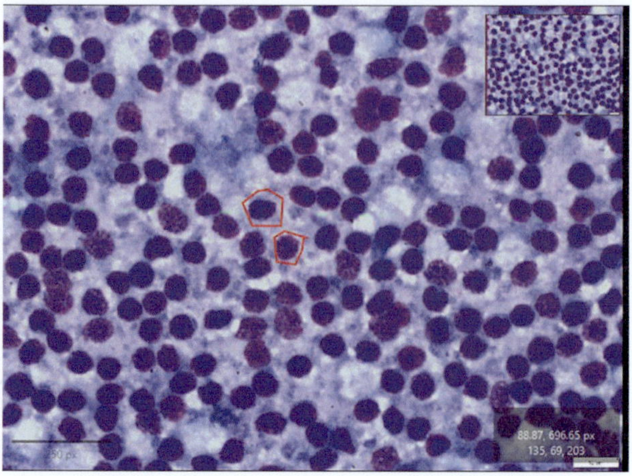

Fig. 6.8 Polygon annotation by drawing polygon around the image of interest

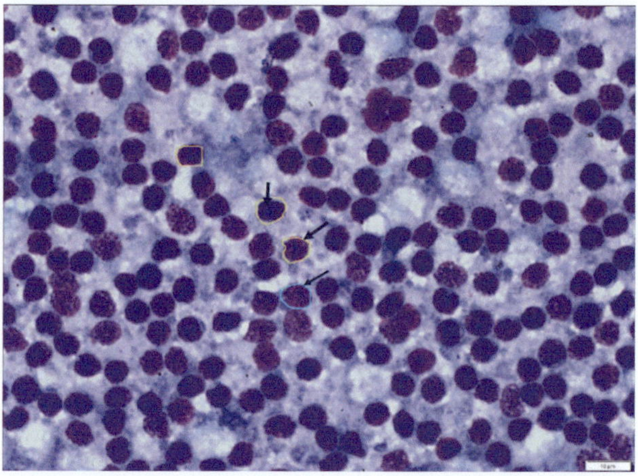

Fig. 6.9 Scribble annotation

Table 6.2 The comparison of different types of annotations

Annotation type	Description	Use in cytology	Advantages	Disadvantage
Image Classification	The whole image is labelled	Whole smear or slide is classified	Fast and simple. It is useful for weak supervision	Unsuitable for detection or segmentation
Bounding Box Annotation	Boxes are drawn around cells or regions of interest	Cell detection	Easier to annotate	Inaccurate for irregularly shaped objects
Polygon Annotation	Detailed outlines of objects using vertices	More precise to delineate the cells or nuclei	High accuracy for irregular shapes	Time-consuming and labour-intensive
Semantic Segmentation	Pixel-wise labelling, where each pixel is assigned to a class	Segmentation of nuclei, cytoplasm and background	Suitable for training a CNN	Extensive effort and expertise are needed
Instance Segmentation	It not only differentiates each pixel by category, but also differentiates between individual objects of the same class.	Counting and analysing individual cells	Enables both localization and classification	Highly complex annotation
Point Annotation	Specific object is annotated by marking those points of interest	Cell counting	Very fast; useful for cell counting	Limited information; unsuitable for segmentation
Scribble Annotation	Rough lines or strokes indicating object boundaries	Weakly supervised segmentation	Faster than full segmentation	Less accurate; needs post-processing or special models

6.4 Methods of Annotations

The methods of annotations are described below:

6.4.1 Fine Annotation

It accurately outlines the object of interest [5].

Characteristics of fine annotation

- High accuracy.
- Subcategories of the objects of interest are also labelled.
- It is a time-consuming process.

Advantages
- High-quality dataset is generated.
- Improved performance is achieved.

Challenges
- Time-consuming
- Expensive

6.4.2 Weak Annotation

The weak annotation identifies the object of interest without the complete separation from the adjacent tissue. It is incomplete and coarse. However, it saves time [6, 7].

Characteristics of weak annotation
- Low precision.
- Less details of information.
- Rapid and cheap.

Advantages
- Rapid and cheap.
- Useful for developing pre-trained models.

Challenges
- The model may not be perfect due to weak annotation.

6.4.3 Sparse Annotation

In sparse annotation, only a small part of the image is annotated and the substantial part of the image is not annotated.

Characteristics
- Annotation is partial.
- Only the important area is annotated.
- Faster and cheaper.

Advantages
- Faster and cheaper, but the necessary information remains intact.
- It is used in a large dataset.

Challenges
- At times, the model may need dense and complete annotation and then sparse annotation may not be useful.

6.5 Image Segmentation

Purpose and Importance The segmentation of the image is very important to identify the ROI and to extract the features for diagnosis and classification. The ROI may be individual cells, nuclei, gland or any other structures.

- *Traditional Methods*: The traditional method includes adjusting optical density or by watershed algorithms (Fig. 6.10). These are limited by inconsistent intensity of the stain, cellular overlapping, complex arrangements, etc.
- *Deep Learning Approaches*: Convolutional Neural Networks (CNNs) are a type of deep learning technique. The trained CNN model can directly identify the ROI from the image with high accuracy.

6.6 Feature Extraction

Traditional feature extraction Traditional feature extraction involves the measurement of morphometric data (diameter, perimeter, area) and textural data.

Deep learning CNN extracts the features itself to classify the image and diagnosis.

6.7 Conclusions

Image processing is an important component of model building and diagnosis. There may be various barriers to get a satisfactory image. Proper selection of the slides is an important step of digitalization. The slide should be free of artefact and stain should be optimum. Digital images are often affected by noise that needs reduction. The pathologists should be aware of these hurdles to overcome them.

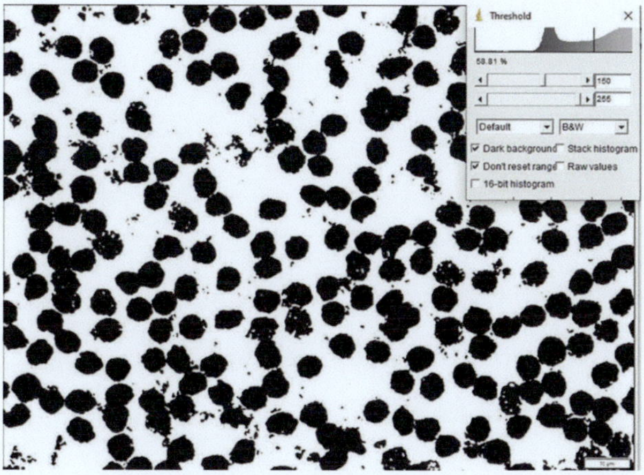

Fig. 6.10 Detection of cells of interest by adjusting the threshold

References

1. Roy S, Kumar Jain A, Lal S, Kini J. A study about color normalization methods for histopathology images. Micron. 2018;114:42–61. https://doi.org/10.1016/j.micron.2018.07.005. Epub 2018 Aug 1.
2. Macenko M, Niethammer M, Marron JS, Borland D, Woosley JT, Xiaojun G. A method for normalizing histology slides for quantitative analysis. In: 2009 IEEE International Symposium on Biomedical Imaging: from Nano to Macro, Boston, 2009. p. 1107–10.
3. Ke J, Shen Y, Lu Y. Style normalization in histology with federated learning. In: Proceedings of the 2021 IEEE 18th International Symposium on Biomedical Imaging (ISBI), Nice, France, 13–16 April 2021. p. 953–6.
4. Goodfellow I, Pouget-Abadie J, Mirza M, Xu B, Warde-Farley D, Ozair S, Courville A, Bengio Y. Generative adversarial nets. Cambridge, MA: MIT Press; 2014. p. 2672–80.
5. Khened M, Kori A, Rajkumar H, Krishnamurthi G, Srinivasan B. A generalized deep learning framework for whole-slide image segmentation and analysis. Sci Rep. 2021;11(1):11579. https://doi.org/10.1038/s41598-021-90444-8. PMID: 34078928; PMCID: PMC8172839.
6. Chen Z, Chen Z, Liu J, Zheng Q, Zhu Y, Zuo Y, Wang Z, Guan X, Wang Y, Li Y. Weakly supervised histopathology image segmentation with sparse point annotations. IEEE J Biomed Health Inform. 2021;25:1673–85.
7. Dai J, He K, Sun J. BoxSup: exploiting bounding boxes to supervise convolutional networks for semantic segmentation. In: Proceedings of the 2015 IEEE International Conference on Computer Vision (ICCV), Santiago, Chile, 7–13 December 2015. p. 1635–43.

7 Artificial Neural Network: An Overview

Abstract

Artificial intelligence (AI) is a branch of computer science that simulates the human brain and performs various challenging and complicated tasks. An artificial neural network (ANN) is a computational model that simulates the human brain. ANN is composed of multiple nodes that simulate the biological neurons. The ANN model is multi-layered and is composed of an input layer, a hidden layer and the output layer. The model learns from the experience or training data. In each learning session, the strength of the inter-nodal connection is changed. The ANN model mainly learns by supervised learning, unsupervised learning, reinforcement learning and transfer learning. The ANN model building is a multistep process and needs attention in each step. The current chapter discusses the various fundamental aspects of ANN.

Keywords

Artificial intelligence · Artificial neural network · Supervised learning · Unsupervised learning · Transfer learning · Reinforcement learning · Activation function · Optimization algorithms

7.1 Introduction

The human brain is composed of a huge number of interconnected neurons. It can perform various functions. The unique characteristics of the human brain are its high learning capacities, parallel data processing and non-linear thinking capabilities. Ordinary computers are unable to do these functions. Here begins the role of the artificial intelligence (AI). AI simulates the human brain and performs various challenging and complicated tasks that are impossible to perform by ordinary computers [1, 2]. In the last few decades, there is a significant progress of AI in the field of pathology. In fact, AI is reshaping the medical field. Artificial intelligence is the

P. Dey, *Computational Cytology*, https://doi.org/10.1007/978-981-95-3272-8_7

cornerstone of computation cytology. It helps to take many important decisions in computational cytology such as screening and detection of malignancy, diagnosis, classification and management of patients [3–8].

7.2 Terminologies Used in AI

There are several terminologies in AI and they deserve to be defined.

Artificial Intelligence (AI): AI is the simulation of human intellect with the help of computer programs.
Artificial Neural Network (ANN): ANN is a computer program that mimics the human brain. It is a key component of machine learning and deep learning.
Machine Learning (ML): ML is the subcategory of AI that executes certain tasks without further program designing.
Deep Learning (DL): DL is a subcategory of ML that utilizes ANN to analyse the complex patterns in the data. DL is mainly used in image classification and diagnosis.
Convolutional network (CNN): CNN is a subset of DL that mainly deals with images. In CNN, multiple filters are used to convolute the images and reduction of the dimensions. So, by repeated convolution operations, the large data is reduced to a small small-dimensional image.

7.3 Basic Principles of Artificial Neural Network

The software program of ANN simulates the organization of the biological neurons of the human brain.

Biological neuron: The biological neuron receives the input information through the dendrites and processes it in the cell body. If the total input exceeds a certain value, then it fires the next neuron through the axon. The synapse is the connection between the axon and the dendrite of the other neuron.
Artificial neuron: An ANN is made of multiple nodes that simulate the biological neurons. Each node receives the signal/information from the other nodes. Each signal has its own weightage (w) and intensity (i). If the total combined signal value supersedes the threshold value, then it activates the next node (Fig. 7.1).

The ANN model is multi-layered and is composed of input, hidden and output layers (Fig. 7.2). These layers are composed of multiple nodes.

Input layer: The inner layer receives the data as numerical values, and text.
Hidden layer: The hidden layer is composed of multiple nodes. It is responsible for analysing the complex data.
Output layer: The Output layer is the final outcome of an ANN model. It is composed of single to multiple nodes, depending on the model's target.

Every node is linked with all the other nodes of the next layer. The input layer receives information from the outer environment which means the dataset. It then

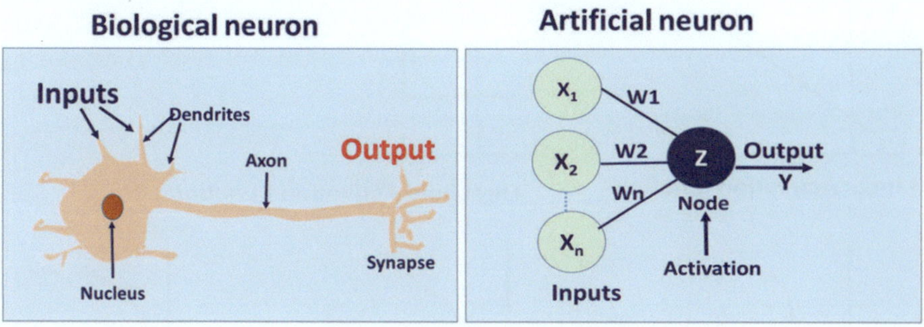

Fig. 7.1 The diagram compares the biological neuron versus artificial neuron

Fig. 7.2 Multilayer perceptron consisting of input, hidden and output layers

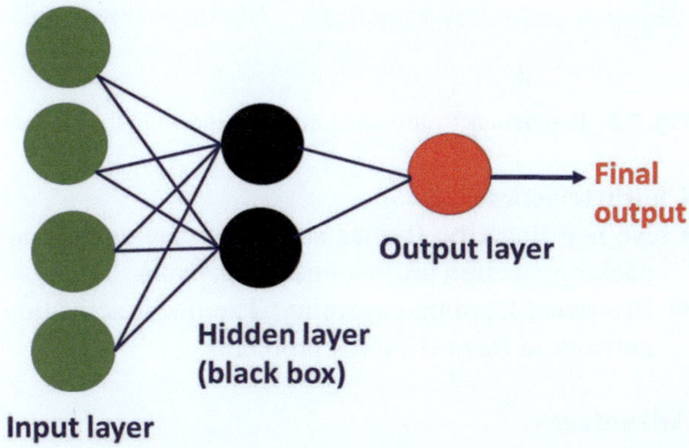

transmits the signal to the hidden layer which processes the signal further and finally hands over the signal to the output layer. The hidden layer helps to make decisions on complex problems. The signal processing activities of the hidden layer are not controlled by the operator and so its other name is "black box". The final output may be single or multiple, depending on the model setup. The above-mentioned architecture of the ANN is known as a multilayer perceptron which is the main building block of any ANN model.

7.4 Activation Functions

The activation function determines the initiation of data processing of the neuron in an ANN. Figure 7.3 shows the diagrammatic representation of various activation functions.

7.4.1 Linear Activation Function

Here, the output is directly proportional to the input data (Box 7.1).

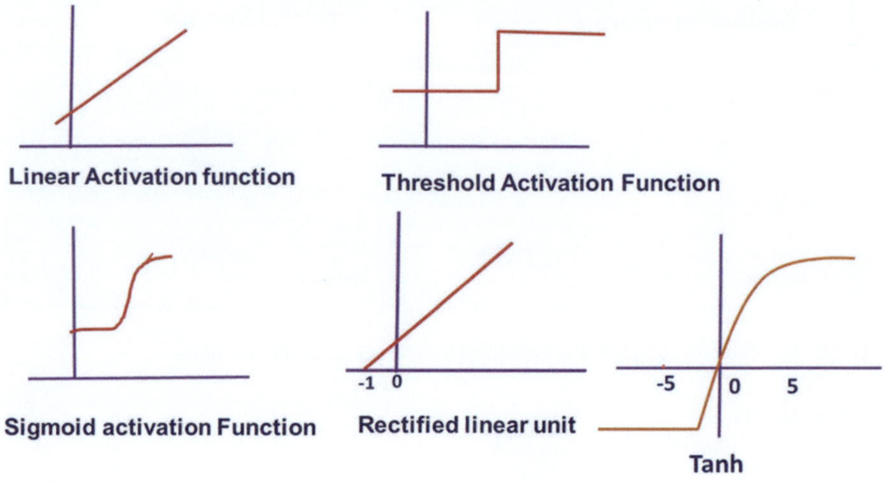

Fig. 7.3 Different activation functions are shown in the diagram

Characteristics:

- No non-linearity: It does not follow any non-linearity, so it is not suitable for a backpropagation artificial neural network.
- Restricted learning capability: The linear activation function does not allow the network to learn complex problems.

Advantages

- Simple and easy to use.
- Suitable for getting the continuous output data.

Disadvantages

- It is unable to use complex data.

Box 7.1: Linear Activation Function

Here. the output is directly proportional to the input data.

Characteristics:

- No non-linearity: As It does not follow any non-linearity, so it is not suitable for a backpropagation artificial neural network.
- Restricted learning capability: The network does not learn the complex problems.

Advantages

- Simple and easy to use.
- Suitable for getting the continuous output data.

Disasdvantages

- Not fit to use complex data.

7.4.2 Threshold Activation Function

Threshold activation function is also a simple function. If the input value crosses a threshold value, then the node is activated and sends the signal to the next node (Box 7.2).

Characteristics:

- Binary output: The threshold activation function is a step function and the output is binary means either 0 or 1.
- Used in back propagation: The transition is sharp in this type of activation function and it can be used in a back propagation model.

Advantages:

- Threshold activation function is most suitable where a strict differentiation is required such as in binary classification.
- It is simple and easy to use.

Disadvantages

- Threshold activation function is not suitable for a deep learning network.
- It cannot handle the complex data.

Box 7.2: Threshold Activation Function

In the case of threshold activation, if the input value crosses a certain threshold value, then the neuron is activated and sends the signal to the next neuron.

Characteristics

- Binary output: The output is binary means either 0 or 1.
- Used in back propagation: It can be used in a back propagation model.

Advantages

- It is best suitable for binary classification.
- It is simple and easy to use.

Disadvantages

- Unsuitable for a deep learning network.
- Unable to handle the complex data.

7.4.3 Sigmoid Activation Function

It is widely used in the activation of the ANN and a smooth gradient is obtained (Box 7.3).

Characteristics:

- Smooth and continuous function.
- Monotonic: In the case of a sigmoid activation function, the large input value provides larger outputs and the value is continuously increasing.
- Non-linear: It helps in learning complex data.

Advantages

- *Binary interpretation*: It is useful in binary classification as the output is either 0 or 1.
- *Smooth and Non-Linear*: Sigmoid activation helps in learning a non-linear dataset.
- Disadvantages of Sigmoid Activation
- *Vanishing Gradient Problem*: The gradient may be 0 for very small or large values of input. This may be responsible for the slowing of the ANN.
- *Computationally Expensive*: It is computationally expensive compared to the ReLu function.

Box 7.3: Sigmoid Activation Function

In the sigmoid activation function, a smooth gradient is obtained.

Characteristics

- Smooth and continuous function.
- Monotonic: The value is continuously increasing.
- Non-linear: It helps in learning complex data.

Advantages

- Binary interpretation: It is useful in binary classification as the output is either 0 or 1.
- Smooth and Non-Linear: It helps in learning a non-linear dataset.

Disadvantages of Sigmoid Activation

- *Vanishing Gradient Problem*: The gradient may be 0 in very small or large values of input which may be responsible for the slowing of the ANN.
- *Computationally Expensive*: It is computationally expensive compared to the ReLu function.

7.4.4 Rectified Linear Units (ReLU)

ReLU activation is widely used in deep learning neural networks. It avoids the vanishing gradient problem and is speedy in training. In ReLu activation, all the negative functions return to 0 and the positive value are retained as the input value (Box 7.4).

So the mathematical representation of ReLu is:

$$f(x) = \max(0,x)$$

x is the input.

If x is negative, then the output is zero.

If x is positive, then the output is x.

Characteristics:

- ReLu is simple and introduces non-linearity.
- It is computationally efficient.

Advantages:

- Vanishing gradient problem: No vanishing gradient problem as it does not saturate the positive input.
- Deep learning: It is the best fit for a deep learning neural network.
- Computational efficiency: It is faster than the sigmoid activation function.

Disadvantages:

- *Dying ReLu problem*: If the neuron receives only the negative input, then the positive output will always be 0. This may make the neuron permanently inactive.
- *Non Zero-Centred*: Outputs are always non-negative, and this may cause suboptimal updates of the weight.

Box 7.4: Rectified Linear Units (ReLU)

In ReLu activation, all the negative functions return to 0 and the positive value will be retained as the input value.

Mathematical representation

$$f(x) = \max(0,x)$$

x is the input
If x is negative, then the output is zero
If x is positive, then the output is x

Characteristics

- Simple and introduces non-linearity.
- Computationally efficient.

Advantages

- No vanishing gradient problem.
- Deep learning: It is the best fit for deep learning neural networks.
- Computational efficiency: It is faster than the sigmoid activation function.

Disadvantages:

- *Dying ReLu problem*: Too many negative inputs may make the neuron permanently inactive.
- *Non Zero-Centred*: Outputs are always non-negative, and this may cause suboptimal updates of the weight.

7.4.5 Hyperbolic Tangent (Tanh) Activation Function

It is similar to sigmoid activation function. However, the range is more centred around zero. It is also commonly used in ANN (Box 7.5).

Characteristics

- Range of the output is between −1 and 1.
- The output of the Tanh function is symmetric around zero and this helps in training.
- It is the best suited for gradient-based optimization.

Advantages
- Tanh gradient function has zero-centred output which balances the gradient.
- The gradient is stronger than the other activation function.
- It is very effective for the hidden layer of ANN.

Disadvantages
- Computationally expensive.
- It also faces the vanishing gradient problem as the large positive or negative values make the derivative close to zero which causes slow learning of the model.

Box 7.5: Hyperbolic Tangent (Tanh) Activation

It is similar to sigmoid activation function. However, in Tanh, the range is more centred around zero.

Characteristics
- Range of the output is between −1 and 1.
- The output of the Tanh function is symmetric around zero.
- It is the best suited for gradient-based optimization.

Advantages
- The zero-centred output balances the gradient.
- The gradient is stronger than the other activation function.
- Very effective for the hidden layer of ANN.

Disadvantages
- Computationally expensive.
- Vanishing gradient problem is present.

Table 7.1 shows a comparison of different activation functions.

Table 7.1 The different activation functions are compared

Activation function	Differentiability	Gradient	Advantages	Disadvantages	Best to use
Linear	Differentiable	No vanishing gradient	It is used in regression problems	Unable to solve a complex problem	Used in regression models
Step threshold	Not differentiable	Vanishing gradient	Simple, used in a perceptron	Cannot handle the complex data	Used in back propagation
Tanh hyperbolic tangent	Fully differentiable	Vanishing gradient	This is zero-centred	Computationally expensive, Unsuitable for gradient-based learning	Good for hidden layer activation
Sigmoid	Fully differentiable	Vanishing gradient	Smooth and continuous function	Slow learning	Binary classification
ReLu	Differentiable except at x = 0	No vanishing gradient	Easy and fast computation	Dying neuron problem	Best for deep learning

7.5 Learning

Learning is a crucial part of the ANN model. The model learns from the experience or training data. In each learning session, the strength of the intermodal connection is changed. The learning of ANN is a dynamic process and it depends on the several factors which are described below.

1. *Input Data*: Several data-related factors influence the learning of ANN such as
   - Quality of data: If the input data is biased or incomplete, then then the learning capability is decreased.
   - Quantity of Data: Scanty input data affects the learning, whereas, large amount of input data helps in better learning and efficiency of the model.
   - Irrelevant feature selection: Irrelevant feature selection may cause a slowdown in learning.
   - Pre-processed data: The standardization of data and removal of the missing data help in better learning of the ANN model.
2. *Training Algorithm*
   - *Weight Initialization*: Weight initialization means the initial weight allotment to the neurons of the ANN model before training. This is important because it influences the learning of the ANN model and prevents vanishing gradients.
   - *Optimization Algorithm*: Optimization Algorithm is an important factor of learning as it prevents the loss of function by adjusting the weights and biases of the ANN model. The commonly used optimization algorithms are Gradient Descent (GD), Stochastic Gradient Descent (SGD), Mini-Batch Gradient Descent, Momentum-Based Optimization and Adaptive Learning Rate Methods.
   - *Loss Function*: The loss function measures the errors between the predicted and actual output of the model. Any ANN model aims to reduce the value of the loss function so that the model works with high performance.
   - Learning *Rate*: Learning rate determines how much the weight of the ANN model is adjusted in each iteration. A well-tuned learning rate determines the efficient training and faster convergence of the model. Too high learning rate leads to overshooting the target, and too low learning rate may take long training time.
3. Hyperparameter Tuning
   - *Batch Size*: The batch size has a significant role in training dynamics. Small batch size may lead to an erratic learning process, whereas, larger batch size gives a stable gradient and so may help in rapid learning.
   - *Epochs*: If the epochs are too many, then there is a high chance of overfitting, whereas, too less number of epochs may lead to under fitting.

Hardware Graphics Processing Unit (GPU) enables a faster training process.

The different types of learning are described below:

7.5.1 Supervised Learning

Here, the network is trained by labelled data with well-defined output (Fig. 7.4). The network receives the feedback and then adjusts the weight to reduce the errors (Box 7.6).

Characteristics:
- Supervised learning needs labelled data with known output or target.
- The Loss function indicates the difference between the predicted and actual output. It guides the adjustment of weight.
- It is applied for the classification, regression, and prediction of disease outcome.

Example:
Classification: Supervised learning can be used to classify the grades of cervical intraepithelial lesions.
Regression: It may help in assessing the prognosis of the carcinoma based on the known output data.

Algorithms Used:
- Backpropagation ANN model.
- Loss functions.

Box 7.6: Supervised Learning
The neural network is trained by a labelled data with well-defined output.

Characteristics:
- The labelled data with known output or target.
- The Loss function guides the adjustment of the weight.
- It helps in the classification, regression and prediction of disease outcome.

Algorithms Used:
- Backpropagation ANN model.
- Loss functions.

7.5.2 Unsupervised Learning

Here, the data is not labelled and no training dataset is available (Fig. 7.5). So, the network discovers the hidden patterns or structures without any external supervision (Box 7.7).

Characteristics:
- The dataset is unlabelled.
- The ANN model is unsupervised and finds the hidden pattern itself.
- *Example*: Classification of cancer depending on the gene expression profile.

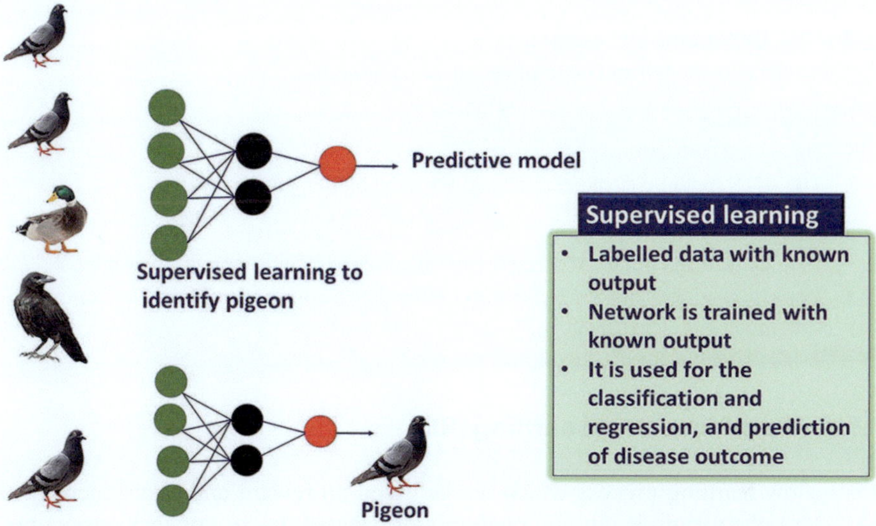

Fig. 7.4 Supervised learning shows that a neural network was trained to identify pigeons

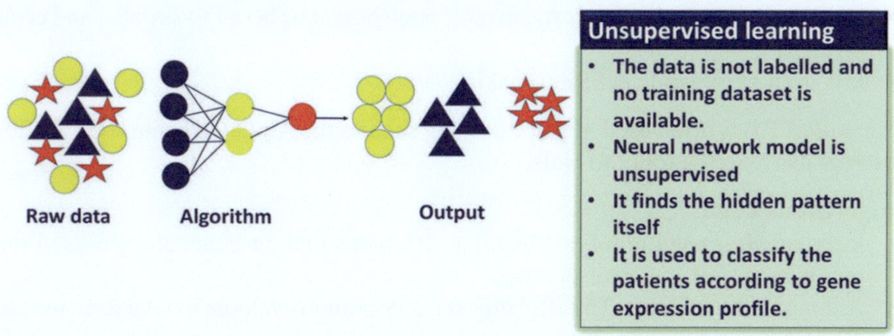

Fig. 7.5 Unsupervised learning: The model works on unlabelled data and itself finds out unsaved patterns

Algorithm used:

- Data clustering: It may help to classify the patients according to gene expression profile.
- Reduction of dimension: Principal Component Analysis (PCA) or t-Distributed Stochastic Neighbour Embedding (t-SNE) are types of unsupervised learning. They reduce the redundant features and make the complex data much simpler to analyse.

Box 7.7: Unsupervised Learning
The data is unlabelled and no training dataset is available.

Characteristics
- Unlabeled dataset.
- The ANN model is unsupervised and finds the hidden pattern itself.

Applications of the Algorithm
- Data clustering: To classify the patients according to gene expression profile.
- Reduction of dimension: Reduce the redundant features and make the complex data much simpler to analyse.

7.5.3 Reinforcement Learning (RL)

It is a slow learning process which works based on reward and punishment (Box 7.8). Here, the weight is initially randomly distributed. In case of each correct prediction, the ANN model is updated (Fig. 7.6).

Characteristics
- Here the ANN model learns by reward/ punishment or better to say trial and error process.
- It is used in dynamic decision-making task.

Examples: RL is often used in game playing such as the AlphaGo game and robotics such as learning the robot to walk.

Algorithms Used
- Robotics: It is used in robotic learning. RL helps in the motion and works of the robots by a trial and error process.
- Autonomous Vehicles: The RL helps the autonomous vehicle to take decisions in the complex environment.
- Treatment Optimization: To plan the optimal dose and timing of medicine by noting the response of the patient.

Box 7.8: Reinforcement Learning
Neural network model works based on the reward and punishment. In case of each correct prediction, the ANN model is updated.

Characteristics
- The model learns by reward/punishment which means by a trial and error process.
- The model helps in dynamic decision-making tasks.

Applications of the Algorithm
- Robotics: It is used in robotic learning.
- Autonomous Vehicles: It helps the autonomous vehicle to take decisions.
- Treatment Optimization: To plan the optimal dose and timing of medicine.

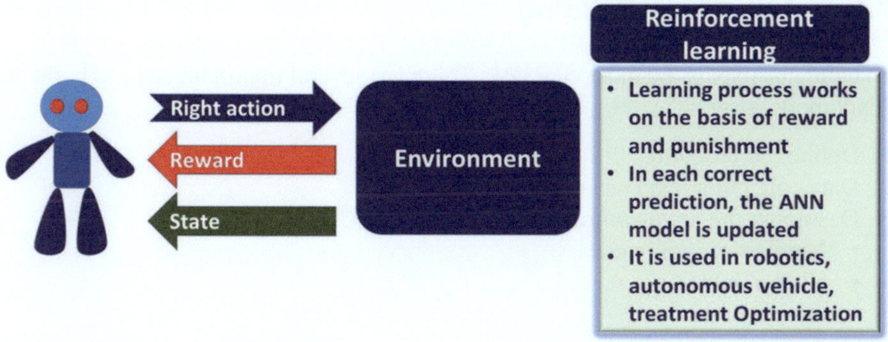

Fig. 7.6 Reinforcement learning model is based on reward and punishment. In each reward, the model is updated

Table 7.2 Comparison of different types of learning

Features	Supervised learning	Un-supervised learning	Reinforcement learning	Transfer learning
Basic principles	Learning from labelled data	Learning from unlabelled data	Learning by reward and punishment and then updating the model	Adopting a pre-trained ANN model for similar types of tasks
Data	Labelled data	Unlabelled data	Experimental data	Pre-trained ANN model
Training	ANN model learns from the input–output pair	Model clustered the data without categorical labels.	Model works based on feedback	It works on a pre-trained ANN model having the source task
Strengths	High accuracy	It is good to work with large amounts of unlabeled data It finds the hidden pattern	Dynamic learning process from the real world	Reduces training time and cost of computation. It is suitable for a small dataset
Weakness	Large amount of labelled data needed.	Results may not always be accurate. Difficult to interpret the result.	Slow learning High computational power needed	Negative transfer may occur

7.5.4 Transfer Learning

In Transfer learning (TL), an already trained ANN model is used for the specific task. The pre-trained ANN model is trained on a large dataset to capture the generalized features. The layers of the ANN with the extracted features are retained and the pre-trained ANN model is fine-tuned for the new task. The TL saves time and computational expense. Moreover, it can work on a small dataset and is beneficial when the cases are rare and data collection is difficult.

The details of transfer learning have been described in Chap. 17.

Table 7.2 compares different types of learning.

7.6 ANN Model Building

To build an ANN is the most vital task. There are several important steps to build an ANN model (Fig. 7.7).

1. Define the problem.
2. Data collection and Data preprocessing.
3. Designing the architecture of the model:
   - Number of input nodes.
   - Hidden nodes.
   - Output node.
   - Activation function.
   - Weight initialization.
   - Selecting loss of function.
   - Number of iterations.
4. Selecting an optimization algorithm.
5. Compiling the model.
6. Training the model.
7. Evaluating the model.
8. Further fine-tuning the model.

7.6.1 Define the Problem

At first, the main aim of the ANN model should be identified. In the case of cervical cancer screening, the detection of dysplastic cells may be the main aim of the model.

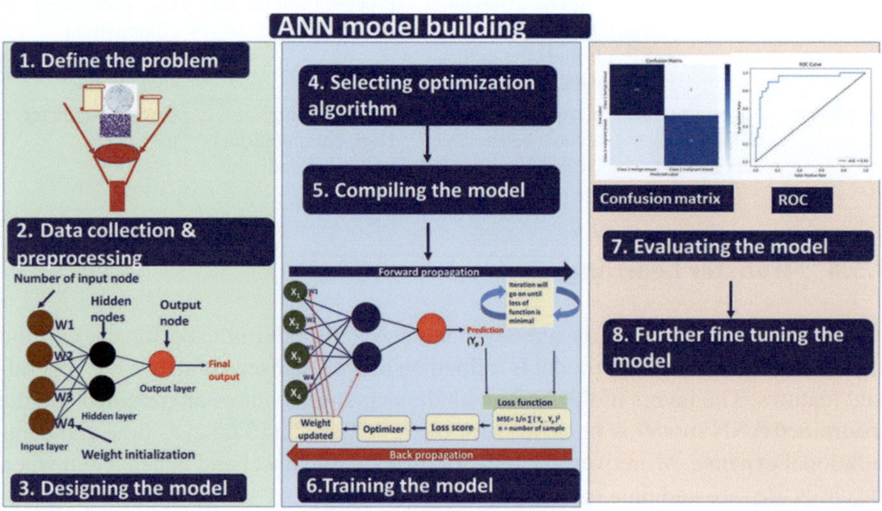

Fig. 7.7 Steps to build an artificial neural network model

7.6.2 Data Collection and Data Pre-Processing

Data collection and pre-processing are the crucial steps of model building. The pre-processed data is used for the training and testing of the ANN model. The details of data collection from the various sources have been described in the previous chapter.

Data pre-processing includes the following main steps:

A. *Data Cleaning*
   - Missing data: The repeated missing data is identified.
   - Data outliers: The extreme variation of data should be removed.
   - Duplicate data: It is important to remove duplicate data.
   - Data formatting: Taking care to format data properly.

B. *Data Transformation*
   - *Feature scaling*: Feature scaling takes care that the numerical values of the input nodes are in the same scale so that the high value of certain features should not influence the others. Feature scaling can be done by Min-Max Scaling, standardization, Robust Scaling and Log Transformation. Optimum feature scaling helps to improve the convergence speed, reduces vanishing gradient and improve the efficiency of the activation function.
   - *Encoding Categorical Variables*: It means to encode categorical values to numerical values such as female = 0, male = 1.
   - *Feature Engineering*: Feature Engineering means the manipulating the raw data into the meaningful input data to increase the efficiency of ANN model. It is done by generating new features from the raw data, modifying the existing data, and selecting the most relevant features.

C. *Data Augmentation*: It includes augmenting the image or text data by various transforming methods to the raw data.

D. *Reduction of the dimension*: The dimension reduction can be done by removing the redundant features.

E. *Data splitting*: The input data is split into training, validation and test sets. The data splitting is one of the crucial steps in ANN model building. Its prime function is to assess the function of the model, avoiding overfitting and fine tuning of the hyperparameters.

Types of subset of data:

Training set: This set of data is for training the model so that the weights of the nodes and also the biases are optimized by the back propagation process. The training set should be large enough to identify the pattern.

Validation set: This dataset is applied for tuning the hyperparameters and preventing overfitting. It does not help the ANN model directly in the learning process. However, the validation set adjusts the learning rate, number of layers etc. It also halts the training when the loss begins to increase.

Test set: After initial training, the performance of the network model is tested on the test set of data.

Splitting ratio: The ratio of the splitting is commonly used as training set: validation set: test set = 70:15:15. In a small set of data, to have the robust validation, the ratio can be used as 60:20:20.

Method of splitting: The data can be divided by the following techniques:

Random splitting: Here, the dataset is randomly shuffled and it is fine when the dataset is uniformly distributed.

Stratified Splitting: It is used when the dataset is imbalanced. In the case of Stratified Splitting the class proportion is consistent in each set of data. For example, in the dataset, the first 90% cases are normal healthy people and last 10% cases have cancer. If we use random splitting of data, then the cancer cases will be in either the training or validation dataset and therefore the dataset will give rise to poor generalization and low diagnostic accuracy.

Time-Based Splitting: It is used for time-series data and past data is used to predict the future.

7.6.3 Designing the Architecture of the Model

Designing the architecture of the network includes the following steps (Fig. 7.8).

7.6.3.1 The Number of Layers and Neurons

Input layer: The number of nodes in the input layer equals the number of features of the dataset.

Hidden layer: One or two hidden layers are sufficient for the simple problem. However, for the complex problems, multiple hidden layers are needed. Choosing the right number of nodes in the hidden layer is crucial, as too less number of nodes may cause underfitting and too many nodes may cause overfitting.

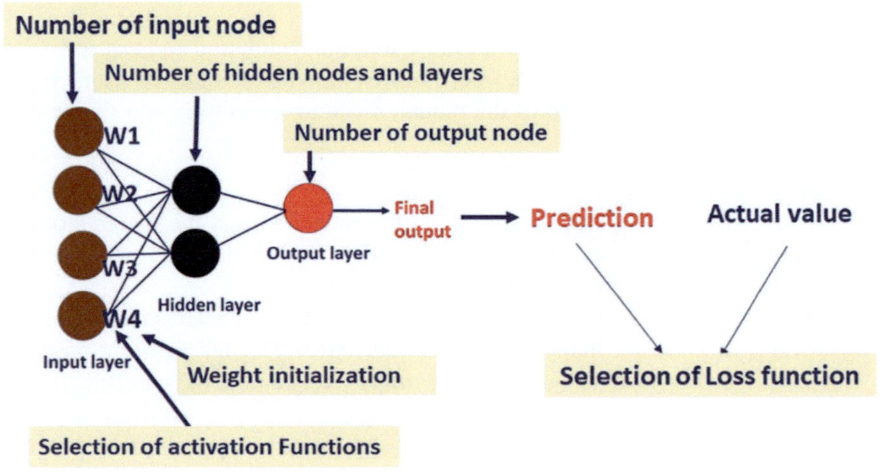

Fig. 7.8 Schematic diagram showing the design of network architecture

Determining the number of hidden nodes:

- Half of the sum of input and output nodes.
- Or, 2/third of the number of input nodes.
- *Based on the complexity of the problem*:

  Shallow network: Only 1–5 nodes are sufficient.

  Deep networks: Multiple hidden layers with 5 to 50 nodes or more than that, depending on the complexity.

Practical Approach Practically, the optimum number of nodes are determined by Bayesian optimization, cross-validation or by random search techniques.

7.6.3.2 Selecting Activation Functions

- For binary classification: Sigmoid activation.
- Hidden layer: ReLU activation function.
- For multi-classification output: Softmax.

7.6.3.3 Initializing Weights and Biases

Initializing weights and biases is an important step to make an ANN model as it helps in rapid convergence and eliminates the vanishing gradient problem. It can be done by these methods.

(i) *Random Initialization*

Here, random small values of weight are assigned. It is used in the simple ANN that consists only a few layers.

(ii) *Xavier/Glorot Initialization*

Xavier Initialization is also known as Glorot initialization. In this weight initialization technique, the stable variance of activations and gradients are maintained in all the layers. The main advantage of Xavier initialization is to avoid vanishing gradient and maintain a constant flow of gradient.

Use: It is commonly applied when the ANN model uses the sigmoid and Tanh activation function.

(iii) *He Initialization*

He Initialization is also known as Kaiming Initialization based on the proposition by Kaiming He et al. It is designed to avoid vanishing or exploding gradients in ReLU activation. Here, based on the number of input nodes, the initial weight is scaled [9].

Use: It is applied when the network uses the ReLu activation function.

(iv) *Lecum Initialization*

In the Lecum initialization technique, a smaller variance is used compared to Xavier initialization.

Use: When the ANN model uses Tanh activation function.

Table 7.3 shows the comparison of different weight initialization techniques.

Table 7.3 The comparison of different weight initialization techniques

Technique	Used in Activation	Use in deep networks	Prevents vanishing gradient	Prevents exploding gradient
Random	Any	Unstable	No	No
Xavier/ Glorot	Sigmoid, Tanh	Shallow	Yes	To some extent
He	ReLU,	Yes	Yes	Yes
Lecum	Sigmoid, Tanh	Shallow	Yes	No

7.6.3.4 Selecting Loss Function

The loss function quantifies the error. It is the difference between the predicted and actual output in the neural network (Box 7.9). The high loss function means that the model is working poorly and low loss function means that the model is working fine and its prediction ability is good.

(i) Loss Functions for Regression Problems:

Mean Squared Error (MSE): It is the average of the squared difference between the target and predicted value. It is good when the errors are normally distributed. But penalize the large errors more than the small errors.

$$\text{MSE} = \frac{1}{n}\Sigma\left(Y_a - Y_p\right)^2$$

Y_a is the actual value, Y_p is the predicted value and n is the number of observations.

Mean Absolute Error (*MAE*): MAE is the average of the absolute difference between the actual and predicted values. It does not penalize the large errors more.

Huber Loss: It combines MSE and MAE. Compared to MSE, the sensitivity to outliers is low in Huber loss.

(ii) Loss Functions for Classification Problems:

Binary Cross-Entropy: It is mainly used for binary classification. Binary Cross-Entropy keeps the correct prediction closer to 1 in and the incorrect prediction closer to 0. It works best in sigmoid activation.

Categorical Cross-Entropy (*CCE*): It is used for multi-class classification. It works best in the case of softmax activation in the final layer.

Sparse Categorical Cross-Entropy (*SCCE*): SCCE is almost similar to CCE. However, the class labels are integer encoded in SSCE. It is used for multi-class classification problems.

Table 7.4 shows the comparison of different types of loss function.

Box 7.9: Loss Function

The loss function quantifies the error by measuring the difference between the predicted and actual output of the model.

A. Loss Functions for Regression Problems
   - *Mean Squared Error* (MSE): It is the average of the squared difference between the actual and predicted value.
   - *Mean Absolute Error* (*MAE*): It is the average of the absolute difference between the actual and predicted value.
   - *Huber Loss*: It combines MSE and MAE.

B. Loss Functions for Classification Problems
   - *Binary Cross-Entropy*: It keeps the correct prediction closer to 1 and the incorrect prediction closer to 0. It works best in sigmoid activation.
   - *Categorical Cross-Entropy* (*CCE*): It is used for multi-class classification and it works best in the case of softmax activation.
   - *Sparse Categorical Cross-Entropy* (*SCCE*): Here, the class labels are integers. It is used for multi-class classification problems.

Table 7.4 Comparison of different types of loss function

Loss function	Best for	Outliers problem to solve	Output activation function
Binary Cross-Entropy	Binary classification	No	Sigmoid
Categorical Cross-Entropy (CCE)	Multi-class classification	No	Softmax
Sparse Categorical Cross-Entropy (SCCE)	Multi-class classification (integer labels)	No	Softmax
Mean Squared Error (MSE)	Regression, predicting continuous values	No, affected by a large number outliers	Any
Mean Absolute Error (MAE)	Regression	Yes	Predicting continuous values
Huber Loss	Regression	Yes, a balance between MSE and MAE for outlier handling	It works best with regression and ReLu

7.6.3.5 Number of Iterations

The number of iterations in the ANN model means the number of times the network is trained by the training data and the parameters (weight and bias) of the model are altered.

The terminology

Epoch: Epoch means the one complete pass of the total training set data in the training process. So one epoch means one full cycle of the entire training dataset.

Batch size: Batch size measures the number of the training samples that are passing through the network at each time.

Iterations: The number of updates per epoch.

Iterations per Epoch = Total Training Samples/Batch Size

For example, if there is 100,000 training sample and the batch size is 1000, then Iterations per epoch: 100000/1000 = 100

If training of 5 epochs, then total iterations will be 5 × 100 = 500

Factors Influencing the Number of Iterations

- *Dataset size*: Large datasets need more iterations and small datasets may work with fewer iterations.
- *Batch size*:
  - Small batch size: more number of iterations
  - Large batch size: Less number of iterations
- *Epochs*: More epochs help in better learning; however, it may cause overfitting.
- *Computational Power*: Large number of iterations may need high speed and memory of the computer.

7.6.4 Selecting an Optimization Algorithm

Optimization algorithms are the crucial components of the network building as they adjust the weights and biases to reduce the loss function and increase the efficiency of the ANN model.

The commonly used Optimization algorithms are described below:

7.6.4.1 Gradient-Based Algorithm

Gradient Descent-Based Optimization

In gradient descent: optimization the weight is adjusted iteratively by applying the gradient of loss function.

(a) Stochastic Gradient Descent (SGD): In SGD, the weight is updated at each iteration. It is relatively faster and good for a large dataset (Fig. 7.9).
(b) Batch Gradient Descent (BGD): In BGD, the weight is adjusted after the iteration of the entire dataset (Fig. 7.10). It is slow and computationally extensive for a large dataset. However, BGD provides a smooth and stable update.
(c) Mini-Batch Gradient Descent: It uses small batches of data to upgrade the weights. So it gives the benefit of BGD and SGD.

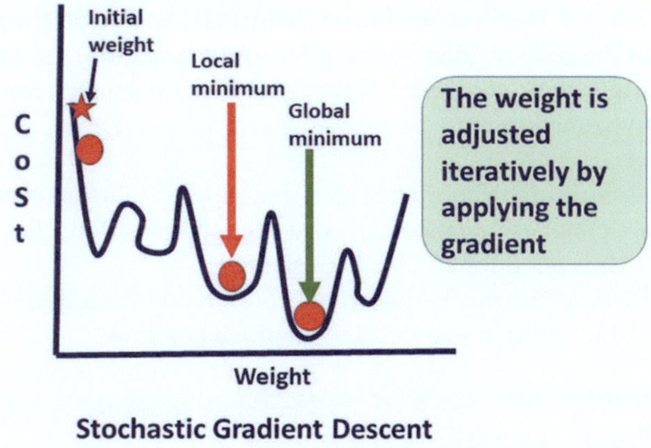

Fig. 7.9 Stochastic gradient descent: Here, the weight is updated at each iteration

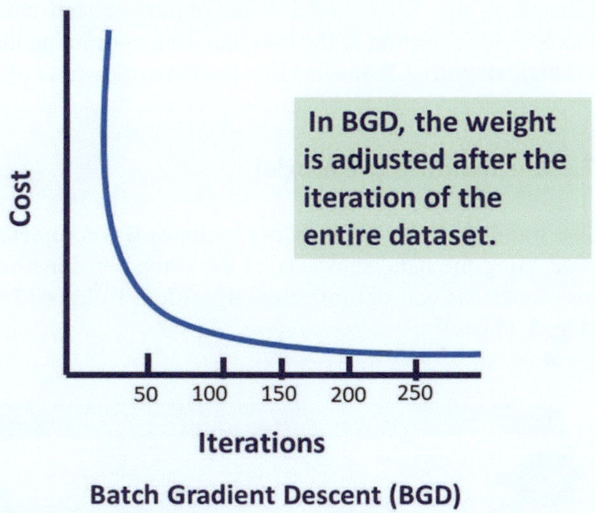

Fig. 7.10 Batch gradient descent: the weight is adjusted after iteration of the entire dataset

7.6.4.2 Momentum-Based Optimization

It is a variant of the gradient descent algorithm that adds momentum in the updating of weights. Nesterov Accelerated Gradient is a commonly used Momentum-Based Optimization algorithm.

7.6.4.3 Adaptive Learning Rate Optimization

Here, the learning rate is dynamically adjusted for each parameter. Unlike the gradient descent, the learning rate is not fixed. The commonly used algorithms in this category are the Adaptive Gradient Algorithm, Root Mean Square Propagation and Adaptive Moment Estimation.

7.6.4.4 Derivative-Free Optimization Algorithm

In the case of unavailable gradient information, the Derivative-Free Optimization Algorithms are used. These algorithms are suitable for noisy or non-smooth objective functions.

Genetic algorithm: The Genetic algorithm follows the natural selection process and it applies mutation and crossover operations to adjust the neural network weight. It is good for architectural search.

Particle Swarm Optimization (*PSO*): It considers neurons as particles that swarm in the space to search for the optimal position.

7.6.5 Compiling the Model

Compiling the ANN model is an important step before the training process. It includes the selection of the loss function, optimizing the algorithm and defining the evaluation matrix. It ensures that the network works efficiently.

7.6.6 Training the Model

The training of the ANN model includes the complete process of data entry, preprocessing the data, selection of the activation function, the number of iterations, loss functions and optimization algorithm, followed by the training of the dataset (Fig. 7.11).

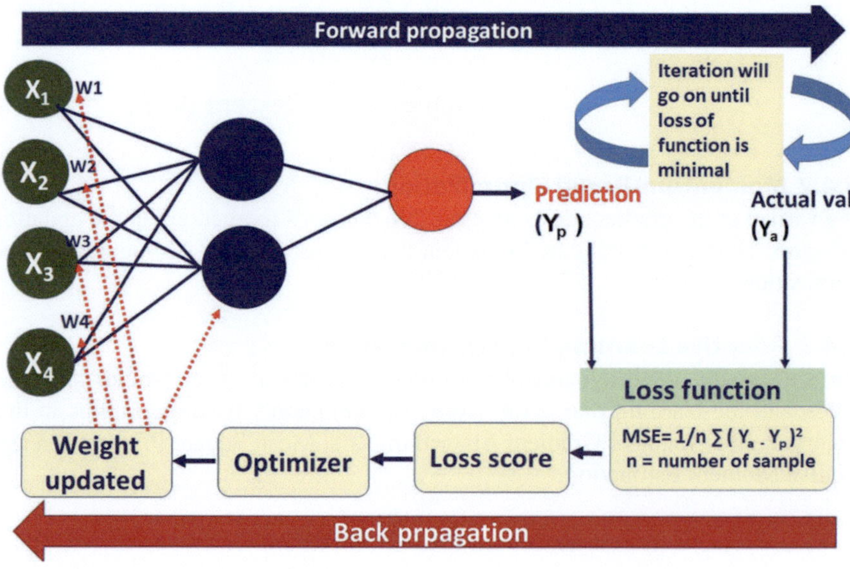

Fig. 7.11 Training of the neural network model

7.6.6.1 Forward Propagation

In the case of forward propagation, data flows from the input layer to the hidden layer to the output layer.

Input layer: It receives the data and then transfers it to the hidden layer.
Hidden layer: It processes the data and then hands over the data to the output layer.
Output layer: The output layer finally generates the prediction.

7.6.6.2 Back Propagation

After forward propagation, the model evaluates the error and calculates the loss function. The network adjusts the weights and biases by a suitable optimization algorithm. After the multiple iterations and updating the parameters (weight and bias), the network reaches the target.

7.6.7 Evaluating the Model

After adequate training, the model is evaluated on a test set of data which was not used in training or validation time.

7.6.7.1 Performance Metrics of Model Evaluation

1. *Accuracy*: It indicates the proportion of correctly classified cases.

$$\frac{TP + TN}{TP + FP + TN + FN}$$

   TP = True positive, TN = True negative, FN = False negative, FP = False positive.

2. *Precision and recall*:

   Precision: It indicates how many predicted positive cases are really positive.

$$\frac{TP}{TP + FP}$$

   Recall or Sensitivity: It indicates how many actual positive cases are correctly predicted.

$$\frac{TP}{TP + FN}$$

3. Confusion matrix (Fig. 7.12a): The confusion matrix provides a detailed summary of the correct (TP, TN) and incorrect (FP, FN) cases (Table 7.5).

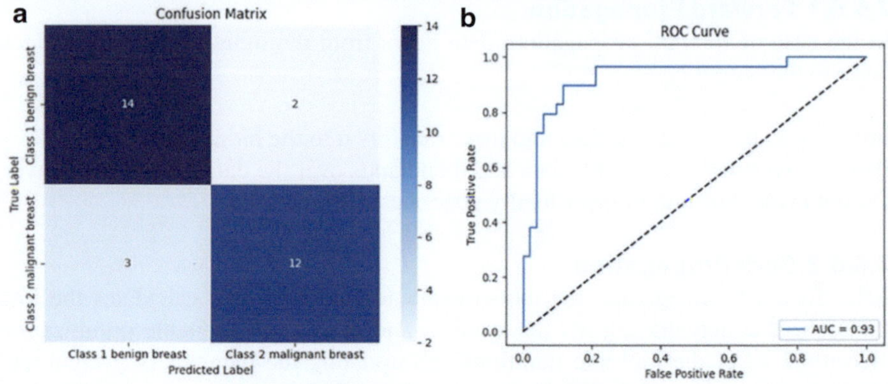

Fig. 7.12 Confusion matrix (**a**) and receiver operating characteristic (ROC) curve (**b**) are two main evaluation parameters

Table 7.5 The format of the confusion matrix

Actual	Predicted positive	Predicted negative
Actual positive	TP	FN
Actual negative	FP	TN

TP True positive, *TN* True negative, *FN* False negative, *FP* False positive

4. *ROC Curve and AUC (Area Under Curve)*

The Receiver Operating Characteristic (*ROC*) *curve*: ROC curve is a graphical plot that shows the diagnostic performance of the binary classifier model (Fig. 7.12b). ROC curve is plotted with the True Positive Rate (Sensitivity) against False Positive Rate (1 - Specificity) at all possible classification threshold.

AUC (*Area Under Curve*): AUC means the area under ROC curve. AUC measures the capability of the binary classification model to identify the positive and negative cases correctly.

High AUC (near1): The model is efficient to distinguish positive and negative cases.

Low AUC (near 0.5): The model marginally separates the cases.

AUC near 0: The model is worse than random guessing.

7.6.7.2 Regression Metrics

In case of regression problems, the MSE and MAE are used (discussed before).

7.7 Conclusion

The concept of ANN is very basic to make further building of the complex neural network model. The traditional ANN consists of three layers input, hidden and output layer. The hidden layer solves the complex problem and we do not have much control on this layer (black box). Due to the black box problem the pathologists often are critical on the decision of neural network. Any ANN model should be properly evaluated before clinical applications The model should be validated with external data. The further tuning should be done after the initial launching of the model.

References

1. Dey P, Dey R. Artificial neural network--mechanism and application in pathology. Indian J Pathol Microbiol. 2002;45(3):371–4.
2. Dey P. Artificial neural network in diagnostic cytology. Cytojournal. 2022;19:27. https://doi.org/10.25259/Cytojournal_33_2021. PMID: 35510103; PMCID: PMC9063555.
3. Saini T, Saikia UN, Dey P. An artificial neural network for the prediction of the risk of malignancy in category III Bethesda thyroid lesions. Cytopathology. 2023;34(1):48–54. https://doi.org/10.1111/cyt.13180. Epub 2022 Oct 6.
4. Subbaiah RM, Dey P, Nijhawan R. Artificial neural network in breast lesions from fine-needle aspiration cytology smear. Diagn Cytopathol. 2014;42(3):218–24. https://doi.org/10.1002/dc.23026. Epub 2013 Aug 1.
5. Savala R, Dey P, Gupta N. Artificial neural network model to distinguish follicular adenoma from follicular carcinoma on fine needle aspiration of thyroid. Diagn Cytopathol. 2018;46(3):244–9. https://doi.org/10.1002/dc.23880. Epub 2017 Dec 20.
6. Kapatia G, Dey P, Saikia UN. Artificial neural network model to distinguish pleomorphic adenoma from adenoid cystic carcinoma on fine needle aspiration cytology. Cytopathology. 2020;31(5):445–50. https://doi.org/10.1111/cyt.12784. Epub 2019 Dec 22.
7. Barwad A, Dey P, Susheilia S. Artificial neural network in diagnosis of metastatic carcinoma in effusion cytology. Cytometry B Clin Cytom. 2012;82(2):107–11. https://doi.org/10.1002/cyto.b.20632. Epub 2011 Nov 10.
8. Dey P, Logasundaram R, Joshi K. Artificial neural network in diagnosis of lobular carcinoma of breast in fine-needle aspiration cytology. Diagn Cytopathol. 2013;41(2):102–6. https://doi.org/10.1002/dc.21773. Epub 2011 Oct 11.
9. He K, Zhang X, Ren S, Sun J. Delving deep into rectifiers: surpassing human-level performance on imagenet classification, 2015 IEEE International Conference on Computer Vision (ICCV), Santiago, Chile, 2015, pp. 1026–34. https://doi.org/10.1109/ICCV.2015.123.

Deep Learning in Computational Cytology

8

Abstract

Deep learning (DL) is a branch of machine learning that has reshaped the field of cytology. Convolutional neural network (CNN) is a part of deep learning which has the ability to extract features without any external help. The whole scanning images (WSI) contain huge data and it can be handled only by CNN. The DL system mainly contains a feedforward neural network, convolutional neural network, recurrent neural network, autoencoders, generative adversarial networks and a transformer. There are certain limitations of DL. It needs a huge amount of data for proper training. The training process in DL is relatively slow. More powerful computational processing is needed to implement DL. Moreover, the data storage may be another problem in DL because WSI may take huge computer space. The present chapter discusses the basic principles of different DL systems and their potential applications.

Keywords

Deep learning · Feedforward neural network · Convolutional neural network · Recurrent neural network · Autoencoders · Generative adversarial networks · Transformer · Whole slide scanning images

8.1 Introduction

Deep learning (DL) is a branch of machine learning. It is a revolutionary technology that has reshaped the field of cytology [1]. Convolutional neural network (CNN) is a part of deep learning. Unlike traditional artificial neural networks, CNN has the ability to do feature extraction by itself. Moreover, whole slide scanning images (WSI) contain huge data and they cannot be handled by traditional artificial neural network (ANN). DL has the unique ability to cope with huge image data. This new branch of artificial intelligence (AI) is now an integral part of computational cytology (CCyt).

P. Dey, *Computational Cytology*, https://doi.org/10.1007/978-981-95-3272-8_8

Table 8.1 Traditional artificial neural network versus deep learning

Features	Traditional artificial neural network	Deep learning
Complexity of the model	Simple	Highly complex architecture
Number of hidden layers	1–2 hidden layers	Multiple hidden layers, more than 3
Feature extraction	Manual feature extraction	Automatic feature extraction
Computational power	Relatively low	High
Data requirement	Smaller dataset	Large volume of data is needed
Training time	Less training time and faster	Slow
Use	Basic classification	Image recognition

In the present chapter, the basic principles, different types and potential of DL have been discussed.

8.2 Deep Learning: A Bird's Eye View

Deep learning (DL) is a subfield of machine learning. It contains many layers and so the term "deep" is introduced. DL network is made by getting inspired by the human brain. Multiple layers of DL help to learn hierarchical representations of data. DL performs its task by processing a huge amount of unstructured data such as image recognition from WSI. Unlike traditional ANN, it automatically extracts the essential features and no manual input is required (Table 8.1). Moreover, DL is free of selection bias. The performance of DL depends on a large amount of data and higher computational power.

8.3 Types of Deep Learning Models

The DL system mainly contains the following types of the neural network:

- Feedforward neural network (FNN).
- Convolutional neural network (CNN).
- Recurrent neural network (RNN).
- Autoencoders.
- Generative Adversarial Networks (GANs).

8.4 Feedforward Neural Networks (FNNs)

FNN is one of the simplest forms of DL which is also known as a Multi-Layer Perceptron.

Basic Principle: In this network, the data moves only in the forward direction from the input to the hidden layer to the output layer (Box 8.1).

Basic network structure (Fig. 8.1):

Input layer: It receives input data.
Hidden layer: It performs the complex non-linear function by weighted connections.
Output layer: It provides the final prediction.

8.4.1 Computational Flow

In FNN, the data flow in one direction: Input to hidden layer to output

Steps:

- Input values: x_1, x_2, x_3-------x_n are incorporated into the input layer.
- Each hidden layer neuron computes a weighted sum of its inputs:

$$y = \sum w_i x_i \ + \ b$$

- y is a weighted sum, w_i is the weight, b is the bias.
- Next, the activation function is introduced: ReLu, sigmoid or Tanh.
- The output of one layer becomes the input to the next.
- Final layer is the output.

Training: FNN is trained by backpropagation and gradient descent.

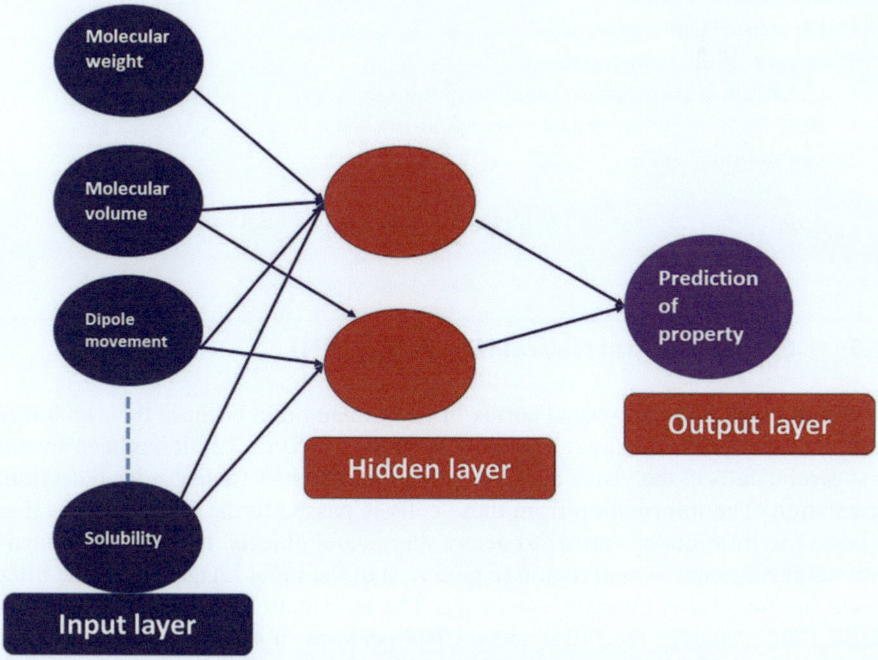

Fig. 8.1 The network architecture of feedforward neural networks

8.4.2 Main Characteristics of FNN

- Direction: One way.
- Layers: Fully connected.
- Learning: Backpropagation and gradient descent.
- Activation function: It introduces non-linearity.
- Limitation: Unable to handle sequential data.

Applications: It is used in simple classification or regression tasks.

Box 8.1: Feedforward Neural Networks
The simplest form of deep learning.

Basic Principle: The data moves only in the forward direction from the input to the hidden layer to the output layer.

Basic network structure:
- Input layer: It receives input data.
- Hidden layer: It performs the complex non-linear function.
- Output layer: It provides the final prediction.

Training: FNN is trained by backpropagation and gradient descent.

Main Characteristics
- Direction: One way.
- Layers: Fully connected.
- Learning: Backpropagation and gradient descent.
- Activation function: It introduces non-linearity.
- Limitation: Unable to handle sequential data.

Applications: It is used in simple classification or regression tasks.

8.5 Convolutional Neural Network (CNN)

CNN are inspired by the visual cortex of the human brain because their architecture and function mimic the functioning of the visual cortex [2]. It has been shown that certain cells in the visual cortex perform simple tasks such as edge detection, orientation. The information from these cells is passed to the complex cells that process the information further to detect shapes and objects. In CNN, the convolutional layer notes a small region (e.g., 3 × 3) of the input image. The same filter works on the different parts of the image. The information of the different layers of the CNN provides the full objects. CNN performs a series of operations that include (a) convolution, (b) ReLU and (c) pooling. By doing these operations repeatedly, the dimension reduction happens and a large image with a vast number of pixels is converted into a significantly less number of pixels [1]. Finally, a fully converted traditional ANN is made from the flattened layer containing a handful of pixels (Box 8.2).

8.5.1 Steps of CNN

1. *Input*: An image is incorporated (e.g., 100 × 100 × 3).
2. *Convolution Layer*: Here, the filter with a smaller matrix (3*3 or 9*9) is superimposed on the original image (Fig. 8.2). Usually, multiple filters are used to extract features. A convolutional operation is done. It means the multiplication of the pixel values of the original image and the superimpose filter, followed by addition. The filter is placed systematically in a sliding manner and the convolution operation makes the original image into a simple, simplified feature map. This simplified image is considered an input layer. In convolution operation, multiple filters are applied to get multiple feature maps. These feature maps are stacked together to form the output layers.
3. *Activation Function*: Rectified Linear Unit (ReLU) activation function is commonly used in CNN (Fig. 8.3). In ReLU activation, all the negative values are replaced by 0.

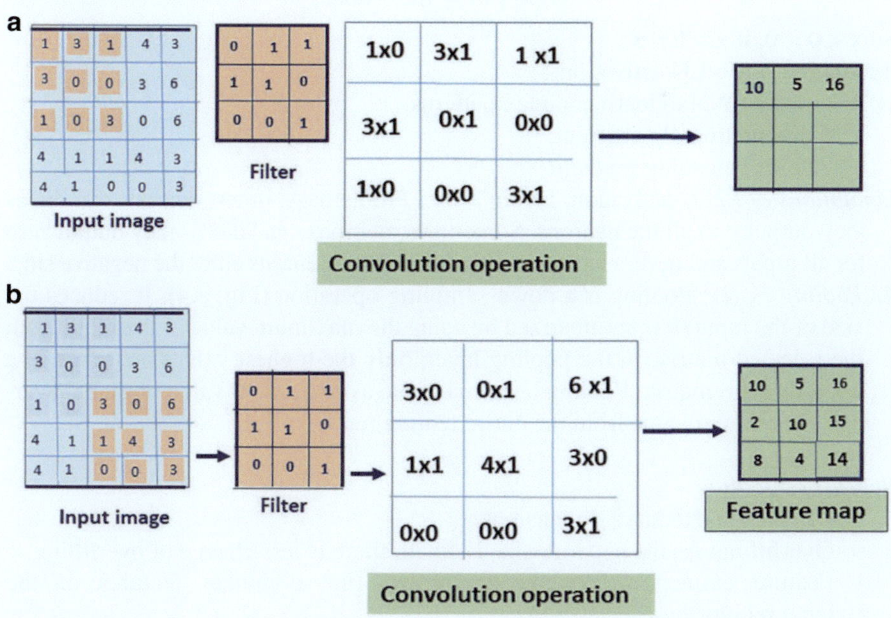

Fig. 8.2 Convolution operation: A filter is sequentially superimposed on the original image (**a** and **b**). The value of a pixel of the filter is multiplied by the same of the original image and then added. The 5 × 5 image is ultimately converted into a 3 × 3 image

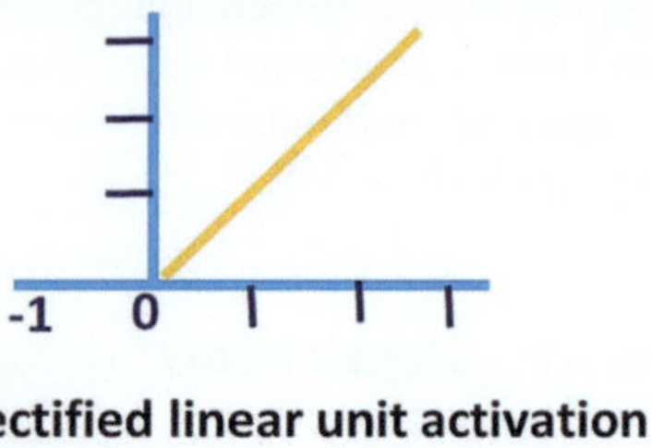

Fig. 8.3 Activation by the rectified linear unit activation function which takes only positive values of x

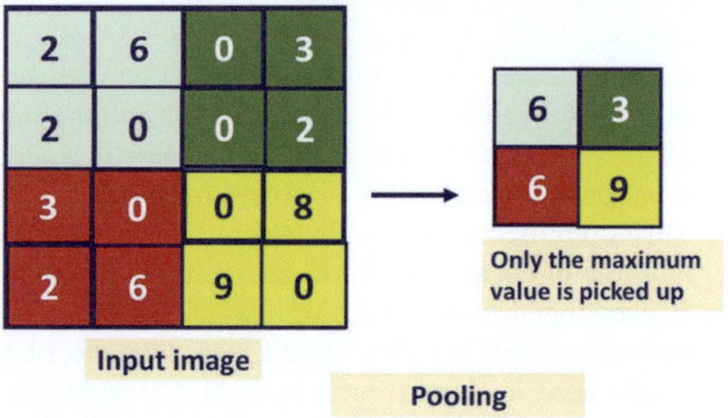

Fig. 8.4 Pooling operation takes only the maximum pixel value

$$\text{ReLU}(\text{x}) = \max(0,\text{x})$$

So x < 0 = 0, if x > 0 = x.

Advantages of ReLU activation:

- Allows CNN to learn complex patterns.
- Computationally efficient.
- Avoids vanishing gradient.

Limitations of ReLU activation: Dying ReLU Problem: At times, neurons can die as they output 0 to all the neurons. Sometimes, neurons can "die"—they output zero for all inputs and never recover. It may occur if the neurons enter the negative side.

4. *Pooling Layer*: Pooling is a down-sampling operation (Fig. 8.4). It reduces the size of the input. It is summarized by using the maximum value of the input from the selected matrix. In the pooling layer, only the highest values are taken in a 2 × 2 or 3 × 3 matrix. Pooling layer may note average pixel value or global average / maximum value from the entire feature map.

Benefits of pooling

- Dimension: Reduces dimensions.
- Overfitting: As the network size is small, there is less chance of overfitting.
- Feature extraction: Pooling emphasizes the dominant features of the local region.

Hyperparameters in pooling

- *Pooling window*: The size of the pooling window is usually 2 × 2 or 3 × 3.
- *Stride size*: The step size is equal to the pool size.
- *Padding*: Around the border, zero is added to control the output size.

5. *Repeat*: Convolution, ReLU and pooling operations are repeated several times.
6. *Flattening*: The 2D data is converted into 1D vector.
7. *Fully Connected Layers*: Now traditional ANN is made from the input data of the fully connected layer.
   Activation function:
   Sigmoid function: It is used for binary classification.
   Softmax: Softmax is used for multiclass classification.
   Linear: For regression.
   The total operation is highlighted in Fig. 8.5.
8. Output Layer: The final prediction comes from the output layer.

8.5.2 Advantages of CNNs

CNN has following advantages:

- *Automatic Feature Extraction*: Traditional ANN needs manual data extraction. This is time-consuming and labour-intensive. Whereas, from the original raw data (image), CNN automatically extracts the features such as shape, texture, edges.
- *Parameter Sharing*: CNN uses shared weights because the same filter is used in the different parts of the images. This significantly reduces the number of parameters.

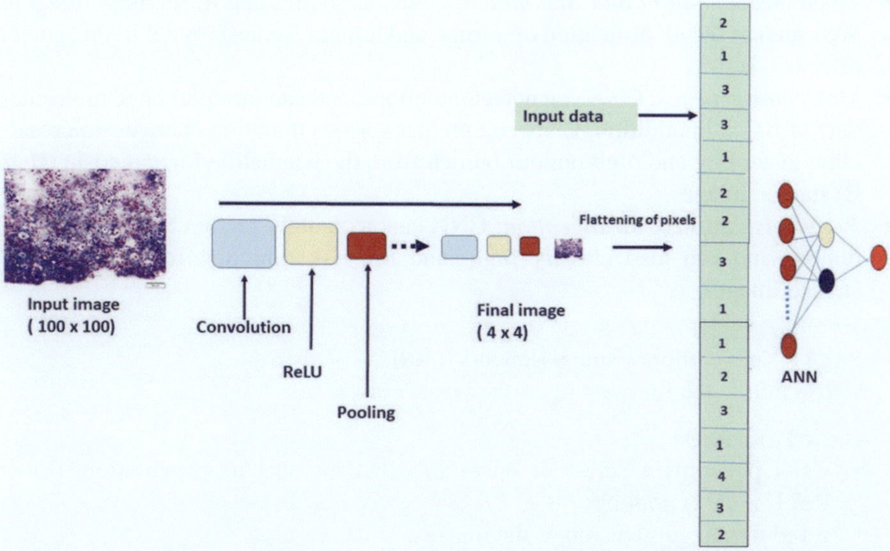

Fig. 8.5 Total operation is highlighted. Repeated convolution, ReLU and pooling operation convert higher higher-dimensional image into a lower dimension image. The pixel value of the image is flattened and is used as input data to make a traditional artificial neural network (ANN)

- *Translation Invariance*: CNN can recognize an object regardless of its position in the image.
- *Computation and Memory*: CNN has less computation time and memory usage.
- *Scalable and Deep*: CNN contains many layers and learn in a hierarchical way. The early layers of CNN detect the primitive nature of the object, such as edges, middle layers detect shapes and deep layers detect specific objects.

8.5.3 Limitations of CNNs

- Data hungry: CNN is data hungry and needs huge datasets for proper functioning
- Non-image data: It is not effective in non-image data.
- Black box problem: The decision of the black box (hidden layer) can not be explained by rationality.
- It is computationally expensive.

8.5.4 Applications

CNN has a wide range of applications such as:

- *Imaging in Cancer*: Image classification and detection:
  - Screening of cancer.
  - Cancer detection, classification and grading.
- *Tissue Segmentation and Annotation*: CNN can be trained to segment tissue in WSI such as the identification of normal and tumour tissue, stromal tissue, nuclei of cells.
- *Molecular genetics*: CNN can detect mutations, and can interpret huge molecular data of NGS. In addition, CNN can predict various mutation changes, microsatellite instability and high tumour burden from the haematoxylin and eosin (H & E) stained images.
- *Prognosis and Risk Stratification*: CNN can accurately predict the prognosis of tumour and can also classify high- and low-risk tumours from the H & E stained images.

Box 8.2: Convolutional Neural Network (CNN)
CNNs mimic the functioning of the visual cortex.

Basic Principles:

- CNN performs a series of operations that include (a) convolution, (b) ReLU and (c) pooling.
- It reduces the dimension of the images.
- Finally, a fully converted traditional ANN is made from the flattened layer containing a handful of pixels.

(continued)

Box 3.2 (continued)

Steps of CNN:

- *Input*: Image is loaded.
- *Convolution Layer*: The filter with a smaller matrix is superimposed on the original image and a convolutional operation is done.
- *Activation Function*: Rectified Linear Unit (ReLU) activation function.
- *Pooling Layer*: Pooling takes the maximum value of the input from the selected matrix.
- *Repeat*: Convolution, ReLU and pooling operations are repeated several times.
- *Flattening of the final layer.*
- *Fully Connected Layers*: Now, traditional ANN is made.

Advantages of CNN

- *Automatic Feature Extraction.*
- *Parameter Sharing.*
- *Translation Invariance*: Recognize an object regardless of its position.
- *Computation and memory*: less computation time and memory usage.
- *Scalable and Deep.*

Limitations

- *Data hungry*: CNN needs huge datasets.
- *Non-image data*: It is not effective in non-image data.
- *Black box problem.*
- Computationally *expensive.*

Applications

- *Imaging in Cancer*: Image classification and detection.
- *Tissue Segmentation and Annotation.*
- *Molecular genetics*: CNN can detect mutations, and can interpret huge molecular data
- Prognosis and Risk Stratification

8.6 Recurrent Neural Networks (RNNs)

RNN is designed to process temporal dynamic data (Box 8.3). It has an input layer, a hidden layer and an output layer. Here, the output of the previous sequence is considered as the input of the next sequence (Fig. 8.6). Unlike FNN, the RNN is not independent as it maintains an internal state (memory) over time.

Variants of RNN

- *Long Short-Term Memory (LSTM)*: It introduces gates to control the flow of information. LSTM is used in text and speech data.
- *Gated Recurrent Units (GRUs)*: It has few parameters and are faster. It is simpler than LSTM.

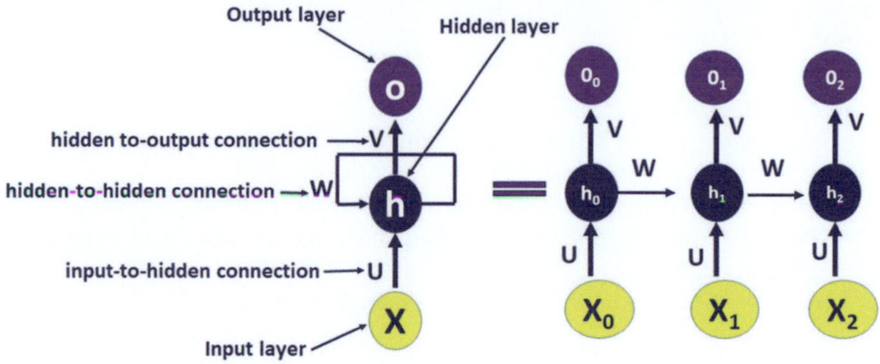

Fig. 8.6 Schematic diagram of recurrent neural network

Applications of RNNs

- Natural language processing.
- Health care: Patient monitoring.
- Molecular genetics: RNN can interpret raw electrical signals from Oxford Nanopore Technologies into nucleotide sequences.

Box 8.3 Recurrent Neural Network (RNN)

Basic principle: RNN is designed to process temporal dynamic data. Here, the output of the previous sequence is considered as input of the next sequence. RNN is not independent as it maintains an internal state (memory) over time.

Variants of RNN:

- *Long Short-Term Memory (LSTM)*: It introduces gates to control the flow of information.
- *Gated Recurrent Units (GRUs)*: It has few parameters and is faster.

Applications of RNNs

- Natural language processing.
- Health care: Patient monitoring.
- Molecular genetics: RNN can interpret raw electrical signals from Oxford Nanopore Technologies into nucleotide sequences.

8.7 Autoencoders

Autoencoder is a type of unsupervised neural network that is used mainly for reduction of dimension and denoising purposes (Box 8.4). The autoencoder has two components (Fig. 8.7):

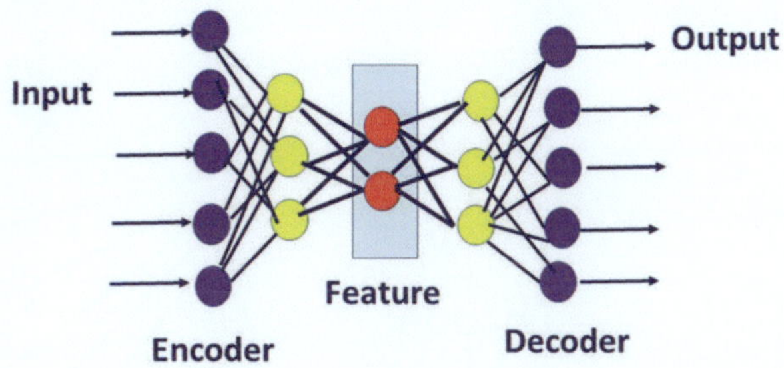

Fig. 8.7 Autoencoder The encoder reduces the dimensions of the dataset, however, it retains the salient features. The decoder reconstructs the data and produces the output

Encoder: It compresses input data and reduces multidimensional data into a lower dimension. Encoder represents the input data in a latent space.

Decoder: It reconstructs the original data from the compressed latent representation.

Applications:

- Reduction of the dimension of input data.
- Image denoising.
- Natural language processing.
- Anomaly detection: It can detect anomalies in molecular patterns.

Box 8.4: Autoencoders

Autoencoder is a type of unsupervised neural network that is used mainly for reduction of dimension and denoising purposes.

Components

Encoder: It compresses input data and reduces multidimensional data into lower dimension.

Decoder: It reconstructs the original data.

Applications:

- Reduction of the dimension of input data.
- Image denoising.
- Natural language processing.
- Anomaly detection: It can detect anomaly in molecular pattern.

8.8 Generative Adversarial Networks (GANs)

The detailed discussion on GAN has been done in Chap. 16

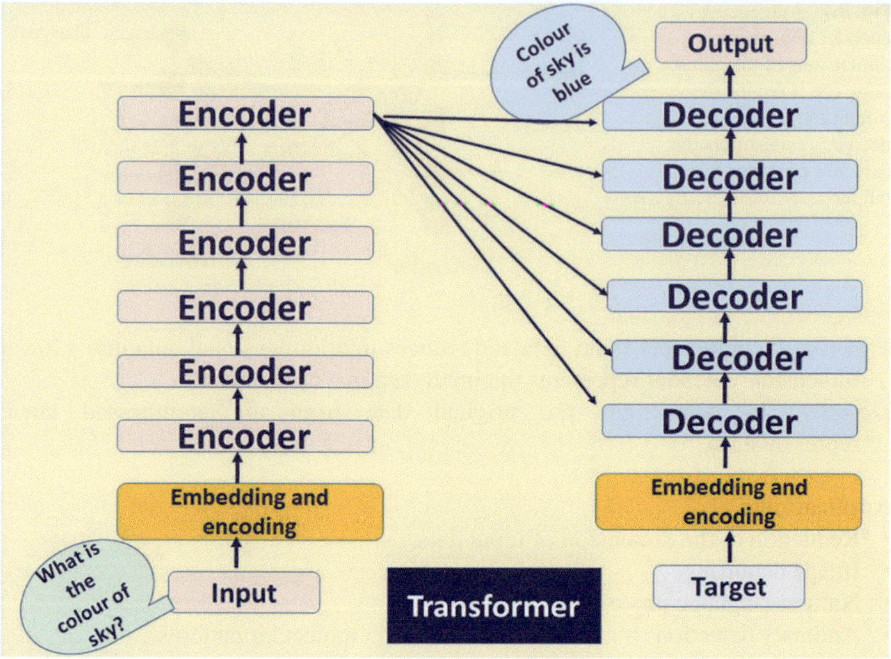

Fig. 8.8 Each transformer has an encoder and a decoder. The output of the encoder is fed into the decoder to generate the output

8.9 Transformer

Transformer is a type of deep learning technique that can process sequential data without relying on recurrence [3, 4]. It transforms the input sequence into an output sequence (Fig. 8.8). Transformer uses a self-attention mechanism to process text data (Box 8.5).

8.10 Key Architecture of Transformers

- *Encoder–decoder stacks*
  Encoder: Encoder is composed of layers and sublayers that process the input sequence.
  Decoder: It generates the output sequence based on the output of the encoder.
- *Self-attention mechanism*: The transformer allows the model to focus on different parts of the input sequence and weigh the importance of each element. Self-attention helps to know the context and relationship between words in a sentence.
- *Parallel processing*: Multiple sequences are processed in parallel and so the transformer is faster than RNN.
- *Feedforward layer*: After self-attention, fully connected layers is used for additional transformation.

8.10.1 Strength of the Transformer

The transformer has certain characteristics that make it a powerful DL technique.

- Parallel Processing makes it faster to work.
- Transformer is scalable and can work with a huge number of parameters.
- It is versatile and can work in text, speech and image data.

8.10.2 Applications

- Translation of one language to another can be done by a transformer.
- It can answer questions.
- Image classification
- It can summarize text data
- A transformer can generate code.

Box 8.5: Transformer

Transformer can process sequential data without relying on recurrence. It transforms the input sequence into an output sequence.

Key architecture of Transformers:

- *Encoder–decoder stacks*:
  - Encoder: Encoder is composed of layers and sublayers that process the input sequence.
  - Decoder: It generates the output sequence based on the output of the encoder.
- *Self-attention mechanism*: It allows the model to focus on different parts of input sequence and weigh the importance of each element.
- *Parallel processing.*
- *Feed forward layer*: After self-attention, fully connected layers are used for additional transformation.

Strength of the Transformer

- Parallel Processing makes it faster to work.
- Scalable.
- It is versatile and can work in text, speech and image data.

Applications

- Translation of one language to other.
- It can answer questions.
- Image classification.
- It can summarize text data.
- Transformer can generate code.

Table 8.2 compares different types of DL techniques.

Table 8.2 Comparison of different types of deep learning techniques

Type of model	Aim to apply	Data type	Key architecture	Strengths	Common applications
Feedforward Neural Network	Supervised learning	Structured data	Input, hidden and output layers	Simple	Classification and regression
Convolutional Neural Network	Feature extraction from images	Image	Convolution layer, ReLU activation and pooling layer	Good for image data	Image recognition
Recurrent Neural Network	Sequence modelling	Time series	Recurrent connections	Captures temporal dynamic data	Language processing
Autoencoder	Data compression and reconstruction	Any data, predominantly images	Encoder and decoder	Learning from unsupervised data	Reduction of dimension
Generative Adversarial Network	Fake data generation	Text data, video	A generator and a discriminator	Produces highly realistic synthetic data	Synthetic or fake data generation
Transformer	Parallel sequence	Text, audio, video	Self-attention mechanism	Handles long-range dependencies	Natural language processing

8.11 Conclusions

Deep learning has immense potential in pathology (cytology). In CCyt, we need a WSI of the cytology to analyse for various purposes. CNN, a type of DL, can help us to handle huge data of the images and automatic feature extractions. CNN plays an important role in diagnosis, grading, therapy response and prognosis prediction. RNN helps to analyse the sequential data. GAN is a relatively recent type of DL that can synthesize new data for a training set in rare or uncommon diseases. There are certain limitations of DL. It needs a huge amount of data for proper training. The training process is relatively slow. More powerful computational processing is needed. Moreover, the data storage may be another problem in DL because WSI may take huge computer space. Hopefully, in future, all the hurdles will be overcome. An earnest collaboration of software and hardware engineers, bioinformatics and pathologists may help to apply DL successfully.

References

1. Dey P. The emerging role of deep learning in cytology. Cytopathology. 2021;32(2):154–60. https://doi.org/10.1111/cyt.12942. Epub 2020 Dec 17.
2. LeCun Y, Bengio Y, Hinton G. Deep learning. Nature. 2015;521(7553):436–44. https://doi.org/10.1038/nature14539.
3. Goodfellow IJ, Pouget-Abadie J, Mirza M, et al. Generative adversarial nets. Adv Neural Inf Process Syst. 2014;27:2672–80.
4. Vaswani A, Shazeer N, Parma N et al. Attention is all you need. 31st Conference on Neural Information Processing Systems (NIPS). Advances in Neural Information Processing Systems. Vol. 30. Curran Associates, Inc. arXiv:1706.03762.

Part III

Applications of Computational Cytology

9 Applications of Artificial Intelligence in Computational Cytology

Abstract

The applications of computational cytology and artificial intelligence are rapidly evolving. Its major applications are in digital slide analysis, screening of cancer, accurate diagnosis, classifying the diseases, prognosis prediction, prediction of mutational changes from haematoxylin and eosin staining slides and management of diseases. Currently, the integration of clinical data, molecular data, radiological imaging and text data along with whole slide imaging data, has made major breakthroughs in this field. In the present chapter, details of clinical applications of computational cytology and artificial intelligence are discussed.

Keywords

Computational cytology · Artificial intelligence · Digital slide analysis · Screening of cancer · Diagnosis · Classifying the diseases · Prognosis prediction · Prediction of mutational change · Management of diseases

9.1 Introduction

Computational cytology has immense potential in the diagnosis and management of diseases. Its major applications will be in accurate diagnosis, classifying the diseases and guiding of management of diseases. The applications of computational cytology are rapidly evolving [1]. Currently, the integration of clinical data, molecular data, radiological imaging and text data along with whole slide imaging (WSI) data has made major breakthroughs in this field. In the present chapter, the clinical applications of computational cytology (CCyt) are discussed.

P. Dey, *Computational Cytology*, https://doi.org/10.1007/978-981-95-3272-8_9

9.2 Applications of Computational Cytology

The various applications of computational cytology are described here (Fig. 9.1):

9.2.1 Digital Slide Analysis

WSI gives a complete digitization of the cytology slides with Z-axis scanning into high-resolution images [2]. The digital slides can be processed with the extraction of data.

9.2.1.1 Key Applications

- *Automated Image Segmentation*: With the help of AI, it is possible to identify and delineate the target areas. The cells, nuclei, glands, etc. can be identified successfully.
- *Feature Extraction*: The essential morphological features such as shape, size, nuclear pleomorphism can be quantified [3, 4].
- *Textural analysis*: Textural analysis of the cells can be done which may further help in diagnosis [5]. Satyadhas J et al. [5] extracted the shape and texture of cervical cancer cells on Papanicolaou's stained smear by applying neural network.
- *Image pre-processing* [6]: AI can help in image processing by:
  1) Colour normalization of the slides.
  2) Removing the folds, air bubbles and other artefacts from the slides.

9.2.2 Screening of Cancer on Cytology Smears

CNN in WSI is applied to screen cancer cells in different samples including cervical, urine and effusion fluid [7–9].

Fig. 9.1 Applications of computational cytology

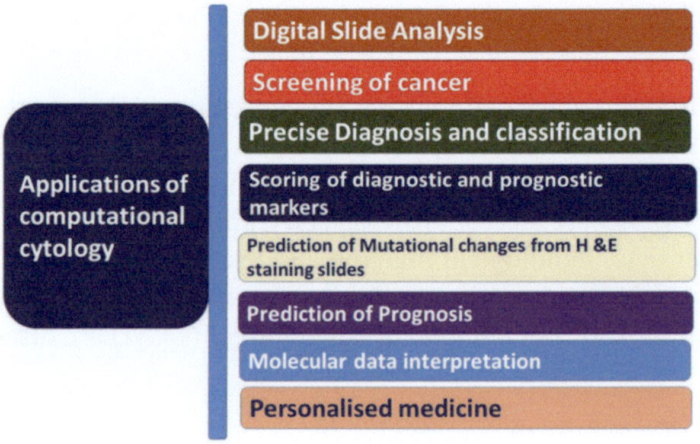

9.2.2.1 Cervical Cancer Screening

Cervical cancer screening is usually done on CNN of WSI of cervical smears (Fig. 9.2).

Li X et al. [10] successfully made a deep convolutional neural network (DCNN) model to diagnose carcinoma cells in cervical smears. However, they did not attempt to classify the cervical intraepithelial neoplasia.

Kanavati F et al. [11] used a convolutional and recurrent neural network model in 1605 WSIs of cervical smears. The model was able to detect the malignant cells with high accuracy (AUC 0.96). The model discriminated only the neoplastic and normal cells. It did not classify cells into low-grade squamous intraepithelial lesions (LSIL) and high-grade squamous intraepithelial lesions (HSIL). However, the model had promising potential in cervical cancer screening process.

Tan X et al. [12] constructed a DCNN model to screen the cervical intraepithelial lesions (CIN). The model showed 99.4% sensitivity and 99.4% specificity (AUC is 0.67). The sensitivity of detection of high-grade squamous intraepithelial lesions (HSIL) was 73.9%, however, the specificity of the model was remarkably low to (34.8%) apply it in routine screening.

Cheng S et al. [13] made a recurrent neural network-based model on 3545 WSIs of cervical smears to classify cells. The model had 93.5% specificity and 95.1% sensitivity. The study showed only 0.8% false-negative cases. It indicates that the system can exclude a good number of negative cases and can reduce the workload of the cytotechnologists.

9.2.2.2 Multilevel Classification of Cervical Cells

Rahaman MM et al. [14] developed a hybrid deep feature fusion (HDFF) technique based on DL to classify the cervical cells. The model showed 99.14% accuracy in classification of the cells in five classes that includes superficial, parabasal, koilocytotic, metaplastic and dyskeratotic cells. Wang CW et al. [15] used a DL model on WSIs of conventional Pap smear samples to detect HSILs or squamous cell carcinoma. The model showed a high precision of 0.93%. The DL model had high

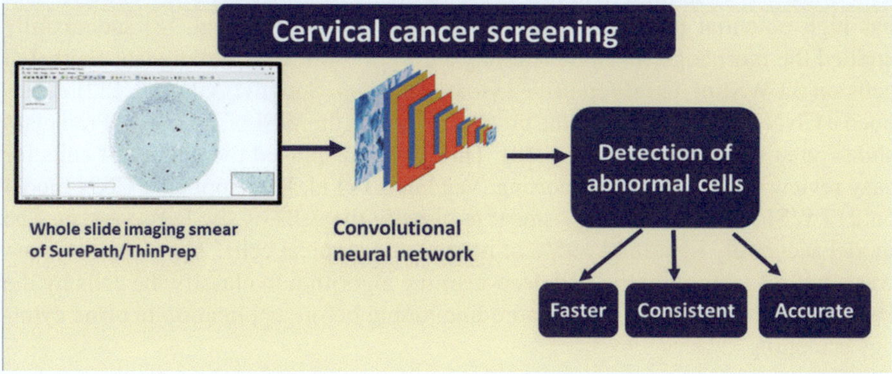

Fig. 9.2 Cervical smear screening

sensitivity (90%) and specificity (100.0%) and so can be used for a routine cervical screening program. Holmström O et al. [16] used a cloud-based deep learning system (DLS) on 740 WSI for the detection of atypical cervical cells. The DL model had 95.7% sensitivity and 100% specificity compared to 84.7% and 78.4% respectively for the pathologists. The authors had the opinion that AI-based screening can reduce the workload of the cytotechnologists.

Hussain E et al. [17] used six different DCNNs for multi-class diagnosis of cervical lesions. The classes include no intraepithelial lesion and malignancy (NILM), LSIL, HSIL and Squamous cell carcinoma (SCC). The study showed 98.90% accuracy with 79.80% sensitivity and 97.90% specificity. A Graph Convolutional Network was applied by Shi J et al. [18] for cervical cell classification in a 5-class including superficial, parabasal, koilocytotic, dyskeratotic and metaplastic. The model had 98.37% accuracy and 99.80% sensitivity. It is unfair and confusing to classify the cells in this manner. Bao H et al. [19] trained a supervised DL model based on 188,542 digital cytological images. The AI model detected 92.6% of CIN 2 and 96.1% of CIN 3 which was much higher compared to experienced cytopathologists. They concluded that DL model may help with the primary cytology screening.

Zhang L et al. [20] developed CNN to classify the cervical cells into seven layers including normal cells, dysplastic cells and squamous cell carcinomas. The model showed 98.3% accuracy. The CNN model automatically learns from the images and bypasses the problems of cell segmentation or feature design.

Table 9.1 highlights the salient features of different studies of cervical cancer screening based of artificial intelligence.

9.2.2.3 Urothelial Carcinoma Screening

Urothelial cell carcinoma is successfully screened by deep learning technique applied in urine cytology smears (Fig. 9.3). The results are consistent, with high accuracy. Lebret T et al. [21] used a digital medical device labelled as (VisioCyt®) based on DL to detect malignant urothelial cells on WSIs of cytology smears. This was a multicentric study that included 14 centres. The system showed 93.7% and 66.7% sensitivity in high- and low-grade tumours, respectively. The VisioCyt® tool has high potential to diagnose urothelial cancer. Zhang Z et al. [8] successfully applied the morphogo machine learning algorithm to identify malignant urothelial cells on 37 WSI of ThinPrep urine cytology smears. Sanghvi AB et al. [22] developed a CNN model to identify the urothelial cells in the WSI of 2405 ThinPrep glass slides (area under the curve of 0.88). The system displayed the gallery of cells for easy review of the cells for reporting. Vaickus LJ et al. [23] applied a CNN model on 217 WSIs of urine cytology smear to classify the cells by the Paris system. The model accurately identified >95% of normal and atypical cells. The current system was a hybrid morphometric and deep-learning algorithm to classify the cells by the Paris system. The system needs more fine-tuning before application in urine cytology screening.

Table 9.1 Cervical cancer screening by deep learning model

Author	Year	Number of smears	Technology	Cervical sample	Accuracy	Comments
Li X [10]	2023	Total 400 smears (211 cervical cancer and 189 normal smears)	DCNN	WSI of ThinPrep smears	Sensitivity: 96.21%, Specificity: 98.95%, Accuracy: 97.5%	Insufficient data to predict LSIL and HSIL.
Kanavati F [11]	2022	1605	CNN (EfficientNetB0 architecture) and RNN model	WSIs of ThinPrep smears	AUC 0.96 Accuracy: 0.907 Sensitivity: 85% Specificity: 91%	Model classified only negative and neoplastic cells. It may reduce the workload of the cytotechnologists.
Tan X [12]	2021	16,000	DCNN	WSI of ThinPrep smears	Sensitivity: 99.4% specificity: 34.8%	Model classified the smear in 5 classes: normal, ASCUS, LSIL and HSIL cells as well as squamous cell carcinoma
Cheng S [13]	2021	3545	Both CNN and RNN on Applied integrated strategy of low- and high-resolution combination	WSI of ThinPrep smears.	Sensitivity: 95.1% Specificity: 93.5%	Only focused on positive and negative cases rather than subclasses.
Rahaman MM [14]	2021	917 single-cell images	Hybrid deep feature fusion technique based on Deep learning	Publicly available single-cell images	Accuracy: 99.14%	Classified in five classes: superficial, parabasal, koilocytotic, metaplastic and dyskeratotic cells. Some classes are unnecessary.

(continued)

Table 9.1 (continued)

Author	Year	Number of smears	Technology	Cervical sample	Accuracy	Comments
Wang CW [15]	2021	143	DL model	WSIs of a conventional pap smear	Sensitivity: 90% specificity: 100%	Detect HSILs or SQC from NILM
Holmström O [16]	2021	361	Deep learning	WSI of conventional pap smear of HIV-positive women	*AI* Sensitivity: 95.7% Specificity: 100% *Manual* Sensitivity: 84.7% Specificity: 78.4%	AI classified atypia, low-grade atypia and high-grade atypia. AI had good sensitivity. The system can be used for routine screening.
Hussain E [17]	2020	1670	Six different deep CNN: Alexnet, Vggnet (vgg-16 and vgg-19), Resnet (resnet-50 and resnet-101) and Googlenet architecture	Both conventional and liquid-based cytology	Accuracy: 98.90% sensitivity: 79.80% specificity: 97.90%	Four classes: NILM, LSIL, HSIL and SQC
Shi J [18]	2020	Total 13,852 smears (two datasets: 4049 and 9803)	Graph convolutional network	Cervical cell image dataset SIPaKMeD	Accuracy: 98.37% sensitivity: 99.80% Specificity: 99.60	Cervical cell classification in 5-class including superficial, parabasal, koilocytotic, dyskeratotic and metaplastic
Bao H [19]	2020	2145	DL model-based WSI of cytological images	WSI of images LBC of cervical sample	Sensitivity: 97% Overall AUC: 0.762 CIN2+: 0.755 CIN3+: 0.726	DL model may help with the primary cytology screening
Zhang L [20]	2017	Total 917 smears (242 normal and 675 abnormal)	CNN	Publicly available dataset of cervical lesions	Accuracy: 98.3% Sensitivity: CIN2: 81% CIN3: 85.1% Specificity: CIN2: 67.1% CIN3: 56.8%	Total of seven classes. However, AI provides only normal or abnormal categories.

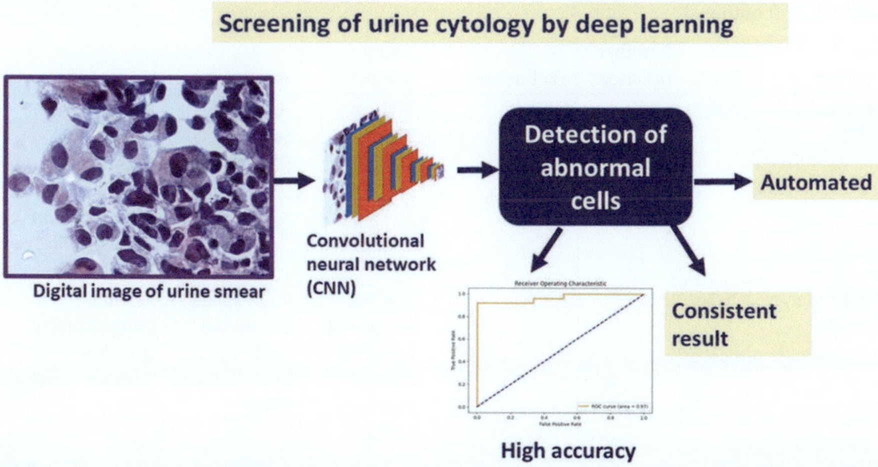

Fig. 9.3 Urothelial carcinoma screening

Table 9.2 Urothelial carcinoma screening from urine cytology

Author	Year	Number of cases	Technology	Urine sample	Accuracy	Comments
Lebret T [21]	2023	319	Medical device labelled as (VisioCyt®) based on DL on WSI of urine smear	Voided urine samples prepared by ThinPrep	Sensitivity of high grade tumour: 93.7% Sensitivity of low grade tumours: 66.7%	Overall higher sensitivity of AI model than manual screening. It can be used for routine screening
Zhang Z [8]	2021	37	CNN	Void urine samples prepared by ThinPrep	Not mentioned	The study needs more number of cases.
Sanghvi AB [22]	2019	2405	CNN	WSI of ThinPrep smears	AUC: 0.88 High grade Urothelial carcinomas Sensitivity: 79.5% Specificity: 84.5%	The system displayed the gallery of cells for easy review

(continued)

Table 9.2 (continued)

Author	Year	Number of cases	Technology	Urine sample	Accuracy	Comments
Vaickus LJ [23]	2019	217	CNN	WSI of ThinPrep smears	AUC:0.92 accuracy: 95%	The system needs more fine-tuning before application in urine cytology screening
Muralidaran C [24]	2016	117	ANN	Digital images of Milipore filtered cytology smear	High grade Urothelial carcinomas Specificity: 100%	Manual morphometry was done. Tedious process.

Abbreviations: *CNN* convolutional neural network, *ANN* Artificial neural network, *AUC* Area under the curve

Muralidaran et al. [24] developed an artificial neural network (ANN) model to detect urothelial cell carcinomas. The model had 100% sensitivity and specificity. However, the data extraction in this study was manual and cumbersome.

Table 9.2 shows the summary of the different studies on urothelial carcinoma screening from urine cytology samples.

9.2.3 Precise Diagnosis and Classification

AI helps in the confirmation of diagnosis of various tumours. It gives precise and consistent diagnosis with minimal error.

9.2.3.1 Breast Carcinoma [25, 26]

Tumour Detection and Grading CNN can detect invasive carcinoma, ductal carcinoma in situ (DCIS) and benign lesions with high sensitivity and accuracy (Fig. 9.4).

AI is widely used in the diagnosis and subtyping of carcinoma of the breast from the cytological smears [27] (Table 9.3). Subbaiah RM et al. [28] applied an ANN model on the digitized smears of FNAC samples of 52 cases of fibroadenomas and 60 cases of infiltrating ductal carcinomas. They had 100% accuracy in the detection of malignant lesions of the breast.

El Agouri H et al. [29] developed a Resnet50 and Xception models to classify benign lesions, in situ carcinoma and invasive carcinoma on 328 WSIs from 116 surgically resected breast tissue. The model correctly classified the carcinoma cases with 88% accuracy and 95% sensitivity. The study highlighted that the ANN model can be used to assist the pathologists in reporting.

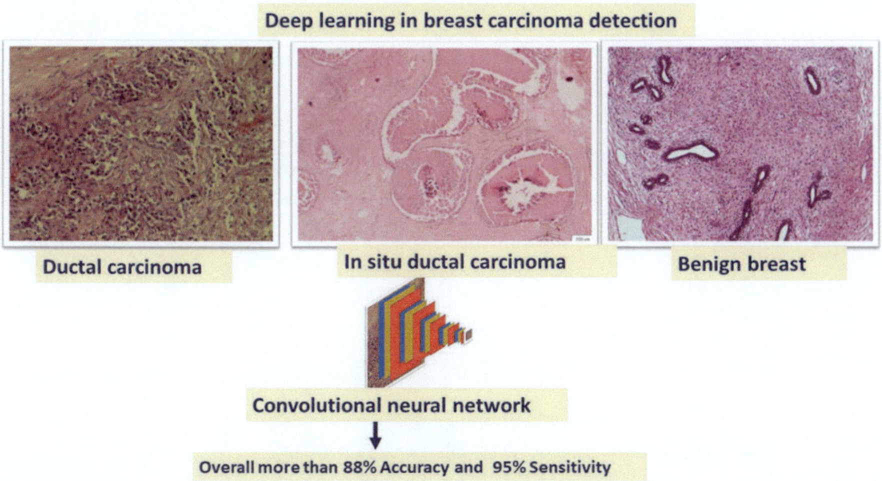

Fig. 9.4 Breast carcinoma identification by convolutional neural network

Cruz-Roa A et al. [30] developed a unique method of High-throughput Adaptive Sampling for whole-slide Histopathology Image analysis (HASHI) to detect invasive breast cancer on histopathology of WSIs. The accuracy of the detection rate of invasive carcinoma was 61.1–75%.

Yamamoto Y et al. [31] analysed 11,661 nuclei of 22 cases of breast lesions including normal cases, usual ductal hyperplasia and low/high grade ductal carcinoma in situ (DCIS). They quantitated morphological information of myoepithelial cells instead of studying tumour cells. Applying machine learning, support vector machine (SVM) on the WSI of histopathology images, they were able to subclassify these lesions with 90.9% accuracy.

Spanhol FA et al. [32] identified 80% breast carcinoma cases by applying computer-aided diagnosis on histopathological images. The accuracy of detection of malignancy was quite low 80% to 85%.

9.2.3.2 Lung Carcinoma Diagnosis

Deep learning plays an important role in screening, and precise diagnosis of lung carcinomas by interpreting complex molecular data of liquid biopsy, interpreting radiological imaging data, risk factor assessment and interpreting cytological and histopathological images (Fig. 9.5).

Lung carcinomas can be successfully diagnosed and classified on WSI images by CNN [33, 34]. Kanavati F [34] applied CNN with transfer learning on 3554 WSI images. They were successful in diagnosing and classification of lung carcinomas with an AUC of the ROC curve from 0.975 to 0.988. The work is highly promising and indicates that the CNN model can be used in routine reporting.

Civit-Masot J et al. applied a CNN model on 15,000 images that include images of 5000 from healthy tissue, 5000 adenocarcinomas, and 5000 squamous cell

Table 9.3 Diagnosis of carcinoma of breast

Author	Year	Number of cases	Technique	Sample type	Main findings	Accuracy/ sensitivity/ specificity	Comments
El Agouri [29]	2022	116 cases with 328 images	Resnet50 and Xception models	WSIs from surgically resected breast tissue	They classified the cases as: Normal tissue/ benign lesions, in situ carcinoma or invasive carcinoma.	Accuracy: 88% sensitivity: 95%	The study had good discriminatory power to differentiate benign from carcinoma cases.
Cruz-Roa A [30]	2018	695 cases from cancer genome atlas	CNN-based high-throughput adaptive sampling for whole-slide histopathology image analysis (HASHI)	WSI of invasive breast cancer		Accuracy: 61.1–75%.	The system can help pathologists for the rapid detection and localization of breast carcinomas
Yamamoto Y [31]	2017	11,661 nuclei of 22 cases	Support vector machine (SVM)	Histopathology images of breast	The system classified four histological types: Normal cases, usual ductal hyperplasia and low−/ high-grade Ductal carcinoma in situ.	Accuracy: 90.9%	They studied quantitative morphological information of myoepithelial cells instead of tumour cells.
Spanhol FA [32]	2016	7909 images from 82 patients	Computer-aided diagnosis	Digitized histopathology images of breast	Automated classification of these Images in benign and malignant	Accuracy: 85%	Feature extraction is time-consuming
Subbaiah RM [28]	2014	112 cases (52: Fibroadenomas and 60: Infiltrating ductal carcinoma	ANN	Digitized FNAC smears of breast	Semi-quantitative cytology data, morphometric, nuclear densitometric data and grey level co-occurrence matrix were extracted to identify the malignant cells.	Accuracy: 100%	The feature extraction is a tedious job and there is a chance of bias in the cell selection

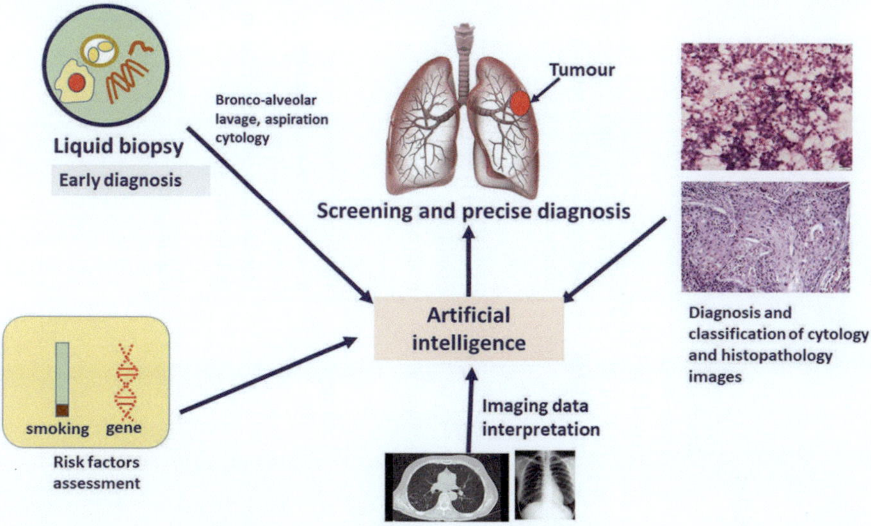

Fig. 9.5 Lung cancer screening and precise diagnosis

carcinoma. They successfully classified benign and malignant components of ling with 99.69% accuracy [35].

Jain DK et al. [36] applied Kernel PCA integrated with a convolutional neural network on the 15,000 publicly available histopathology images of lung carcinomas to identify the neoplastic and non-neoplastic cells. It had 97.1%accuracy. Jiao Y et al. [37] applied a promising Deep Embedding-based Logistic Regression in multi-organ datasets that include colorectal, lung and breast cancers. They showed high accuracy in the identification of malignancy (AUC of over 0.95 in all three organs).

Table 9.4 shows features of different studies that diagnose carcinoma of the lung by applying a neural network.

9.2.3.3 Lung Cancer Classification

Yang et al. [38] applied the ResNet-152 VGG-19 Xception model to classify lung cancers such as adenocarcinoma (ADC), squamous cell carcinoma (SCC), small cell carcinoma (SCC), large cell neuroendocrine carcinomas and non-neoplastic lung lesions on H&E-stained slides. They annotated the cancer regions on 205 WSIs. From these 205 WSI images, a total of 10,049 sample patch images were generated. These patches include different subtypes of lung carcinomas along with non-neoplastic lesions. The authors achieved high accuracy with AUC of ROC 0.97. They highlighted the high performance and consistency of the ANN model compared to the experienced pathologists. Kosaraju, S et al. [39] applied a Deep Learning-Based Framework on 113 WSI images of lung lesions including carcinomas and non-neoplastic lesions. They generated 160,000 patches from the cancer slides and 140,000 patches from the

Table 9.4 Neural network in lung carcinoma diagnosis

Author	Year	Number of cases	Technique	Sample type	Main findings	Accuracy/ sensitivity/ specificity (%)	Comments
Kanavati F [34]	2023	3554	CNN with transfer learning	WSI images of lung carcinomas	The system differentiated carcinoma and non-neoplastic lesions of the lung	AUC of ROC curve 0.988.	The model has high accuracy and can be used in a routine laboratory.
Civit-Masot J [35]	2022	15,000	CNN	Publicly available dataset of lung carcinoma	Model identified squamous cell carcinoma, adenocarcinoma and benign areas of lung	SQC:97.2% ADC: 97.1% Benign: 99.9%	The model is helpful in identifying and classifying the malignant lung tumour.
Jain D.K. [36]	2022	15,000 digital images	Kernel PCA integrated with a convolutional neural network	Publicly available dataset of lung carcinoma	Model identified squamous cell carcinoma, adenocarcinomaand benign areas of the lung	Accuracy: 97.1%	The model removed noise, resized and normalized the image. It was a successful identification and classification of lung tumours
Jiao Y [37]	2021	Not mentioned	Deep Embedding-based Logistic Regression	Multi-organ datasets that include colorectal, lung and breast cancers	Identified lung carcinoma	AUC: 0.95	Rapid speed

non-neoplastic slides. The model successfully classified lung cancer (ADC, SQC, SCC, large cell neuroendocrine carcinomas(LCNE) and non-neoplastic lung lesions (AUC 0.96 of ROC).

Chen CL et al. [40] used a deep learning model on WSI images of 9662 cases to classify the lung carcinomas. They were able to classify squamous cell carcinoma and adenocarcinoma successfully with the area under the receiver operating curve of 0.9594 and 0.9414, respectively.

Table 9.5 highlights salient features of different studies that used AI to classify lung carcinomas.

9.2.3.4 AI on Cytology of Lung Carcinomas

The subtyping between ADC and SQC from cytological material is difficult as it often needs complete immunocytochemistry including CK 5/6, CK 7, p40/p63, TTF-1 and napsin. However, DCNN can classify lung carcinomas with high sensitivity and specificity (Fig. 9.6).

In a multi-institutional study, Kim T et al. [41] applied a DL-based model on 1273 WSIs of cytology smears of lung lesions. A total of 30,590 image patches were developed. The sensitivity, specificity and accuracy of malignancy detection were 95.9%, 98.2%, and 96.9%, respectively. The result was comparable to the performance of the experienced pathologists.

Tsukamoto T et al. [42] worked on the cytological images of lung cancer to classify ADC, SQC and SCC. They used multiple DCNN technique including AlexNet, GoogLeNet (Inception V3), VGG16 and ResNet50, having accuracy rates of 74.0%, 66.8%, 76.8% and 74.0%, respectively. Unfortunately, the accuracy rate in their study was low. Probably, the model needed fine-tuning.

Teramoto A et al. [43] applied a DCNN model on the cytology smears of lung carcinomas. The smears were prepared from liquid-based cytology (LBC). They included 306 benign and 315 malignant image patches. The sensitivity and specificity of identification of malignant cells were 89.3% and 83.3%, respectively.

Table 9.6 shows the salient features of different convolutional neural network studies on the cytology of lung carcinoma cases.

9.2.3.5 Prostate Cancer

Huang W et al. [44] applied a CNN-based model on 1000 WSI images of prostate biopsy for prostate cancer grading and quantification. The AI model was able to distinguish carcinoma from benign prostatic epithelium with high accuracy (AUC in ROC of 0.92). The performance of the CNN was in good agreement with the training pathologist. The study showed that AI-based platform can accurately and efficiently detect and grade prostate cancer.

Pantanowitz L et al. [45] developed a multi-layered CNN-based model on histopathology of the core needle biopsy of prostate to predict the probability of cancer. The CNN models were trained on 1,357,480 image patches developed from 549 WSIs images of the slides. The model showed a high level of accuracy (AUC of 0·997) for cancer detection. They concluded that an

Table 9.5 Artificial intelligence in classification of lung carcinomas

Author	Year	Number of cases	Technique	Sample type	Main findings	Accuracy/ sensitivity/ specificity (%)	Comments
Yang J.W [38]	2022	205	Four pre-trained CNN models used: ResNet15, VGG19, Xception and NASNETLarge	WSIs images of histopathology of lung carcinomas	Classified ADC, SQC, SCC, LCNC and non-neoplastic lung lesions	AUC: 0.97	Successfully classified into different types of lung carcinomas. A set of CNN models was used.
Kosaraju S [39]	2022	113	Weakly supervised learning, Class Activation Maps generated from CNN	WSI images of lung cancer biopsies	Successfully classified lung cancer ADC, SQC, SCC, LCNE and non-neoplastic lung lesions	AUC: 0.96 of ROC	The authors developed a novel slide visualization of WSI, named HipoMap. The model can be used in other cancers also
Chen CL [40]	2021	9662 cases	Deep learning model	WSI of histopathology of lung carcinomas	Classified squamous cell carcinoma and adenocarcinoma of lung	AUC: 0.9594	The model showed good classification performance

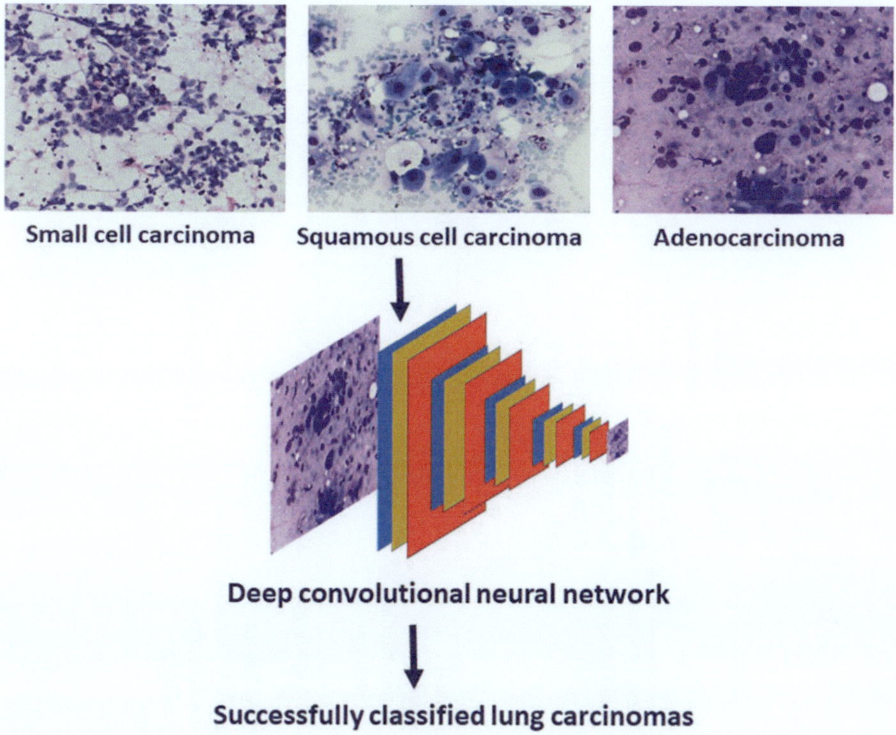

Fig. 9.6 Deep convolutional neural network to classify lung carcinomas

AI-based algorithm can be used clinically to accurately detect and grade carcinoma of the prostate.

Ström P et al. [46] made an AI model on 6682 digitized slides from needle core biopsies of the prostate to predict the presence, extent, and Gleason grade of carcinoma. The study showed 0.997 AUC of the receiver operating characteristic curve to distinguish between benign and malignant tissues compared to 0.96 for the expert pathologist. AI system and pathologists had equal performance regarding the Gleason grades. They concluded that an AI system can be a useful aid for the pathologists.

Table 9.7 highlights characteristic features of different AI-based studies on prostate.

9.2.3.6 Colorectal Carcinoma

Uddin AH et al. [47] applied a neural network model to identify colonic cancer from the haematoxylin and eosin (H&E) stained histological images. The study showed 99.96% accuracy. The proposed model was considered effective in colonic cancer detection.

Dabass M et al. [48] used a CNN model to identify and grade in H & E stained histopathological images of the colon. The model showed 97.5% accuracy in

Table 9.6 Convolutional neural network on cytology samples of lung

Author	Year	Number of cases	Technique	Sample type	Main findings	Accuracy/ sensitivity/ specificity (%)	Comments
Kim T [41]	2023	1273 cytology smears	Multiple CNN models: VGG19, ResNet50, ResNext50, InceptionV3, DenseNet121, and EfficientNetB7.	WSI of cytology smears of sputum and bronchial washing,	Detected benign and malignant cells	Accuracy: 96.9%, Sensitivity: 95.9%, Specificity: 98.2%,	Large dataset collected from multiple centres. High performance of the model. AI model augmented the performance of the students.
Tsukamoto T [42]	2022	55	Four DCNN techniques: AlexNet, GoogLeNet (Inception V3), VGG16 and ResNet50	Exfoliative and bronchoscopy or CT-guided fine-needle aspiration cytology smear	Classified ADC, SQC and SCC	Accuracy: 66.8–76.8%	Total number of cases were low. The accuracy rate in the study is low
Teramoto A [43]	2019	621 images	DCNN	Liquid-based cytology (BD SurePathTM Liquid-based Pap Test) smear of fine-needle aspiration Cytology of lung carcinomas	Detected benign and malignant cells	Sensitivity: 89.3 Specificity: 83.3% Accuracy: 87%	The model is efficient in detecting malignancy in cytology samples.

Table 9.7 Convolutional neural network of prostate carcinoma

Author	Year	Number of cases	Technique	Sample type	Main findings	Accuracy/ sensitivity/ specificity (%)	Comments
Huang W [44]	2021	1000	CNN	WSI images of prostate biopsy	Distinguished carcinoma from benign prostatic epithelium	AUC: 0.92	The performance of CNN was in good agreement with the training pathologist
Pantanowitz L [45]	2020	549	Multi-layer CNN-based model	WSI of the H & E-stained core needle biopsy of prostate	Detected prostate adenocarcinoma and did Gleason grading	Benign versus carcinoma; AUC: 0·997 Sensitivity: 99.59 Specificity: 90·14% Gleason score; AUC: 0.941 Sensitivity: 85.9% Specificity: 90.41	High performance both in the detection of carcinoma and in Gleason grading
Ström P [46]	2020	6682	DCN: Inception V3 models pretrained on ImageNet	Digitized slides from needle core biopsies of the prostate	Predicted the presence, extent, and Gleason grade of prostate carcinoma	AI: 0.997 AUC Manual: 0.96	AI system and pathologists had equal performance regarding the Gleason grades

identifying and grading of colonic cancer. The authors concluded that the AI model will work as a secondary referential diagnosis for the pathologists.

Iizuka O et al. [49] developed a CNN and recurrent neural networks (RNNs) models on the histopathology of WSIs of the colon. The models were able to identify the colonic adenocarcinoma and adenoma with AUC of ROC as 0.96 and 0.99, respectively. The model was considered a promising tool in the histopathology reporting.

Table 9.8 highlights the salient features of different AI-based studies to identify colonic carcinoma.

9.2.3.7 Cervical Carcinoma

Li X et al. [10] applied a DCNN model to screen and diagnose cervical cancer. They used the WSI image of ThinPrep preparation slides of 211 cervical carcinomas and 100 normal smears. The sensitivity, specificity, and accuracy of cancer detection were 96.21%, 98.95%, and 97.5%, respectively. The study was promising in the detection of carcinomas.

Hamdi M et al. [50] applied deep-learning (DL) models (ResNet50-VGG19, VGG19-GoogLeNet, and ResNet50-GoogLeNet) on 962 WSIs of smears of LBC slides. The model was able to detect squamous intraepithelial lesions, carcinoma and normal smears. The overall accuracy rate of the model was 99% with an AUC of 98.75% in the ROC.

9.2.3.8 Urothelial Carcinoma

Nojima S et al. [51] applied a deep learning network on the images of Papanicolaou-stained urinary cytology glass slides from 232 patients. The neural network identified the malignant urothelial cells with high accuracy (AUC in ROC was 0.9890). They concluded that the use of the deep learning network will help to detect malignant cells and thereby to decide plan of management.

Awan R et al. [52] applied a CNN model on WSIs of 398 cytology slides prepared by the ThinPrep technique. The system successfully detected the malignant cells with an AUC in the ROC curve of 0.81. The study emphasized the potential promise of an automated detection of malignant cells.

Lilli L et al. [53] used a CNN model on the images of urinary cytology samples of 60 cases. They had 274 images of urothelial normal cells and 416 abnormal cells. The model had weak performance with an accuracy of up to 89.90%.

9.2.3.9 Cytology of Thyroid Lesions

ANN is commonly used in fine needle aspiration cytology of thyroid lesions because preoperative diagnosis of thyroid lesions is important for management. The various studies have successfully identified papillary carcinoma of the thyroid in fine-needle aspiration cytology smears of thyroid [54–56] (Fig. 9.7).

9.2.3.10 Diagnosis of Benign Versus Malignant

Guan Q et al. [54] made a deep convolutional neural network model (VGG-16 model and Inception-v3) on FNAC of 279 thyroid nodules processed by

Table 9.8 Convolutional neural network of colorectal carcinomas

Author	Year	Number of cases	Technique	Sample type	Main findings	Accuracy/ sensitivity/ specificity (%)	Comments
Uddin AH [47]	2024	Colonic ADC 500 images and normal colon 500 images	CNN model (DenseNet201 or ResNet50)	Publicly available dataset of H&E-stained histological images of human colorectal cancer and normal tissue	Identified colonic adenocarcinoma	Accuracy: 99.96%	Efficient and, consistent with high accuracies
Dabass M [48]	2022	Not mentioned	CNN model comprised of Enhanced Convolutional Learning Modules, multi-level Attention Learning Module, and Transitional Modules	H&E-stained histopathological images of colonic carcinoma available as publicly available datasets	Identified and graded colonic carcinoma	Accuracy: 97.5–100%	The AI model may work as a secondary referential diagnosis for the pathologists
Iizuka O [49]	2020	4036 WSIs	CNN and recurrent neural network models	WSI of adenocarcinoma, of adenoma, and non-neoplastic lesions of colonic tissue	Identified colonic adenocarcinoma and adenoma	Colonic adenocarcinoma AUC: 0.96 Adenoma AUC: 0.99	High performance indicates it as a promising tool in the histopathology reporting.

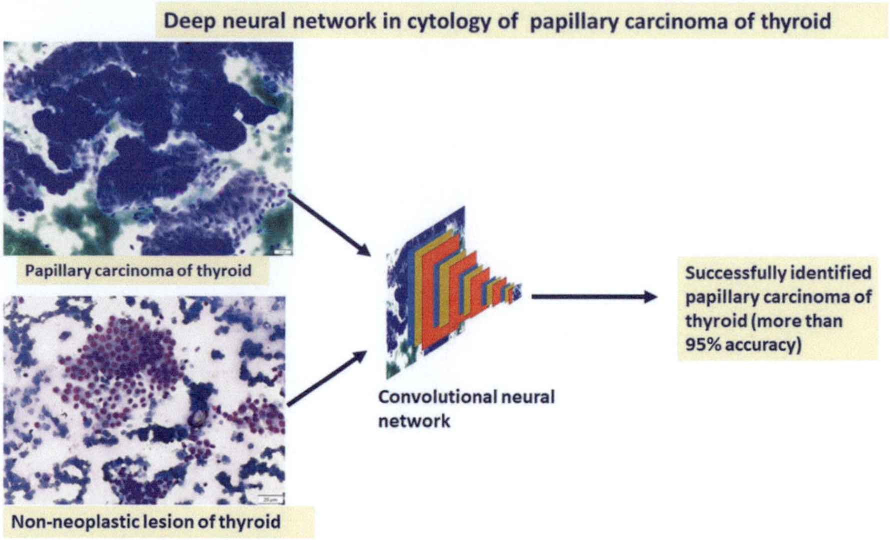

Fig. 9.7 Deep neural network in the identification of papillary carcinoma of thyroid

liquid-based cytology (SurePath). The dataset consists of 159 cases of papillary thyroid carcinoma (PTC) and 120 cases of non-neoplastic lesions of the Bethesda Type II category. The model distinguished PTC from the other non-neoplastic lesions of the thyroid. The accuracy rate, sensitivity and specificity of VGG-16 were 95%, 100%, and 94.91%, respectively. The Inception-v3 model showed 87.5% accuracy, 98.55% sensitivity and 86.44% specificity. This model carries significant potential in the diagnosis of PTC on FNAC samples.

Sanyal P et al. [55] applied a CNN model on Romanowsky/Pap-stained smears of FNAC of 186 cases of papillary thyroid carcinoma and 184 cases of non-neoplastic lesions of thyroid. Their main aim was to distinguish papillary carcinoma thyroid and non-papillary carcinoma thyroid on FNAC slides. The model showed 90.48% sensitivity, 83.3% specificity and 85.06% diagnostic accuracy. The study needs a large, diverse dataset to prove its real-world efficiency.

Gopinath B et al. [56] used a combination of Elman neural network, SVM and k-nearest neighbours classifiers on FNAC images downloaded from the online image atlas of the Papanicolaou Society of Cytopathology. They worked on 80 images (40 benign and 40 malignant). The model detected benign from malignant thyroid cells with good diagnostic accuracy (90%), sensitivity (85%) and specificity (100%). The study was done on downloaded images and so the application of the model is doubtful in the real world.

Cochand-Priollet B et al. [57] applied a computer-assisted system to discriminate benign from malignant thyroid lesions on May Grunwald Giemsa-stained smears of 157 cases of FNAC of thyroid. The study showed low accuracy 50.49%.

9.2.3.11 Follicular Adenoma Versus Carcinoma

Shapiro NA et al. [58] developed an ANN model on the cytology features, morphometric data and Giemsa-stained smears images of the 197 cases of thyroid follicular tumours (adenoma and carcinoma) to distinguish follicular adenoma versus follicular carcinoma of thyroid. Image analysis successfully classified 87% of cases.

Savala R et al. [59] developed an ANN model based on semi-quantitative cytology features, morphometric data and 26 follicular adenomas and 31 follicular carcinomas of FNAC smear. The area under the receiver operating curve was 1 indicating the high accuracy of the model. However, the model needs data extraction which was quite tedious. Moreover, the total number of cases was much less.

Maleki S et al. [60] developed a supervised machine learning algorithm (SVM) to differentiate classic papillary thyroid carcinoma (cPTC) from non-invasive follicular thyroid neoplasm with papillary-like nuclear features (NIFTP) on FNAC smears. The dataset had a total of 59 cases (29 cPTCs and 30 NIFTP). The keywords and phrases from the microscopic descriptions were processed by the Matlab Text Analytics Toolbox. The model correctly classified cPTC from NIFTP in 76.05 ± 0.96% of cases. The model had 72.6% sensitivity and 81.6% specificity in the identification of cPTC cases.

Saini T et al. [61] in a novel study made an ANN model on FNAC smears to predict the risk of malignancy in 61 category III Bethesda thyroid lesions (Atypia of undetermined cases, AUS and follicular lesions of undetermined significance, FLUS). Two pathologists identified semi-quantitative morphologic features of these cases. The ANN model differentiated between malignant and benign cases. The model showed 100% specificity.

Table 9.9 highlights different AI-based studies on fine-needle aspiration cytology of thyroid.

9.2.3.12 Effusion Cytology

DCNN is effective in successfully classifying benign from malignant cells in effusion (Fig. 9.8).

Park HS et al. [62] used a deep convolutional neural network model (DCNN) (Inception-ResNet-V2) model from the WSI of malignant pleural effusion of metastatic breast cancer (569 cytological slides, malignant 152, benign 417) to identify malignant cells. In addition, three pathologists also examined the cases. The DCNN model showed better performance than the pathologist by showing higher accuracy (81.1% vs. 68.7%), sensitivity (95.0% vs. 72.5%) and specificity (98.6% vs. 88.9%), respectively, in detecting malignant cells. The model bears the potential to assist the cytopathologist. However, the study has selection bias as it only involves the metastatic breast carcinoma cases.

Sanyal P et al. [63] applied a CNN model on 90 cases of effusion cytology samples (52 cases of metastatic adenocarcinoma and 38 benign effusion samples). The model showed 88% sensitivity and 96% specificity in the identification of malignant cases in effusion. The present model is promising to assist the cytopathologists. However, the study did not use WSI images and they only had selected digital images.

Table 9.9 AI-based studies on fine-needle aspiration cytology of thyroid

Author	Year	Number of cases	Technique	Key findings	Accuracy/sensitivity/ specificity (%)/AUC	Comments
Guan Q [54]	2019	279	Deep convolutional neural network model (VGG-16 model and Inception-v3)	The model distinguished PTC from the other non-neoplastic lesions of thyroid.	*VGG-16* Sensitivity: 100%, specificity: 94.91%, diagnostic accuracy: 95% *Inception-v3* Sensitivity: 98.55%, specificity: 86.44%, diagnostic accuracy: 87.5%	A successful model with high accuracy
Sanyal P [55]	2018	370	CNN	The model distinguished papillary carcinoma thyroid and non-papillary carcinoma thyroid on FNAC slides	Sensitivity: 90.48%, specificity: 83.3%, diagnostic accuracy: 85.06%	The study needs a large diverse dataset to prove its real world efficiency
Gopinath B [56]	2015	80 images	Elman neural network (ENN), support vector machine (SVM) and k-nearest neighbours (k-NN) classifiers	The model detected benign from malignant thyroid cells	Accuracy: 90%, Sensitivity:85% Specificity: 100%	The study is done on downloaded images and so the application of the model is doubtful in real world
Cochand-Priollet [57]	2006	157	Computer assisted system	The system discriminated benign from malignant thyroid lesions	Accuracy: 50.49%	Low accuracy
Shapiro NA [58]	2007	197	ANN	Distinguished follicular adenoma versus follicular carcinoma of thyroid	The model successfully classified 87% of cases	The model is promising

Savala R, Dey P [59]	2018	57	ANN	Distinguished follicular adenoma versus follicular carcinoma of thyroid	AUC:1	The model needs data extraction which is quite tedious. The total number of cases are very less
Maleki et al. [60]	2019	59	Supervised machine learning algorithm (SVM)	The model differentiated classic papillary thyroid carcinoma (cPTC) from non-invasive follicular thyroid neoplasm with papillary-like nuclear features(NIFTP)	To identify cPTC cases Sensitivity: 72.6% specificity: 81.6%	The model used only the microscopic description that includes key words and phrases
Saini T, Dey P et al. [61]	2023	61	ANN	The ANN model differentiated between malignant and benign cases of category III Bethesda thyroid lesions	Specificity:100%	This is a unique study. However, total number of cases are less.

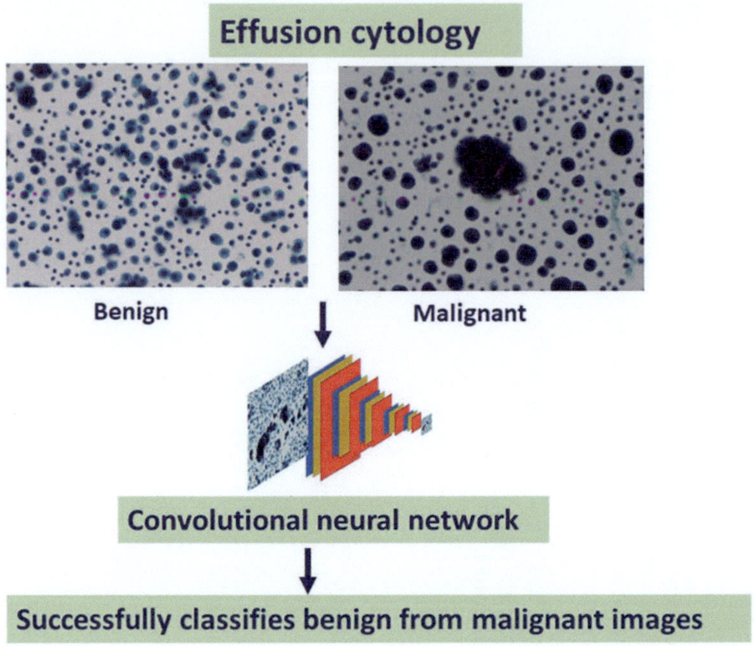

Fig. 9.8 Convolutional neural network to differentiate benign from malignant cells in effusion

Xie X et al. [9] built a deep convolutional neural network model on the WSI of effusion cytology smears prepared by liquid-based cytology (CytoRich Non-gyn, BD). The study included the WSIs of 234 benign and 170 malignant slides. All the malignant cells were confirmed as metastasis from the lung. The model showed 91.67%, 87.50% and 94.44% of accuracy, sensitivity, and specificity, respectively, in identifying malignancy. The study included a large number of cases. However, they included only metastatic lung carcinomas. The model should also be applied in real-world cases for its efficiency.

Barwad A et al. [64] built an ANN model on 114 cytology smears of effusion based on semi-quantitative cytological features, along with morphometric, densitometric and chromatin textural data of the individual nuclei of the cells. They successfully detected malignant cells with 100% sensitivity and specificity. The data collection of the cases needs lot of time and there is also a chance of bias in the selection of cells.

Truong H et al. [65] developed an ANN model on effusion cytology (112 cases) smears to detect malignant cells. They quantitated densitometric and morphometric data of the individual cells. The ANN model had 95.3%, sensitivity of 85.7%, specificity in the detection of malignant cells. The data extraction is a tedious process in this study.

Table 9.10 shows salient features of various AI-based studies on effusion cytology.

Table 9.10 AI-based studies on effusion cytology

Author	Year	Number of cases	Technique	Key findings	Accuracy/sensitivity/ specificity (%)/AUC	Comments
Park HS [62]	2023	569 cytological slides(malignant 152, benign 417)	DCNN(Inception-ResNet-V2)	Detected malignant cells from WSI of malignant pleural effusion of metastatic breast cancer	AI model versus Pathologists Accuracy:81.1% vs. 68.7%,). Sensitivity:95.0% vs. 72.5%, and specificity 98.6% vs. 88.9%	The study has selection bias as it only involves the metastatic breast carcinoma cases.
Sanyal P [63]	2023	90 cases of effusion cytology samples (52 cases of metastatic adenocarcinoma and 38 benign effusion samples)	CNN	Detected malignant cells in effusion samples	Sensitivity: 88%, specificity: 96%	The study did not use WSI images and they only had selected digital images
Xie X [9]	2022	404 (234 benign and 170 malignant slides)	DCNN	Detected metastatic lung carcinomas in WSI of effusion cytology smears prepared by liquid-based cytology (CytoRich non-gyn, BD).	Accuracy: 91.67%, sensitivity: 87.50%, specificity: 94.44%	Large number of cases. Included only metastatic lung carcinomas. Model should be tested in real-world cases.
Barwad A [64]	2012	114	ANN	Detected malignant cells based on semi-quantitative cytological features, along with morphometric, densitometric and chromatin textural data of the individual nuclei of the cells	Sensitivity: 100% and specificity:100%	Data collection is tedious and time-consuming
Truong H [65]	1995	112	ANN	Detected malignant cells by quantifying densitometry and morphometric data of the individual cells	Sensitivity: 95.3% Specificity: 85.7%,	Data extraction is a tedious process

9.2.4 Scoring of Diagnostic and Prognostic Markers

AI enables scoring various biomarkers. Automated scoring by a convolutional neural network is overall superior to manual scoring due to high accuracy and consistency (Fig. 9.9).

The detection of biomarkers in breast carcinoma is of vital importance both for management and prognostic assessment. The commonly used biomarkers in breast carcinoma include HER2, progesterone receptor (PR), estrogen receptor (ER) and proliferative marker Ki67.

Various studies have shown a strong correlation between digital image analysis and manual scoring of various biomarkers [66–71]. The digital scoring is superior to manual due to high reproducibility.

In a large study by Abele N et al. [66], scoring by AI on WSI images of ER, PR and Ki67 was compared with manual scoring of 10 pathologists. There were high agreement rates between the pathologists and the AI system (87.6%for Ki67 and 89.4% for ER/PR). The results are promising and suggest the integration of an AI system in the routine laboratory workflow.

HER2 scoring in breast carcinoma cases is important due to the administration of anti-HER2 therapies, such as trastuzumab. Brügmann et al. [67] validated a new software, HER2-CONNECT(TM), to score HER2 in 167 breast carcinoma tissue core images. The software quantified HER2 immunostaining and was compared with the manual screening of 5 pathologists. The software scoring was in perfect agreement with the pathologist's scoring (92.1%) (Kappa: 0.859).

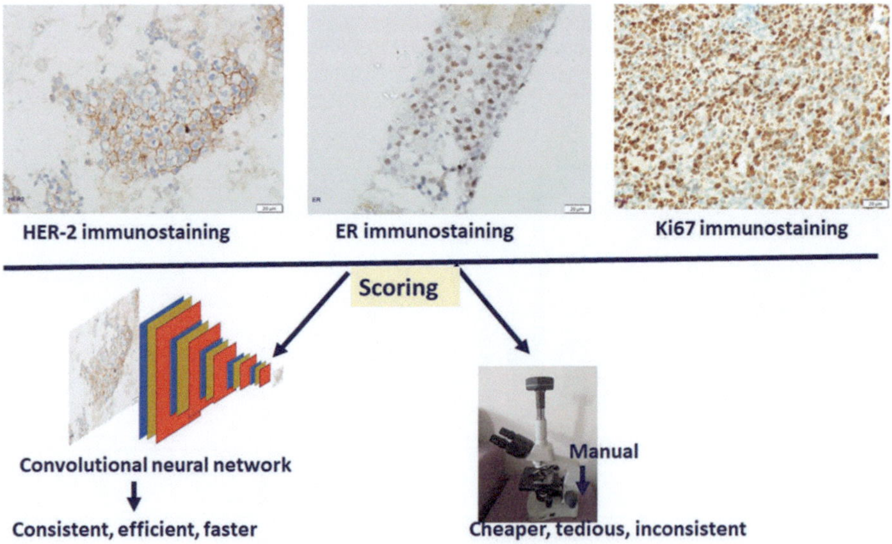

Fig. 9.9 Automated scoring by the convolutional neural network is effective, consistent and faster than manual scoring of various biomarkers

HER2 gene expression in immunohistochemistry detected by an AI model and the gene amplification status in FISH was correlated by different studies. Xue et al. [68] correlated HER2 scoring by AI and consecutive FISH images of invasive breast carcinomas. The study showed moderate accuracy in classification (85.3%). The correlation was highest in group 5 (95.90%) which was the commonest group. The study showed that, regarding assessing the HER2 amplification, AI is a reliable tool.

FISH is a reliable technique for the demonstration of HER2 gene amplification in carcinoma of the breast. The manual counting of the signal is time-consuming. Furrer D et al. [69] detected an automated fluorescence signal by using the MetaSystems™ image analysis system. The overall concordance between manual scoring and the automated signal analyser was 98.4%. The study concluded that the Metafer 4 classifier can be used for HER2 amplification by FISH in breast cancer.

Table 9.11 highlights the salient features of various studies that quantified ER/PR and HER2 by automated scoring:

9.2.4.1 PD-L1 Scoring

Programmed cell death ligand-1 (PDL-1) is expressed in tumour cells and its receptor, Programmed cell death-1 (PD1), is present in T lymphocytes. The interaction of PDL1 in tumour cells with PD1 in T lymphocytes prevents the destruction of tumour cells [72]. The assessment of PDL1 expression in NSCLC is important for management. PDL1 expression can be assessed from the cell block samples of the cytological materials collected during endoscopic brushing or FNAC samples [73]. Immunohistochemistry/ immunocytochemistry is well well-accepted technique for the PDL1 scoring. Inter-observer variation of PDL1 expression scoring often occurs that may affect the treatment. It is necessary to have a consistent and reliable PDL1 scoring. Digital image analysis plays an important role in PDL1 scoring.

Hondelink LM et al. [74] developed a novel automated deep learning model based on 199 whole slide images (WSIs) of stage IV NSCLC. The system assessed tumour proportion score (TPS) for PD-L1 with similar concordance with the reference score (79%) generated by the three pathologists. The model misclassified 21% cases and 80% of those cases, the pathologists were also in disagreement. The mistakes of the model are due to weak staining or incomplete staining.

Cheng G et al. [75] generated a deep learning based model (MobileNetV2 architecture) on WSI images of PD-L1 immunostaining of 84 samples of lung cancer cases for scoring. The model showed 96.4% and 96.8% accuracy and specificity, respectively. This AI-based Model can be applied for PD-L1 quantitation in WSI of lung cancer.

Choi S et al. [76] developed an AI model based on a total of 802 WSI images of NSCLC to score PDL1. The model had good performance with (AUC of 0.889 in ROC) in classifying PD-L1 positive and negative tumour cells. The AI model helped to improve the performance of the pathologists in case of disagreement.

Table 9.11 Automated scoring of HER2 and ER/PR

Biomarker	Author	Year	Number of cases	Technique	Sample type	Key findings	Accuracy/ sensitivity/ specificity (%)/ agreement	Comments
ER/PR/ Ki67	Abele N [66]	2023	204 breast carcinomas	CNN	WSI images of immunohistochemistry slides of ER, PR and Ki67	The biomarkers scoring was compared with manual scoring of 10 pathologists	95.8% of Ki-67 cases and 93.2% of ER/ PR cases are confirmed by pathologists	AI scoring was reliable and AI system can be used in routine laboratory.
HER2	Brügmann A [67]	2012	167 breast carcinomas	HER2-CONNECT(TM) software	HER2 stained digital image	The software quantified HER2 immunostaining and the scoring was in perfect agreement with pathologists	Agreement with the pathologist's scoring 92.1% with Kappa: 0.859	It was a promising supplementary diagnostic tool
HER2 (FISH image)	Xue T [68]	2023	320 breast carcinomas	DCNN, model (Aitrox AI model)	Digitized FISH images of HER2 in invasive breast carcinomas	HER2 scoring by AI was successfully correlated with consecutive FISH images of invasive breast carcinomas	Overall accuracy in all classification: 85.3%	A promising tool for automatically evaluating HER2 amplification
HER2 (FISH image)	Furrer D [69]	2013	32 clearly nonamplified and 32 clearly amplified cases of breast carcinomas	MetaSystems™ image analysis system	Digitized FISH images of HER2	Detected automated fluorescence signal of HER2	Concordance between manual scoring and automated signal analyser: 98.4%	Metafer 4 classifier can be used for HER2 amplification by FISH in breast cancer

ER/PR	Rexhepaj E [70]	2008	743	Image analysis algorithms were developed using MatLab 7	WSI images of ER/PR IHC of breast cancer tissue microarray slides	Automated quantification of the ER/PR was done	Spearman's $\rho = 0.9$ between automated scoring and selected cases of manual scoring	The system can be used in quantification of ER/PR on tissue sections
ER	Diaz LK [71]	2004	70	Computer-assisted techniques	ER IHC of invasive breast carcinomas	Detected automated scoring of ER	Kappa value of agreement with the ER score and manual score: 0.8	High interobserver agreement with automated scoring and manual scoring of ER

Aitrox AI Model based on WSI images of 115 cases of NSCLC was correlated strongly with the TPS Gold Standard determined by three trained pathologists (79.13% accuracy for all subsets). The authors concluded that the Aitrox AI Model had good potential in assisting pathologists in routine laboratory [77].

Kapil A et al. [78] used Auxiliary classifier generative adversarial networks and CNN on WSI images of PDL1 IHC of 270 NSCLC patients. The microscopic visual TPSs are done on WSI images of two pathologists. Pearson correlation coefficient of the automated score was 0.90, indicating good correlation between the automated scoring and the visual scoring.

Table 9.12 highlights the salient features of quantitation of PDL1 biomarkers by an AI model:

9.2.4.2 Ki67 Scoring

Ki67 evaluation in the digital platform also has good performance. Acs B et al. [79] used QuantCenter (3DHistech) and QuPath (open source software) to evaluate Ki67 expression. There was good reproducibility between the different digital platforms.

Saha M et al. [80] made a CNN model that can score Ki67-positive nuclei automatically with 93% precision in breast carcinoma cases. They concluded that the CNN model is highly reliable and helpful for fast and efficient Ki-67 scoring.

9.2.5 Prediction of Mutational Changes from H &E Staining Slides

The AI model can detect the sub-visual changes and can accurately predict the mutational changes of various biomarkers on routinely stained slides. This prediction is very important for targeted therapy. So, an AI model can bypass the costly and time-consuming tests to detect mutational changes.

Pao JJ et al. [81] used the ResNet50 CNN model to predict EGFR mutational status. They included H&E-stained slides of 2099 adenocarcinoma patients. The model predicted EGFR expression status from the H&E slides with relatively good accuracy (AUC 0.870).

Mayer C et al. [82] applied Deep Learning Algorithms to predict ALK and ROS1-fusions from the WSIs images of H&E-stained slides of 234 advanced-stage non-small cell lung carcinoma (NSCLC). The model demonstrated 100% and 98.6% specificities for ALK and ROS1, respectively. The study highlights the ability of an AI model to predict ALK and ROS1 mutations and to guide which cases need the mutational changes to assess.

Tomita N et al. [83] applied ResNet-18, EfficientNet-B0 neural networks on WSIs images of H&E-stained slides of 747 non-squamous cell lung carcinoma (NSCLC) to predict five gene mutations (BRAF, EGFR, KRAS, STK11, and TP53) of lung carcinomas. The model showed good performance (AUC in ROC of 0.799) indicating that there are certain sub-visual changes in H&E-stained slides that can be picked up by the CNN model.

Table 9.12 The salient features of quantitation of PDL1 biomarkers by AI model

Author	Year	Number of cases	Technique	Sample type	Key findings	Accuracy/sensitivity/ specificity (%)/ agreement	Comments
Hondelink L.M [74].	2022	199 WSIs NSCLC	DCNN	WSI of PDL1 stained slides	The system successfully assessed tumour proportion score (TPS) for PD-L1	Concordance with the reference score: 79%	The model can assist the pathologists in routine laboratory.
Cheng G [75]	2022	84 samples of lung cancer	Deep learning based model (MobileNetV2 architecture)	WSI of PDL1 stained images of lung carcinomas	The system successfully scored PDL1 of lung carcinoma cases.	Accuracy: 96.4% specificity: 96.8%	The model can be applied for the quantitative scoring of PD-L1 WSI of lung cancer.
Choi S [76]	2022	802 WSI images of NSCLC	AI model	WSI of PDL1-stained images of lung carcinomas	AI-powered model quantified PDL1 scoring and increased the consensus between the pathologists	AUC of 0.889 in ROC	AI model improves the consensus between the pathologists
Huang Z [77]	2022	115 cases	U-Net based architecture	WSI of PDL1-stained images of lung carcinomas	AI model successfully did TPS of PDL1	Accuracy: 79.13% for all subsets Accuracy: 85.29% for negative TPS subset	AI model had good potential in assisting pathologists in routine laboratory
Kapil A [78]	2018	270	Auxiliary classifier generative adversarial networks (AC-GAN) and CNN	WSI of PDL1-stained images of NSLC	Successful PDL1 scoring by the model	Pearson correlation coefficient of the automated score and expert pathologists was 0.90	Good correlation between the automated scoring and the visual scoring indicates that the model is reliable

Huang K et al. [84] applied a CNN model on 180 WSIs of H&E-stained images of lung carcinomas to predict mutated AKT1, FGFR1, FGFR2, HRAS and MET. The accuracy rate was 72.00% for AKT1, 83.00% for FGFR1, 82.00% for FGFR2, 79.00% for HRAS and 86.00% for MET.

Wang Y et al. [85] developed an automated deep learning-based framework (HEAL Platform). They applied this model on WSIs of lung and colon cancer to predict the mutation of STK11, KEAP1, NF1, TP53, EGFR, FAT1, LRPAB, SETBP1 and KRAS. AUC of the various markers ranged from 0.54 to 0.82.

Coudray N et al. [86] trained a CNN model (Inception v3) on whole-slide images of H&E-stained slides of lung carcinoma (ADC and SQC) to predict the mutations of STK11, EGFR, FAT1, SETBP1, KRAS and TP53 genes (with AUCs from 0.733 to 0.856). They suggested the use of CNN model to predict the genetic mutations from H&E-stained slides.

Table 9.13 showed the salient features of different AI-based studies to predict mutational changes from H&E-stained slides.

9.2.5.1 Prediction of Biomarkers from Haematoxylin and Eosin-Stained Images

HER2 Prediction

Several AI models are developed to predict the HER2 receptor status from simple haematoxylin and eosin (H&E)-stained images [87–90].

Conde-Sousa E et al. [87] developed a CNN model on a 509 WSI dataset of H&E-stained breast carcinoma cases and predicted HER2 overexpression from H&E-stained breast carcinoma cases. The AUC was 0.50 indicating poor performance of the model.

Farahmand et al. [88] made a CNN model on WSI images of 188 H&E breast carcinomas (93 HER2+ and 95 HER2− slides). The model predicted the HER2 expression from H&E-stained images (AUC 0.90). Bypassing the simple prediction of overexpression of HER2, the CNN model was also able to predict the response to trastuzumab therapy from the H&E-stained slides (AUC 0.80).

Naik N et al. [89] applied a multiple instance learning-based deep neural network on 3474 H&E-stained WSI of breast carcinoma from the publicly available datasets to predict ER expression from H&E-stained breast carcinoma cases. (AUC: 0.92). The model had high accuracy and can be used in a routine laboratory to assist pathologists.

Anand D et al. [90] developed a CNN model based on the WSI images of 97cases (26 each HER2 positive and negative cases and 45 independent cases comprising 23 HER2+ and 22 HER2− cases). The model showed high concordance (AUC of 0.82) to predict HER2 expression. The study highlights the importance of AI in the prediction of HER2 expression on H&E-stained images.

Table 9.13 Mutational prediction by applying deep learning

Mutation	Author	Year	Number of cases	Technique	Sample type	Key findings	Accuracy/ sensitivity/ specificity (%)/ Agreement	Comments
EGFR	Pao J.J [81]	2023	2099 adenocarcinoma	ResNet50 CNN model	Haematoxylin and eosin (H&E) stained NSLC	Predicted EGFR expression status from the H&E slides	AUC 0.870 NPV: 0.954 PPV: 0.410	The model can be used for predicting EGFR mutation from H&E-stained slide.
ALK and ROS1 fusions	Mayer C [82]	2022	234	CNN	WSI images of H&E-stained slides of advanced-stage non-small cell lung carcinoma (NSCLC)	Predicted ALK and ROS1-fusions status from the H&E slides	Sensitivity: of 100% for both genes Specificity: 100 for ALK1 and 98.6% for ROS1, respectively	The model guides which cases need the mutational changes to assess.
BRAF, EGFR, KRAS, STK11, and TP53	Tomita N [83]	2022	747	CNN (ResNet-18, EfficientNet-B0 neural networks)	WSIs images of H&E-stained *NSCLC*	Predicted BRAF, EGFR, KRAS, STK11, and TP53 mutations from the H&E slides	AUC in ROC of 0.799	Overall good performance

(continued)

Table 9.13 (continued)

Mutation	Author	Year	Number of cases	Technique	Sample type	Key findings	Accuracy/ sensitivity/ specificity (%)/ Agreement	Comments
AKT1, FGFR1, FGFR2, HRAS and MET	Huang K [84]	2021	180	CNN and residual network (ResNet)	WSIs of H&E-stained images of lung carcinomas were downloaded from The Cancer Genome Atlas (TCGA)	Predicted AKT1, FGFR1, FGFR2, HRAS and MET mutations from the H&E slides	Accuracy: AKT1: 72.00% FGFR1: 83% FGFR2: 82% HRAS:79 and MET: 86.00%	The AI model did not include an independent verification subset to evaluate. The insufficient number of H&E-stained whole slide images used.
STK11, KEAP1, NF1, TP53, EGFR, FAT1, LRPAB,SETBP1 and KRAS	Wang Y [85]	2021	Not mentioned	16 different deep learning architectures are combined to develop HEAL program	WSIs of H&E-stained images of lung carcinomas (ADC, SQC) and normal lung were downloaded from TCGA	Predicted mutations of STK11, KEAP1, NF1, TP53, EGFR, FAT1, LRPAB,SETBP1 and KRAS	Predicted mutations of STK11, KEAP1, NF1, TP53, EGFR, FAT1, LRPAB,SETBP1 and KRAS	HEAL is an open-source framework
STK11, EGFR, FAT1, SETBP1, KRAS and TP53	Coudray N [86]	2018	1634 WSI (1176 tumour tissues and 459 normal)	CNN model (inception v3)	WSI of H&E-stained slides of lung carcinoma (ADC and SQC) downloaded from TCGA	Predicted the mutations of STK11, EGFR, FAT1, SETBP1, KRAS and TP53 genes	AUCs from 0.733 to 0.856	The use of this model is promising to predict gene mutations from H&E-stained slides

PDL1 Scoring Prediction

Sha L et al. [91] successfully classified the positive and negative PDL1 cases (AUC: 0.80 for all cases) on 130 H&E-stained WSI images. The model was robust and useful in the prediction from simple H&E-stained images.

Table 9.14 show the characteristic features of AI-based model to predict the different biomarkers from H& E slides.

9.2.6 Prediction of Prognosis

AI plays an important role in the prognosis prediction of various carcinomas.

9.2.6.1 Tumour-Infiltrating Lymphocytes (TIL)

TIL represents an immune response and is commonly associated with increased survival in different carcinomas [92].

There is lack of standardization and reproducibility regarding the quantification of TIL [93].

The International TILs Working Group has recommended the evaluation protocol of TIL [94].

The salient features of the recommendations are:

- TIL should be measured in the stromal part.
- TIL should be scored along the border of the invasive tumour margin.
- All mononuclear cells (including plasma cells) should be scored.
- TIL should be assessed as a continuous variable and the percentage of TIL should be mentioned clearly.

AI can accurately and reliably assess the quantitation of TIL.

Bai Y et al. [95] applied a CNN model to quantitate TIL in triple-negative breast cancer cases. The proportion of TIL is measured and noted that TIL variables had significant prognostic outcomes.

Thagaard J et al. [96] applied a fully automated CNN to quantitate stromal TIL in Triple-Negative Breast Cancers. The TIL score measured by the CNN model was well correlated with the manual score derived by the pathologist. They also noted that TIL scoring was directly related to the prognosis of the patients.

Barmpoutis P et al. [97] applied DeepLab v3+ network with Inception-ResNet-v2 to automatically quantify tumour-infiltrating lymphocytes on H&E slides of lung carcinomas. The model had 92.87% specificity at 95% sensitivity. The proposed method was fast, reproducible and reliable. The study suggests that the model can be used in a routine laboratory for the quantification of TIL and to assess the prognosis.

9.2.6.2 Tumour–Stromal Ratio

Tumourigenesis consists of three stages: initiation, progression and metastasis. The tumour is surrounded by a microenvironment known as the tumour microenvironment (TME). The TME is intimately related to every stage of tumourigenesis [98].

Table 9.14 Biomarker prediction from H&E-stained images

Biomarker	Author	Year	Number of cases	Technique	Sample type	Key findings	Accuracy/ sensitivity/ specificity (%)/ Agreement	Comments
HER2	Conde-Sousa E [87]	2022	509	CNN	WSI dataset of H&E-stained breast carcinoma	The model predicted HER2 overexpression from H&E-stained breast carcinoma cases	AUC: 0.50	Poor accuracy
HER2	Farahmand S [88]	2022	188	CNN	WSIs images of H&E breast carcinomas (93 HER2+ and 95 HER2− slides)	The model predicted the HER2 expression from H&E-stained images	AUC 0.90	Strong agreement between pathologist and AI model
ER	Naik N [89]	2020	3474	Multiple instance learning-based deep neural network	H&E-stained WSI of breast carcinoma from the publicly available datasets	Predicted ER expression from H&E-stained breast carcinoma	AUC: 0.92	High accuracy in prediction of ER expression
HER2	Anand D [90]	2020	97	CNN	H&E-stained WSI of breast carcinoma from TCGA	The model successfully predicted HER2 overexpression from H&E-stained breast carcinoma cases	AUC of 0.82	The model showed good accuracy in automatically quantifying the overexpression of HER2
PDL1	Sha L [91]	2019	130	CNN	H&E-stained WSIs images of NSCL	CNN model successfully predicted the positive and negative PDL1 cases from H&E-stained WSI images	AUC: 0.80 for all cases	-A robust deep learning model. -PD-L1 expression is correlated with the morphological features

TME consists of fibroblast, adipose tissue, neuroendocrine cells, immune cells, lymphatics and extracellular matrix. Tumour stromal ratio is now recognized as a prognostic biomarker for various carcinomas. Increased stromal component is associated with poor prognosis [99–102].

Micke P et al. [103] used machine learning to objectively quantify the tumour stroma fraction in a variety of solid cancers. However, in multivariate analysis, they did not notice any prognostic impact of TIL in various solid tumours.

Contrary to this study, Zhao K et al. [104] applied a CNN model using transfer learning to quantify tumour-stromal ratio (TSR)on WSI of H&E slides of colorectal carcinomas and showed that TSR was an independent prognostic factor.

9.2.7 Molecular Data Interpretation

This topic is discussed in the *subsequent chapter*.

9.2.8 Precision (Personalized) Medicine

This topic is discussed in the subsequent chapter.

9.3 Conclusions

Computational pathology along with artificial intelligence has immense potential in diagnosis, screening of cancer, prediction of prognosis, personalized medicine and molecular data interpretation. The artificial intelligence can be routinely integrated in a laboratory to quantitate the biomarkers and predict mutational changes from the H & E slides. Multimodal data fusion including clinical text data, WSI data, radiological imaging, and molecular data provides a holistic approach of disease. This may help in precise diagnosis and also understanding the mechanism of the disease. The pathologists should be aware of the potential of computational pathology. There is a need for collaboration between pathologists, bioinformatics and computer software engineers to apply it successfully in the laboratory.

References

1. Dey P. The emerging role of deep learning in cytology. Cytopathology. 2021;32(2):154–60. https://doi.org/10.1111/cyt.12942. Epub 2020 Dec 17.
2. Saini T, Bansal B, Dey P. Digital cytology: current status and future prospects. Diagn Cytopathol. 2023;51(3):211–8. https://doi.org/10.1002/dc.25099. Epub 2023 Jan 3.
3. Öztürk Ş, Akdemir B. Application of feature extraction and classification methods for histopathological image using GLCM, LBP, LBGLCM. GLRLM and SFTA. Proc Comput Sci. 2018;132:40–6.
4. Yamamoto Y, Saito A, Numata Y, et al. A novel method for morphological pleomorphism and heterogeneity quantitative measurement: named cell feature level co-occurrence matrix. J Pathol Inform. 2016;7(1):36.

5. Satyadhas J, Preetha V. Texture based Feature Extraction of Smear Images for Cervical Cancer. Int Res J Eng Technol (IRJET). 2020;07(06):5194–8.
6. Macenko M, et al. A method for normalizing histology slides for quantitative analysis. 2009 IEEE international symposium on biomedical imaging: from nano to macro, Boston, MA, USA. 2009. pp. 1107–10.
7. Liang Y, Pan C, Sun W, Liu Q, Du Y. Global context-aware cervical cell detection with soft scale anchor matching. Comput Methods Prog Biomed. 2021;204:106061.
8. Zhang Z, Fu X, Liu J, Huang Z, Liu N, Fang F, Rao J. Developing a machine learning algorithm for identifying abnormal urothelial cells: a feasibility study. Acta Cytol. 2021;65(4):335–41.
9. Xie X, Fu CC, Lv L, Ye Q, Yu Y, Fang Q, Zhang L, Hou L, Wu C. Deep convolutional neural network-based classification of cancer cells on cytological pleural effusion images. Mod Pathol. 2022;35(5):609–14.
10. Li X, Du M, Zuo S, Zhou M, Peng Q, Chen Z, Zhou J, He Q. Deep convolutional neural networks using an active learning strategy for cervical cancer screening and diagnosis. Front Bioinform. 2023;3:1101667. https://doi.org/10.3389/fbinf.2023.1101667. PMID: 36969799; PMCID: PMC10034408.
11. Kanavati F, Hirose N, Ishii T, Fukuda A, Ichihara S, Tsuneki M. A deep learning model for cervical cancer screening on liquid-based cytology specimens in whole slide images. Cancers (Basel). 2022;14(5):1159. https://doi.org/10.3390/cancers14051159. PMID: 35267466; PMCID: PMC8909106.
12. Tan X, Li K, Zhang J, Wang W, Wu B, Wu J, Li X, Huang X. Automatic model for cervical cancer screening based on convolutional neural network: a retrospective, multicohort, multicenter study. Cancer Cell Int. 2021;21(1):35. https://doi.org/10.1186/s12935-020-01742-6. PMID: 33413391; PMCID: PMC7791865.
13. Cheng S, Liu S, Yu J, Rao G, Xiao Y, Han W, Zhu W, Lv X, Li N, Cai J, Wang Z, Feng X, Yang F, Geng X, Ma J, Li X, Wei Z, Zhang X, Quan T, Zeng S, Chen L, Hu J, Liu X. Robust whole slide image analysis for cervical cancer screening using deep learning. Nat Commun. 2021;12(1):5639.
14. Rahaman MM, Li C, Yao Y, Kulwa F, Wu X, Li X, Wang Q. DeepCervix: a deep learning-based framework for the classification of cervical cells using hybrid deep feature fusion techniques. Comput Biol Med. 2021;136:104649.
15. Wang CW, Liou YA, Lin YJ, Chang CC, Chu PH, Lee YC, Wang CH, Chao TK. Artificial intelligence-assisted fast screening cervical high grade squamous intraepithelial lesion and squamous cell carcinoma diagnosis and treatment planning. Sci Rep. 2021;11(1):16244.
16. Holmström O, Linder N, Kaingu H, Mbuuko N, Mbete J, Kinyua F, Törnquist S, Muinde M, Krogerus L, Lundin M, Diwan V, Lundin J. Point-of-care digital cytology with artificial intelligence for cervical cancer screening in a resource-limited setting. JAMA Netw Open. 2021;4(3):e211740.
17. Hussain E, Mahanta LB, Das CR, Talukdar RK. A comprehensive study on the multi-class cervical cancer diagnostic prediction on pap smear images using a fusion-based decision from ensemble deep convolutional neural network. Tissue Cell. 2020;65:101347. https://doi.org/10.1016/j.tice.2020.101347.
18. Shi J, Wang R, Zheng Y, Jiang Z, Zhang H, Yu L. Cervical cell classification with graph convolutional network. Comput Methods Prog Biomed. 2021;198:105807. https://doi.org/10.1016/j.cmpb.2020.105807. Epub 2020 Oct 22.
19. Bao H, Bi H, Zhang X, Zhao Y, Dong Y, Luo X, Zhou D, You Z, Wu Y, Liu Z, Zhang Y, Liu J, Fang L, Wang L. Artificial intelligence-assisted cytology for detection of cervical intraepithelial neoplasia or invasive cancer: a multicenter, clinical-based, observational study. Gynecol Oncol. 2020;159(1):171–8.
20. Zhang L, Lu L, Nogues I, Summers RM, Liu S, Yao J. DeepPap: deep convolutional networks for cervical cell classification. IEEE J Biomed Health Inform. 2017;21(6):1633–43. https://doi.org/10.1109/JBHI.2017.2705583. Epub 2017 May 19.

21. Lebret T, Paoletti X, Pignot G, et al. Artificial intelligence to improve cytology performance in urothelial carcinoma diagnosis: results from validation phase of the French, multicenter, prospective VISIOCYT1 trial. World J Urol. 2023;41(9):2381–8.
22. Sanghvi AB, Allen EZ, Callenberg KM, Pantanowitz L. Performance of an artificial intelligence algorithm for reporting urine cytopathology. Cancer Cytopathol. 2019;127(10):658–66. https://doi.org/10.1002/cncy.22176. Epub 2019 Aug 14.
23. Vaickus LJ, Suriawinata AA, Wei JW, Liu X. Automating the Paris system for urine cytopathology-a hybrid deep-learning and morphometric approach. Cancer Cytopathol. 2019;127(2):98–115. https://doi.org/10.1002/cncy.22099. Epub 2019 Jan 31.
24. Muralidaran C, Dey P, Nijhawan R, Kakkar N. Artificial neural network in diagnosis of urothelial cell carcinoma in urine cytology. Diagn Cytopathol. 2015;43(6):443–9. https://doi.org/10.1002/dc.23244. Epub 2015 Jan 21.
25. Yousif M, van Diest PJ, Laurinavicius A, Rimm D, van der Laak J, Madabhushi A, Schnitt S, Pantanowitz L. Artificial intelligence applied to breast pathology. Virchows Arch. 2022;480(1):191–209.
26. Katayama A, Aoki Y, Watanabe Y, Horiguchi J, Rakha EA, Oyama T. Current status and prospects of artificial intelligence in breast cancer pathology: convolutional neural networks to prospective vision transformers. Int J Clin Oncol. 2024;29(11):1648–68. https://doi.org/10.1007/s10147-024-02513-3. Epub 2024 Apr 15.
27. Dey P, Logasundaram R, Joshi K. Artificial neural network in diagnosis of lobular carcinoma of breast in fine-needle aspiration cytology. Diagn Cytopathol. 2013;41(2):102–6. https://doi.org/10.1002/dc.21773. Epub 2011 Oct 11.
28. Subbaiah RM, Dey P, Nijhawan R. Artificial neural network in breast lesions from fine-needle aspiration cytology smear. Diagn Cytopathol. 2014;42(3):218–24. https://doi.org/10.1002/dc.23026. Epub 2013 Aug 1.
29. El Agouri H, Azizi M, El Attar H, El Khannoussi M, Ibrahimi A, Kabbaj R, et al. Assessment of deep learning algorithms to predict histopathological diagnosis of breast cancer: first Moroccan prospective study on a private dataset. BMC Res Notes. 2022;15(1):66.
30. Cruz-Roa A, Gilmore H, Basavanhally A, Feldman M, Ganesan S, Shih N, et al. High-throughput adaptive sampling for whole-slide histopathology image analysis (HASHI) via convolutional neural networks: application to invasive breast cancer detection. PLoS One. 2018;13(5):e0196828.
31. Yamamoto Y, Saito A, Tateishi A, Shimojo H, Kanno H, Tsuchiya S, et al. Quantitative diagnosis of breast tumors by morphometric classification of microenvironmental myoepithelial cells using a machine learning approach. Sci Rep. 2017;7:46732.
32. Spanhol FA, Oliveira LS, Petitjean C, Heutte L. A dataset for breast cancer histopathological image classification. IEEE Trans Biomed Eng. 2016;63(7):1455–62.
33. Davri A, Birbas E, Kanavos T, Ntritsos G, Giannakeas N, Tzallas AT, Batistatou A. Deep learning for lung cancer diagnosis, prognosis and prediction using histological and cytological images: a systematic review. Cancers (Basel). 2023;15(15):3981.
34. Kanavati F, Toyokawa G, Momosaki S, Rambeau M, Kozuma Y, Shoji F, Yamazaki K, Takeo S, Iizuka O, Tsuneki M. Weakly-supervised learning for lung carcinoma classification using deep learning. Sci Rep. 2020;10(1):9297.
35. Civit-Masot J, Bañuls-Beaterio A, Domínguez-Morales M, Rivas-Pérez M, Muñoz-Saavedra L, Rodríguez Corral JM. Non-small cell lung cancer diagnosis aid with histopathological images using explainable deep learning techniques. Comput Methods Prog Biomed. 2022;226:107108. https://doi.org/10.1016/j.cmpb.2022.107108.
36. Jain DK, Lakshmi KM, Varma KP, Ramachandran M, Bharati S. Lung cancer detection based on kernel PCA-convolution neural network feature extraction and classification by fast deep belief neural network in disease management using multimedia data sources. Comput Intell Neurosci. 2022;2022:3149406. https://doi.org/10.1155/2022/3149406.
37. Jiao Y, Yuan J, Qiang Y, Fei S. Deep embeddings and logistic regression for rapid active learning in histopathological images. Comput Methods Prog Biomed. 2021;212:106464. https://doi.org/10.1016/j.cmpb.2021.106464. Epub 2021 Oct 13.

38. Yang JW, Song DH, An HJ, Seo SB. Classification of subtypes including LCNEC in lung cancer biopsy slides using convolutional neural network from scratch. Sci Rep. 2022;12:1830.
39. Kosaraju S, Park J, Lee H, Yang JW, Kang M. Deep learning-based framework for slide-based histopathological image analysis. Sci Rep. 2022;12:19075.
40. Chen CL, Chen CC, Yu WH, Chen SH, Chang YC, Hsu TI, Hsiao M, Yeh CY, Chen CY. An annotation-free whole-slide training approach to pathological classification of lung cancer types using deep learning. Nat Commun. 2021;12(1):1193.
41. Kim T, Chang H, Kim B, Yang J, Koo D, Lee J, Chang JW, Hwang G, Gong G, Cho NH, Yoo CW, Pyo JY, Chong Y. Deep learning-based diagnosis of lung cancer using a nationwide respiratory cytology image set: improving accuracy and inter-observer variability. Am J Cancer Res. 2023;13(11):5493–503. PMID: 38058836; PMCID: PMC10695775.
42. Tsukamoto T, Teramoto A, Yamada A, Kiriyama Y, Sakurai E, Michiba A, Imaizumi K, Fujita H. Comparison of fine-tuned deep convolutional neural networks for the automated classification of lung cancer cytology images with integration of additional classifiers. Asian Pac J Cancer Prev. 2022;23(4):1315–24.
43. Teramoto A, Yamada A, Kiriyama Y, et al. Automated classification of benign and malignant cells from lung cytological images using deep convolutional neural network. Inf Med Unlocked. 2019;16:100205.
44. Huang W, Randhawa R, Jain P, Iczkowski KA, Hu R, Hubbard S, Eickhoff J, Basu H, Roy R. Development and validation of an artificial intelligence-powered platform for prostate cancer grading and quantification. JAMA Netw Open. 2021;4(11):e2132554. https://doi.org/10.1001/jamanetworkopen.2021.32554. PMID: 34730818; PMCID: PMC8567112.
45. Pantanowitz L, Quiroga-Garza GM, Bien L, Heled R, Laifenfeld D, Linhart C, Sandbank J, Albrecht Shach A, Shalev V, Vecsler M, Michelow P, Hazelhurst S, Dhir R. An artificial intelligence algorithm for prostate cancer diagnosis in whole slide images of core needle biopsies: a blinded clinical validation and deployment study. Lancet Digit Health. 2020;2(8):e407–16. https://doi.org/10.1016/S2589-7500(20)30159-X.
46. Ström P, Kartasalo K, Olsson H, et al. Artificial intelligence for diagnosis and grading of prostate cancer in biopsies: a population-based, diagnostic study. Lancet Oncol. 2020;21(2):222–32. https://doi.org/10.1016/S1470-2045(19)30738-7. Epub 2020 Jan 8. Erratum in: Lancet Oncol. 2020 Feb;21(2):e70.
47. Uddin AH, Chen YL, Akter MR, Ku CS, Yang J, Por LY. Colon and lung cancer classification from multi-modal images using resilient and efficient neural network architectures. Heliyon. 2024;10(9):e30625. https://doi.org/10.1016/j.heliyon.2024.e30625. PMID: 38742084; PMCID: PMC11089372.
48. Dabass M, Vashisth S, Vig R. A convolution neural network with multi-level convolutional and attention learning for classification of cancer grades and tissue structures in colon histopathological images. Comput Biol Med. 2022;147:105680. https://doi.org/10.1016/j.compbiomed.2022.105680. Epub 2022 Jun 2.
49. Iizuka O, Kanavati F, Kato K, Rambeau M, Arihiro K, Tsuneki M. Deep learning models for histopathological classification of gastric and colonic epithelial tumours. Sci Rep. 2020;10(1):1504. https://doi.org/10.1038/s41598-020-58467-9. PMID: 32001752; PMCID: PMC6992793.
50. Hamdi M, Senan EM, Awaji B, Olayah F, Jadhav ME, Alalayah KM. Analysis of WSI images by hybrid systems with fusion features for early diagnosis of cervical cancer. Diagnostics (Basel). 2023;13(15):2538. https://doi.org/10.3390/diagnostics13152538. PMID: 37568901; PMCID: PMC10416962.
51. Nojima S, Terayama K, Shimoura S, Hijiki S, Nonomura N, Morii E, Okuno Y, Fujita K. A deep learning system to diagnose the malignant potential of urothelial carcinoma cells in cytology specimens. Cancer Cytopathol. 2021;129:984–95. https://doi.org/10.1002/cncy.22443.
52. Awan R, Benes K, Azam A, Song TH, Shaban M, Verrill C, Tsang YW, Snead D, Minhas F, Rajpoot N. Deep learning based digital cell profiles for risk stratification of urine cytology images. Cytometry A. 2021;99(7):732–42. https://doi.org/10.1002/cyto.a.24313. Epub 2021 Feb 20.

53. Lilli L, Giarnieri E, Scardapane S. A calibrated multiexit neural network for detecting urothelial cancer cells. Comput Math Methods Med. 2021;2021:5569458. https://doi.org/10.1155/2021/5569458. PMID: 34234839; PMCID: PMC8216797.
54. Guan Q, Wang Y, Ping B, Li D, Du J, Qin Y, Lu H, Wan X, Xiang J. Deep convolutional neural network VGG-16 model for differential diagnosing of papillary thyroid carcinomas in cytological images: a pilot study. J Cancer. 2019;10(20):4876–82. https://doi.org/10.7150/jca.28769. PMID: 31598159; PMCID: PMC6775529.
55. Sanyal P, Mukherjee T, Barui S, Das A, Gangopadhyay P. Artificial intelligence in cytopathology: a neural network to identify papillary carcinoma on thyroid fine-needle aspiration cytology smears. J Pathol Inform. 2018;9:43. https://doi.org/10.4103/jpi.jpi_43_18. PMID: 30607310; PMCID: PMC6289006.
56. Gopinath B, Shanthi N. Development of an automated medical diagnosis system for classifying thyroid tumor cells using multiple classifier fusion. Technol Cancer Res Treat. 2015;14(5):653–62. https://doi.org/10.7785/tcrt.2012.500430. Epub 2014 Nov 26.
57. Cochand-Priollet B, Koutroumbas K, Megalopoulou TM, Pouliakis A, Sivolapenko G, Karakitsos P. Discriminating benign from malignant thyroid lesions using artificial intelligence and statistical selection of morphometric features. Oncol Rep. 2006;15 Spec no.:1023–6. https://doi.org/10.3892/or.15.4.1023.
58. Shapiro NA, Poloz TL, Shkurupij VA, Tarkov MS, Poloz VV, Demin AV. Application of artificial neural network for classification of thyroid follicular tumors. Anal Quant Cytol Histol. 2007;29(2):87–94.
59. Savala R, Dey P, Gupta N. Artificial neural network model to distinguish follicular adenoma from follicular carcinoma on fine needle aspiration of thyroid. Diagn Cytopathol. 2018;46(3):244–9. https://doi.org/10.1002/dc.23880. Epub 2017 Dec 20.
60. Maleki S, Zandvakili A, Gera S, Khutti SD, Gersten A, Khader SN. Differentiating noninvasive follicular thyroid neoplasm with papillary-like nuclear features from classic papillary thyroid carcinoma: analysis of cytomorphologic descriptions using a novel machine-learning approach. J Pathol Inform. 2019;10:29. https://doi.org/10.4103/jpi.jpi_25_19. PMID: 31579155; PMCID: PMC6767786.
61. Saini T, Saikia UN, Dey P. An artificial neural network for the prediction of the risk of malignancy in category III Bethesda thyroid lesions. Cytopathology. 2023;34(1):48–54. https://doi.org/10.1111/cyt.13180. Epub 2022 Oct 6.
62. Park HS, Chong Y, Lee Y, Yim K, Seo KJ, Hwang G, Kim D, Gong G, Cho NH, Yoo CW, Choi HJ. Deep learning-based computational cytopathologic diagnosis of metastatic breast carcinoma in pleural fluid. Cells. 2023;12(14):1847. https://doi.org/10.3390/cells12141847. PMID: 37508511; PMCID: PMC10377793.
63. Sanyal P, Dey P. Using a deep learning neural network for the identification of malignant cells in effusion cytology material. Cytopathology. 2023;34(5):466–71. https://doi.org/10.1111/cyt.13260. Epub 2023 Jun 23.
64. Barwad A, Dey P, Susheilia S. Artificial neural network in diagnosis of metastatic carcinoma in effusion cytology. Cytometry B Clin Cytom. 2012;82(2):107–11. https://doi.org/10.1002/cyto.b.20632. Epub 2011 Nov 10.
65. Truong H, Morimoto R, Walts AE, Erler B, Marchevsky A. Neural networks as an aid in the diagnosis of lymphocyte-rich effusions. Anal Quant Cytol Histol. 1995;17(1):48–54.
66. Abele N, Tiemann K, Krech T, Wellmann A, Schaaf C, Länger F, et al. Noninferiority of artificial intelligence-assisted analysis of Ki-67 and estrogen/progesterone receptor in breast cancer routine diagnostics. Mod Pathol. 2023;36:100033.
67. Brügmann A, Eld M, Lelkaitis G, Nielsen S, Grunkin M, Hansen JD, et al. Digital image analysis of membrane connectivity is a robust measure of HER2 immunostains. Breast Cancer Res Treat. 2012;132:41–9. https://doi.org/10.1007/s10549-011-1514-2.
68. Xue T, Chang H, Ren M, Wang H, Yang Y, Wang B, et al. Deep learning to automatically evaluate HER2 gene amplification status from fluorescence in situ hybridization images. Sci Rep. 2023;13:9746.

69. Furrer D, Jacob S, Caron C, Sanschagrin F, Provencher L, Diorio C. Validation of a new classifier for the automated analysis of the human epidermal growth factor receptor 2 (HER2) gene amplification in breast cancer specimens. Diagn Pathol. 2013;8:17. https://doi.org/10.1186/1746-1596-8-17. PMID: 23379971; PMCID: PMC3584735.
70. Rexhepaj E, Brennan DJ, Holloway P, Kay EW, McCann AH, Landberg G, et al. Novel image analysis approach for quantifying expression of nuclear proteins assessed by immunohistochemistry: application to measurement of oestrogen and progesterone receptor levels in breast cancer. Breast Cancer Res. 2008;10:R89.
71. Diaz LK, Sahin A, Sneige N. Interobserver agreement for estrogen receptor immunohistochemical analysis in breast cancer: a comparison of manual and computer-assisted scoring methods. Ann Diagn Pathol. 2004;8:23–7. https://doi.org/10.1016/j.anndiagpath.2003.11.004.
72. Dey P. In: Dey P, editor. Chapter 5: Pancancer biomarker in recent advances in pathology. New Delhi: Jaypee Brothers Medical Publishers Pvt Ltd; 2024.
73. Hopkins E, Moffat D, Parkinson I, et al. Cell block samples from Endobronchial ultrasound Transbronchial needle aspiration provide sufficient material for ancillary testing in lung cancer—a quaternary referral Centre experience. J Thorac Dis. 2016;8:2544–50. https://doi.org/10.21037/jtd.2016.08.74.
74. Hondelink LM, Hüyük M, Postmus PE, Smit VTHBM, Blom S, von der Thüsen JH, Cohen D. Development and validation of a supervised deep learning algorithm for automated whole-slide programmed death-ligand 1 tumour proportion score assessment in non-small cell lung cancer. Histopathology. 2022;80:635–47. https://doi.org/10.1111/his.14571.
75. Cheng G, Zhang F, Xing Y, Hu X, Zhang H, Chen S, Li M, Peng C, Ding G, Zhang D, et al. Artificial intelligence-assisted score analysis for predicting the expression of the immunotherapy biomarker PD-L1 in lung cancer. Front Immunol. 2022;13:893198. https://doi.org/10.3389/fimmu.2022.893198.
76. Choi S, Cho SI, Ma M, Park S, Pereira S, Aum BJ, Shin S, Paeng K, Yoo D, Jung W, Ock CY, Lee SH, Choi YL, Chung JH, Mok TS, Kim H, Kim S. Artificial intelligence-powered programmed death ligand 1 analyser reduces interobserver variation in tumour proportion score for non-small cell lung cancer with better prediction of immunotherapy response. Eur J Cancer. 2022;170:17–26. https://doi.org/10.1016/j.ejca.2022.04.011. Epub 2022 May 14.
77. Huang Z, Chen L, Lv L, Fu CC, Jin Y, Zheng Q, Wang B, Ye Q, Fang Q, Li Y. A new AI-assisted scoring system for PD-L1 expression in NSCLC. Comput Methods Prog Biomed. 2022;221:106829.
78. Kapil A, Meier A, Zuraw A, Steele KE, Rebelatto MC, Schmidt G, Brieu N. Deep semi supervised generative learning for automated tumor proportion scoring on NSCLC tissue needle biopsies. Sci Rep. 2018;8:17343. https://doi.org/10.1038/s41598-018-35501-5.
79. Acs B, Pelekanou V, Bai Y, Martinez-Morilla S, Toki M, Leung SC, et al. Ki67 reproducibility using digital image analysis: an inter-platform and inter-operator study. Lab Investig. 2019;99:107–17.
80. Saha M, Chakraborty C, Arun I, Ahmed R, Chatterjee S. An advanced deep learning approach for Ki-67 stained hotspot detection and proliferation rate scoring for prognostic evaluation of breast cancer. Sci Rep. 2017;7(1):3213.
81. Pao JJ, Biggs M, Duncan D, Lin DI, Davis R, Huang RSP, Ferguson D, Janovitz T, Hiemenz MC, Eddy NR, et al. Predicting EGFR mutational status from pathology images using a real-world dataset. Sci Rep. 2023;13:4404. https://doi.org/10.1038/s41598-023-31284-6.
82. Mayer C, Ofek E, Fridrich DE, Molchanov Y, Yacobi R, Gazy I, Hayun I, Zalach J, Paz-Yaacov N, Barshack I. Direct identification of ALK and ROS1 fusions in non-small cell lung cancer from hematoxylin and eosin-stained slides using deep learning algorithms. Mod Pathol. 2022;35:1882–7. https://doi.org/10.1038/s41379-022-01141-4.
83. Tomita N, Tafe LJ, Suriawinata AA, Tsongalis GJ, Nasir-Moin M, Dragnev K, Hassanpour S. Predicting oncogene mutations of lung cancer using deep learning and histopathologic features on whole-slide images. Transl Oncol. 2022;24:101494.

84. Huang K, Mo Z, Zhu W, Liao B, Yang Y, Wu F-X. Prediction of target-drug therapy by identifying gene mutations in lung cancer with histopathological stained image and deep learning techniques. Front Oncol. 2021;11:642945. https://doi.org/10.3389/fonc.2021.642945.
85. Wang Y, Coudray N, Zhao Y, Li F, Hu C, Zhang YZ, Imoto S, Tsirigos A, Webb GI, Daly RJ, Song J. HEAL: an automated deep learning framework for cancer histopathology image analysis. Bioinformatics. 2021;37(22):4291–5. https://doi.org/10.1093/bioinformatics/btab380.
86. Coudray N, Ocampo PS, Sakellaropoulos T, Narula N, Snuderl M, Fenyö D, Moreira AL, Razavian N, Tsirigos A. Classification and mutation prediction from non-small cell lung cancer histopathology images using deep learning. Nat Med. 2018;24(10):1559–67. https://doi.org/10.1038/s41591-018-0177-5. Epub 2018 Sep 17. PMID: 30224757; PMCID: PMC9847512.
87. Conde-Sousa E, Vale J, Feng M, Xu K, Wang Y, Della Mea V, et al. HEROHE challenge: predicting HER2 status in breast cancer from hematoxylin-eosin whole-slide imaging. J Imaging. 2022;8:213.
88. Farahmand S, Fernandez AI, Ahmed FS, Rimm DL, Chuang JH, Reisenbichler E, et al. Deep learning trained on hematoxylin and eosin tumor region of interest predicts HER2 status and trastuzumab treatment response in HER2+ breast cancer. Mod Pathol. 2022;35:44–51.
89. Naik N, Madani A, Esteva A, Keskar NS, Press MF, Ruderman D, et al. Deep learning-enabled breast cancer hormonal receptor status determination from base-level H&E stains. Nat Commun. 2020;11:5727. https://doi.org/10.1038/s41467-020-19334-3.
90. Anand D, Kurian NC, Dhage S, Kumar N, Rane S, Gann PH, et al. Deep learning to estimate human epidermal growth factor receptor 2 status from hematoxylin and eosin-stained breast tissue images. J Pathol Inform. 2020;11:19.
91. Sha L, Osinski BL, Ho IY, Tan TL, Willis C, Weiss H, Beaubier N, Mahon BM, Taxter TJ, Yip SSF. Multi-field-of-view deep learning model predicts nonsmall cell lung cancer programmed death-ligand 1 status from whole-slide hematoxylin and eosin images. J Pathol Inform. 2019;10:24. https://doi.org/10.4103/jpi.jpi_24_19. PMID: 31523482; PMCID: PMC6669997.
92. Barnes TA, Amir E. HYPE or HOPE: the prognostic value of infiltrating immune cells in cancer. Br J Cancer. 2017;117(4):451–60.
93. Acs B, Ahmed FS, Gupta S, et al. An open source automated tumor infiltrating lymphocyte algorithm for prognosis in melanoma. Nat Commun. 2019;10(1):5440.
94. Salgado R, Denkert C, Demaria S, et al. The evaluation of tumor infiltrating lymphocytes (TILs) in breast cancer: recommendations by an International TILs Working Group 2014. Ann Oncol. 2015;26:259–71.
95. Bai Y, Cole K, Martinez-Morilla S, et al. An open-source, automated tumor-infiltrating lymphocyte algorithm for prognosis in triple-negative breast cancer. Clin Cancer Res. 2021;27(20):5557–65. https://doi.org/10.1158/1078-0432.CCR-21-0325.
96. Thagaard J, Stovgaard ES, Vognsen LG, Hauberg S, Dahl A, Ebstrup T, Doré J, Vincentz RE, Jepsen RK, Roslind A, Kümler I, Nielsen D, Balslev E. Automated quantification of sTIL density with H&E-based digital image analysis has prognostic potential in triple-negative breast cancers. Cancers (Basel). 2021;13(12):3050. https://doi.org/10.3390/cancers13123050. PMID: 34207414; PMCID: PMC8235502.
97. Barmpoutis P, Di Capite M, Kayhanian H, Waddingham W, Alexander DC, Jansen M, Kwong FNK. Tertiary lymphoid structures (TLS) identification and density assessment on H&E-stained digital slides of lung cancer. PLoS One. 2021;16(9):e0256907. https://doi.org/10.1371/journal.pone.0256907. PMID: 34555057; PMCID: PMC8460026.
98. Wang M, Zhao J, Zhang L, Wei F, Lian Y, Wu Y, Gong Z, Zhang S, Zhou J, Cao K, Li X, Xiong W, Li G, Zeng Z, Guo C. Role of tumor microenvironment in tumorigenesis. J Cancer. 2017;8(5):761–73. https://doi.org/10.7150/jca.17648. PMID: 28382138; PMCID: PMC5381164.
99. Wu J, Liang C, Chen M, Su W. Association between tumor-stroma ratio and prognosis in solid tumor patients: a systematic review and meta-analysis. Oncotarget. 2016;7(42):68954–65. https://doi.org/10.18632/oncotarget.12135. PMID: 27661111; PMCID: PMC5356603.

100. Pongsuvareeyakul T, Khunamornpong S, Settakorn J, Sukpan K, Suprasert P, Intaraphet S, Siriaunkgul S. Prognostic evaluation of tumor-stroma ratio in patients with early stage cervical adenocarcinoma treated by surgery. Asian Pac J Cancer Prev. 2015;16:4363–8. https://doi.org/10.7314/apjcp.2015.16.10.4363.
101. Zhang TH, Xu J, Shen HC, Dong W, Ni Y, Du JJ. Tumor-stroma ratio is an independent predictor for survival in NSCLC. Int J Clin Exp Pathol. 2015;8:11348–55.
102. Dekker TJ, van de Velde CJ, van Pelt GW, Kroep JR, Julien JP, Smit VT, Tollenaar RA, Mesker WE. Prognostic significance of the tumor-stroma ratio: validation study in node-negative premenopausal breast cancer patients from the EORTC perioperative chemotherapy (POP) trial (10854). Breat Cancer Res Treat. 2013;139:371–9. https://doi.org/10.1007/s10549-013-2571-5.
103. Micke P, Strell C, Mattsson J, Martín-Bernabé A, et al. The prognostic impact of the tumour stroma fraction: a machine learning-based analysis in 16 human solid tumour types. EBioMedicine. 2021;65:103269. https://doi.org/10.1016/j.ebiom.2021.103269. Epub 2021 Mar 9. PMID: 33706249; PMCID: PMC7960932.
104. Zhao K, Li Z, Yao S, Wang Y, Wu X, Xu Z, Wu L, Huang Y, Liang C, Liu Z. Artificial intelligence quantified tumour-stroma ratio is an independent predictor for overall survival in resectable colorectal cancer. EBioMedicine. 2020;61:103054. https://doi.org/10.1016/j.ebiom.2020.103054. Epub 2020 Oct 8. PMID: 33039706; PMCID: PMC7648125.

Molecular Data Interpretation by Artificial Intelligence

10

Abstract

Recently, there is an explosion of molecular data from genomic, proteomics, metabolomics and structural data. The genomic data are often massive and have complex relationships with clinical responses. Manual handling of genomic and epigenetic data is almost impossible. Artificial intelligence (AI) and deep learning play an important role in interpreting the huge and complex data. AI guides the researchers and clinicians to predict regulatory elements, variant effect, gene expression, splicing, assessing chromatin accessibility, epigenomics, and also to predict the presence, type, and risk of disease from DNA sequencing data. In the present chapter, the details of molecular data interpretation and the key technologies are discussed.

Keywords

Molecular data · Proteomics · Metabolomics · Regulatory elements prediction · Variant effect prediction · Gene expression prediction · Splicing prediction · Assessing chromatin accessibility · Epigenomics

10.1 Introduction

In recent years, there is a massive development of information on molecular data from genomic, proteomics, metabolomics and structural data. The introduction of next-generation sequencing, CLIP-seq, SELEX and RNA compete has given a widely available data source [1–3]. The genomic data are often massive and have complex relationships with clinical responses. Manual handling of genomic and epigenetic data is almost impossible. AI and deep learning play an important role in interpreting the huge and complex data [4]. AI guides the researchers and clinicians to predict molecular behaviours, and to discover new therapeutic approaches [5].

P. Dey, *Computational Cytology*, https://doi.org/10.1007/978-981-95-3272-8_10

AI may take a new role in personalized medicine for individual therapy. In the present chapter, the details of molecular data interpretation and the key technologies will be discussed.

10.2 Types of Molecular Data

The different categories of molecular data include (Fig. 10.1):

- *Genomic Data*: The genomic data includes, whole genome sequences, single nucleotide polymorphisms (SNPs), Structural variations (insertions, deletions) and epigenetic markers.
- *Proteomic Data*: It includes the information on protein sequences, structures, and post-translational modifications of proteins.
- *Transcriptomic Data*: It means data on RNA molecules such as mRNA expression, alternative splicing events and RNA-seq data.
- *Metabolomics Data*: It means the profiles of small molecules (metabolites) in cells, tissues or organisms such as metabolic fluxes, lipid and glucose levels.
- *Epigenetic Data*: It provides information on the chemical modifications to DNA or chromatin such as DNA methylation, Histone modifications.
- *Structural Data*: Three-dimensional conformations of DNA from crystallography, NMR or cryo-EM.
- *Molecular Interaction Data*: It indicates the binding affinities, reaction kinetics and drug–target interactions.
- *Microbiome Data*: It provides information on the living microorganisms in the gut such as 16S rRNA sequencing data, metagenomics data.

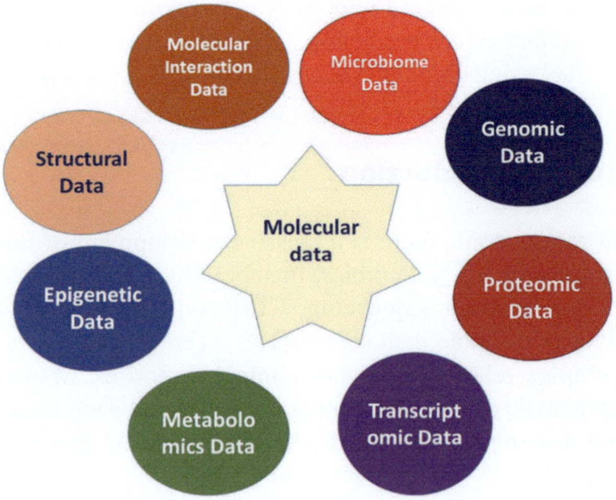

Fig. 10.1 Different categories of molecular data

10.3 AI Methods for Molecular Data Analysis

10.3.1 Feedforward Neural Networks (FNNs)

FNN is the simplest type of neural network (Box 10.1). Here, the data flows from the input layer to the hidden layer and finally to the output layer. In FNN, no loop or feedback connection is used.

Application of FNN

- *Prediction of the molecular properties*: FNN may predict the toxicity, affinity of the molecules.
- *Classification of molecules*: The activity of the molecule against a target can be predicted.
- *Feature-based tasks* are also predicted.

Advantages

- FNN is the simplest neural network and is easy to train.
- It is effective.
- FNN is flexible and can be used for both regression and classification tasks.

Disadvantages

- For proper functioning, FNN needs good molecular representations in the input layer.

Box 10.1: Feedforward Neural Networks (FNNs)

In FNN, the data flows from the input layer to the hidden layer and finally output layer. Here, no loop or feedback connection is used.

Advantages

- Simplest neural network.
- Easy to train.
- Effective.
- Flexible and can be used for both regression and classification tasks.

Disadvantages

- It needs good molecular representations in the input layer.

Application of FNN

- Prediction of the molecular properties.
- Classification of molecules**:** The activity of the molecule against a target can be predicted.
- Feature-based tasks are predicted.

10.4 Convolutional Neural Networks (CNNs)

CNN is originally used for images. In molecular data, CNN processes the molecular images as:

- *Two-dimensional images*: The chemical structure is converted into a 2D image that means molecular structures are drawn as an image.
- *One-dimensional sequences*: The molecule is represented as a 1D sequence by Simplified Molecular Input Line Entry System (SMILES). In SMILES, each atom, connecting bonds, etc., are depicted by simple ASCII characters.
- *Graph Convolutional Networks (GCNs)*: In GCNs, graph-structured data is used (Fig. 10.2) (Box 10.2).

In molecular data, the graph is made of

Node: Node is made of an atom.
Edge: The bond between atoms.

How GCNs Work (Step-by-Step)

1. *Input*:
   - Each molecule is represented by a graph.
   - The node represents an atom with several features such as atomic number, aromaticity.
2. *Message Passing*:
   - The node acquires information from the neighbouring nodes or atoms.
   - It updates the internal feature vector.

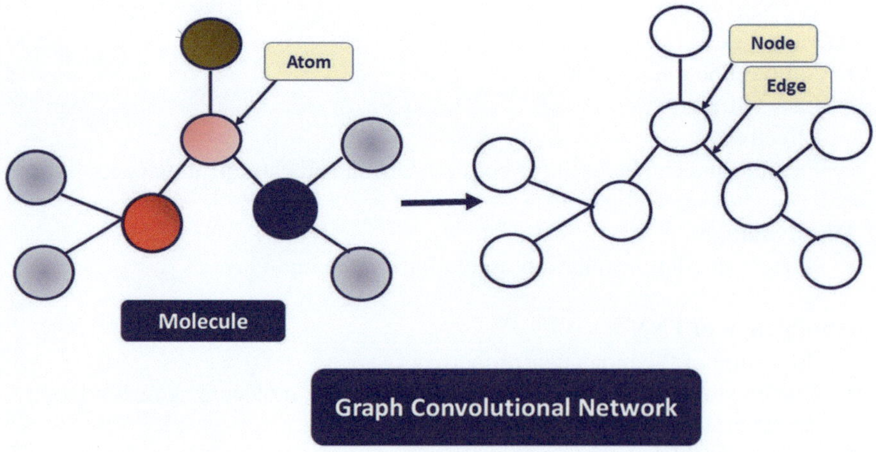

Fig. 10.2 Graph convolutional network. In a molecule, each atom is a node and the connectivity of the atom is the edge

3. *Aggregation*:
   • The overall information is summed and node features get enriched.
4. *Output*:
   • Finally, after passing through multiple layers, the node features are aggregated to give a final prediction.

Advantages of GCN

- Descriptors: No manual description is required.
- *Scalability*: Molecules of variable size and shape can be processed.
- *Structural awareness*: The 3D/2D structures are important.

Box 10.2: Graph Convolutional Networks (GCNs)

In GCNs, graph-structured data is used.

In molecular data of GCN:

Node: Node is made of an atom.
Edge: The bond between atoms.

Step-by-Step GCNs Work:

- *Input*: Each molecule is represented by a graph and the node represents an atom.
- *Message Passing*: The node acquires information from the neighbouring nodes or atoms and updates the internal feature vector.
- *Aggregation*: The overall information is summed and node features get enriched.
- *Output*: Finally, the node features are aggregated to give a final prediction.

Advantages of GCN

- No manual description.
- Molecules of variable size and shape can be processed.
- The 3D/2D structures are important.

10.4.1 How CNN Works

In CNN, the DNA sequences are encoded in 1D image. CNN scan the image to find the local patterns.

In CNN, the convolutional operation is done by the sliding filters. This convolutional operation captures the spatial information of the data [6]. The next steps are the activation by ReLU, followed by pooling. The pooling layer reduces the dimension of the data. Ultimately, a fully connected layer is generated and an ANN is used for the prediction or classification (Fig. 10.3).

DNA sequence is converted into a 1D image. The filters are superimposed on the image for convolution. Activation is done by ReLU followed by pooling. The

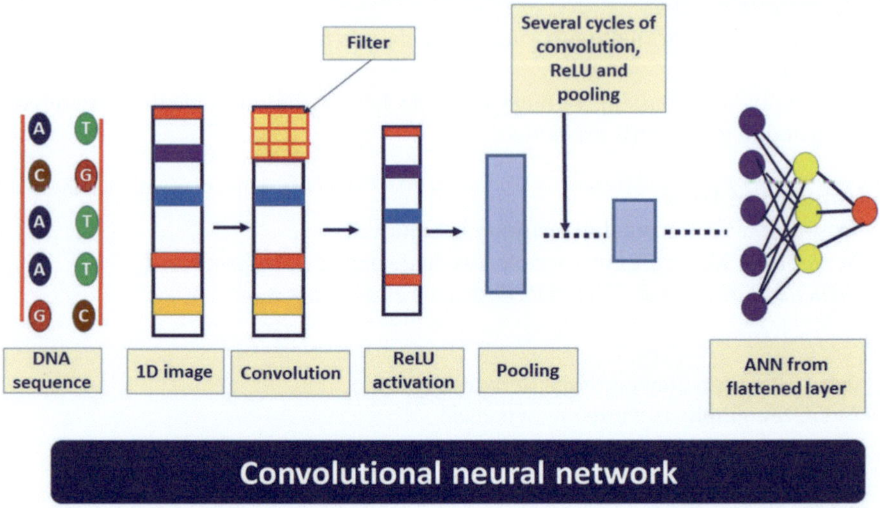

Fig. 10.3 Convolutional neural network

features are self-extracted by CNN. After several cycles of convolution, ReLU and pooling the dimension is reduced significantly. The fully connected neural network is made for final prediction or classification.

10.4.1.1 Advantages of CNN

1. *Automatic Feature Extraction*: In the case of CNN, no manual description is needed. CNN itself captures the important features.
2. *Capture Spatial/Local Relationships*: CNN captures the spatial relationship of the atoms.
3. *Powerful*: CNN is a powerful tool for complex datasets.

10.4.1.2 Applications of CNN

The various applications are described in the following paragraphs (Fig. 10.4).

1. *Predicting Regulatory Elements*: There are short sequences of DNA that control the expression of genes such as enhancers, promoters and silencers. It is costly to identify these regulatory elements experimentally. Moreover, the process is slow. CNN can successfully identify the regulatory elements. DeepSEA [7] program can accurately predict transcription factor (TF) sites and DNA accessibility from genomic sequence. Basset program can accurately predict the regulatory code with deep convolutional neural networks [8].
2. *Variant Effect Prediction*: CNN can directly predict from DNA sequence whether a genetic variant such as a single nucleotide polymorphism (SNP), insertion or deletion of nucleotides (INDEL) will:
   - Influence gene expression.
   - Affect the protein function.
   - Cause disease.

- Predict the sequence change and its effect on altered biological function. DeepSEA and Basset utilize the CNN model to predict about transcription factor binding and chromatin accessibility [8].

3. *Gene Expression Prediction*: CNN can predict how actively a gene is being transcribed into RNA (the gene expression). In addition, CNN gives an overview of the gene regulation [9].
4. *Splicing Prediction*: CNN can accurately predict the slicing sites where two exons are joined after slicing in between introns. SpliceAI is an online open tool for predicting DNA splicing. SpliceAI visual is freely available as a Google Colab notebook [10].
5. *Chromatin Accessibility and Epigenomics*: CNN can predict where DNA is accessible (open) to protein or inaccessible due to histone wrapping (closed). Quang D et al. developed FactorNet that can predict the cell-type-specific transcription factor binding [11].
6. *3D Genome Architecture*: CNN can predict three-dimensional folding and spatial organization of the chromosome within the nucleus. This 3D architecture of the genome helps to assess the gene regulation and enhancer–promoter interactions. DeepC is based on a deep neural network that accurately predicts genome folding from DNA sequence [12].
7. *Disease Classification and disease outcome*: CNN can analyse the DNA and RNA sequence to predict the presence, type and risk of disease [13, 14]· CNN can extract the features related to sequence and function without any manual interference. Moreover, it can detect many non-obvious or cryptic slicing pattern.

Table 10.1 highlights different types of commercial software that are applied in molecular interpretation.

Figure 10.4 shows the applications of CNN.

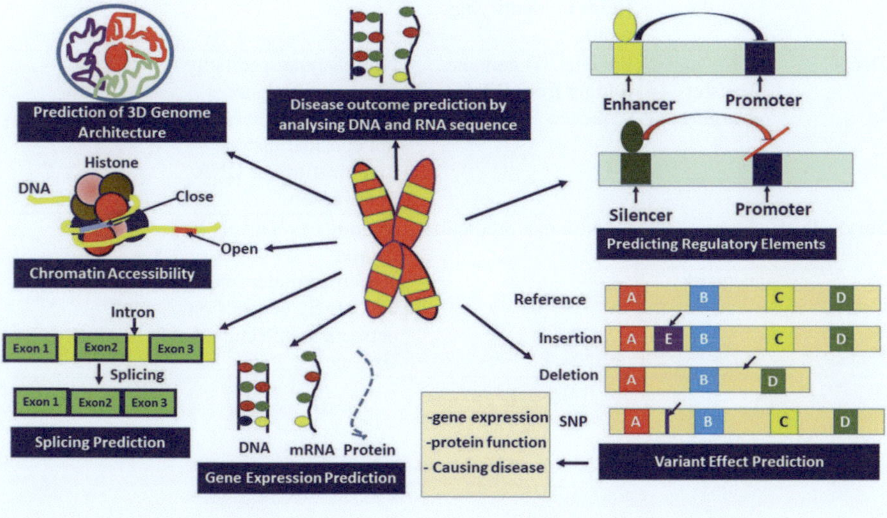

Fig. 10.4 Schematic diagram showing applications of convolutional neural network

Table 10.1 The applications of convolutional neural network in molecular interpretation

Software	Type of neural network	Main applications	Limitations	References
DeepSEA	CNN	To predict transcription factor (TF) sites and DNA accessibility from genomic sequence It learns regulatory sequence code from genomic sequence	The program can only handle limited size of the sequence (up to 1 kbp). Lack of flexibility to read heterogeneous input.	[15]
Basset	CNN	To predict the regulatory code of DNA sequences from genomics data	The model is unable to predict other functional activities	[8]
SpliceAI	CNN	To predict the slicing sites where two exons are joined after slicing between introns	SpliceAI is trained primarily on canonical splice junctions Actual mRNA expression or splicing products are not measured. It does not account for which isoform is predominantly expressed in a tissue	[16]
FactorNet	CNN	To predict cell-type-specific transcription factor binding It is cell-type specific and FactorNet can distinguish TF binding in different cell types Helps in identifying motifs	Large volumes of labelled data are needed Its performance depends on the quality of experimental data Computationally intensive and time-consuming	[11]
DeepC	CNN and transfer learning	Predicts 3D genome folding from DNA sequence	No cell-type specificity The program ignores Epigenetic Signals and does not consider histone modifications or DNA methylation	[12]
SurvivalNet	Deep neural network	Disease risk prediction	Requires a relatively large dataset. Hyperparameter sensitive and largely depends on network architecture, batch size, etc.	[17]

10.5 Recurrent Neural Networks (RNNs)

RNN is used for the processing of the temporal dynamic data [18]. RNNs specially process the sequential data (Box 10.3). It maintains a hidden state that captures information from previous steps. RNN comprises an input layer, a hidden layer and an output layer. It works as a feedback loop mechanism. Here, the output of the previous sequence is considered as input for the next time step. Many molecular datasets have a sequential structure such as SMILES strings, gene expression in course of time. RNN model is best suited for such datasets.

Advantages

- Sequential Data Handling: It handles sequential input by maintaining a memory of previous inputs through hidden states.
- RNNs can process input and output sequences of varying lengths.

Disadvantages

- Vanishing gradient.
- Slow training process as RNN does sequential training.

Application: DeepNano is a RNN-based model which can interpret raw electrical signals from Oxford Nanopore Technologies into nucleotide sequences [19].

ProLanGo is another RNN-based model that can predict the function of proteins [20]. The program can convert protein function prediction into a language translation problem. In fact, the program directly uses the protein sequence by passing any database. The ProLanGo program works in two steps:

1. Conversion of the protein sequence and protein function into the "ProLan" and "GOLan".
2. Building the Neural Machine Translation model from "ProLan" and "GOLan" languages for protein function prediction.

Box 10.3: Recurrent Neural Networks (RNNs).

RNNs specially process the sequential data. It works as a feedback loop mechanism. Here, the output of the previous sequence is passed back as input for the next time step.

Advantages

- Sequential Data Handling.
- RNNs can process input and output sequences of varying lengths.

Disadvantages

- Vanishing gradient.
- Slow training.

(continued)

Box 10.3 (continued)

Applications

- DeepNano: It can interpret raw electrical signals from Oxford Nanopore Technologies into nucleotide sequences.
- ProLanGo: It can predict the function of proteins.
- Natural language processing.

10.6 Autoencoders (AEs)

Autoencoder is one type of unsupervised neural network [21].

It has two components:

1. Encoder: It transforms multidimensional input data into low-dimensional data that comprises the set of latent features.
2. Decoder: It reconstructs the original data from the compressed one.

Applications:

1. Dimension reduction: The gene, protein and metabolomics contain hundreds to thousands of features. The autoencoder diminishes the dimensions; however, it preserves the relevant biological signals.
2. Drug design: Autoencoder can capture chemical and pharmacological properties from the SMILES strings or molecular fingerprint and can generate new molecules.
3. Anomaly detection: Autoencoder can identify the anomalous molecular pattern.

OUTRIDER (Outlier in RNA-Seq Finder) is the program that uses an autoencoder. The program can detect aberrantly expressed genes from the input data of RNA sequencing [22]. OUTRIDER is used in the diagnosis of rare diseases.

There are certain limitations of OUTRIDER. These include: (1) Large cohort of samples is needed., (2) It is basically a statistical program and there is no direct link of gene expression changes. (3) The program only detects anomalous gene expression levels, however, the splicing outliers are not detected.

10.7 Generative Adversarial Networks (GANs)

GAN is an artificial neural network that is used for unsupervised learning. It was first introduced by Goodfellow in the year 2014 [23]. GAN is composed of two networks:

1. Generator: It generates fake data that resembles real data.
2. Discriminator: The discriminator tries to identify the fake data.

The generator and discriminator compete with each other. The generator tries to fool the discriminator and the discriminator tries to identify the fake data. The generator and discriminator are neural networks and they are trained. At one point of time, the discriminator no longer able to recognize the fake data.

10.7.1 Applications of GANs in Molecular Data Interpretation

1. *Molecule Generation*: GAN can generate unique chemical molecules with desirable properties.
2. *Data Augmentation*: GAN can increase the volume of the molecular dataset in case of rare diseases.
3. *Gene Expression Simulation*: GAN can model a disease by generating synthetic gene expression profiles.

10.8 Conclusions

The application of Artificial intelligence in molecular data interpretation has made a paradigm shift. The AI-driven interpretation is rapid and cost-effective. AI not only detects the various anomalies in the gene and its expression but also provides insight into the disease by simulating the disease model. It can also design the chemicals (drugs) with a desirable effect. In future, AI will have a revolutionary effect. However, one should be careful about the quality of the data and its transparency. This needs the collaboration of multiple institutions.

References

1. Licatalosi DD, Mele A, Fak JJ, et al. HITS-CLIP yields genomewide insights into brain alternative RNA processing. Nature. 2008;456(7221):464–9. https://doi.org/10.1038/nature07488. PMID: 18978773.
2. Stoltenburg R, Reinemann C, Strehlitz B. SELEX--a (r)evolutionary method to generate high-affinity nucleic acid ligands. Biomol Eng. 2007;24(4):381–403.
3. Ray D, Kazan H, Chan ET, et al. Rapid and systematic analysis of the RNA recognition specificities of RNA-binding proteins. Nat Biotechnol. 2009;27(7):667–70.
4. Chen Y, Li Y, Narayan R, Subramanian A, Xie X. Gene expression inference with deep learning. Bioinformatics. 2016;32(12):1832–9.
5. Mori Y, Yokota H, Hoshino I, Iwatate Y, Wakamatsu K, Uno T, Suyari H. Deep learning-based gene selection in comprehensive gene analysis in pancreatic cancer. Sci Rep. 2021;11(1):16521. https://doi.org/10.1038/s41598-021-95969-6. PMID: 34389782; PMCID: PMC8363643.
6. Ståhl N, Falkman G, Karlsson A, Mathiason G, Boström J. Deep convolutional neural networks for the prediction of molecular properties: challenges and opportunities connected to the data. J Integr Bioinform. 2018;16(1):20180065. https://doi.org/10.1515/jib-2018-0065. PMID: 30517077; PMCID: PMC6798861.

7. Zhou J, Troyanskaya OG. Predicting effects of noncoding variants with deep learning-based sequence model. Nat Methods. 2015;12(10):931–4. https://doi.org/10.1038/nmeth.3547. Epub 2015 Aug 24. PMID: 26301843; PMCID: PMC4768299.
8. Kelley DR, Snoek J, Rinn JL. Basset: learning the regulatory code of the accessible genome with deep convolutional neural networks. Genome Res. 2016;26:990–9. https://doi.org/10.1101/gr.200535.115.
9. Agarwal V, Shendure J. Predicting mRNA abundance directly from genomic sequence using deep convolutional neural networks. Cell Rep. 2020;31(7):107663. https://doi.org/10.1016/j.celrep.2020.107663.
10. de Sainte Agathe JM, Filser M, Isidor B, Besnard T, Gueguen P, Perrin A, Van Goethem C, Verebi C, Masingue M, Rendu J, Cossée M, Bergougnoux A, Frobert L, Buratti J, Lejeune É, Le Guern É, Pasquier F, Clot F, Kalatzis V, Roux AF, Cogné B, Baux D. SpliceAI-visual: a free online tool to improve SpliceAI splicing variant interpretation. Hum Genomics. 2023;17(1):7. https://doi.org/10.1186/s40246-023-00451-1. PMID: 36765386; PMCID: PMC9912651.
11. Quang D, Xie X. FactorNet: a deep learning framework for predicting cell type specific transcription factor binding from nucleotide-resolution sequential data. Methods. 2019;166:40–7. https://doi.org/10.1016/j.ymeth.2019.03.020. Epub 2019 Mar 26. PMID: 30922998; PMCID: PMC6708499.
12. Schwessinger R, Gosden M, Downes D, Brown RC, Oudelaar AM, Telenius J, Teh YW, Lunter G, Hughes JR. DeepC: predicting 3D genome folding using megabase-scale transfer learning. Nat Methods. 2020;17(11):1118–24. https://doi.org/10.1038/s41592-020-0960-3. Epub 2020 Oct 12. PMID: 33046896; PMCID: PMC7610627.
13. Liu L, Meng Q, Weng C, Lu Q, Wang T, Wen Y. Explainable deep transfer learning model for disease risk prediction using high-dimensional genomic data. PLoS Comput Biol. 2022;18(7):e1010328. https://doi.org/10.1371/journal.pcbi.1010328. PMID: 35839250; PMCID: PMC9328574.
14. Yousefi S, Amrollahi F, Amgad M, Dong C, Lewis JE, Song C, Gutman DA, Halani SH, Velazquez Vega JE, Brat DJ, Cooper LAD. Predicting clinical outcomes from large scale cancer genomic profiles with deep survival models. Sci Rep. 2017;7(1):11707. https://doi.org/10.1038/s41598-017-11817-6. PMID: 28916782; PMCID: PMC5601479.
15. Zhou J, Troyanskaya OG. Predicting effects of noncoding variants with deep learning-based sequence model. Nat Methods. 2015;12:931–4.
16. de Sainte Agathe JM, Filser M, Isidor B, et al. SpliceAI-visual: a free online tool to improve SpliceAI splicing variant interpretation. Hum Genomics. 2023;17(1):7.
17. Yousefi S, Amrollahi F, Amgad M, et al. Predicting clinical outcomes from large scale cancer genomic profiles with deep survival models. Sci Rep. 2017;7(1):11707.
18. Yu Y, Si X, Hu C, Zhang J. A review of recurrent neural networks: LSTM cells and network architectures. Neural Comput. 2019;31(7):1235–70. https://doi.org/10.1162/neco_a_01199. Epub 2019 May 21.
19. Boža V, Perešíni P, Brejová B, Vinař T. DeepNano-blitz: a fast base caller for MinION nanopore sequencers. Bioinformatics. 2020;36(14):4191–2. https://doi.org/10.1093/bioinformatics/btaa297.
20. Cao R, Freitas C, Chan L, Sun M, Jiang H, Chen Z. ProLanGO: protein function prediction using neural machine translation based on a recurrent neural network. Molecules. 2017;22(10):1732. https://doi.org/10.3390/molecules22101732. PMID: 29039790; PMCID: PMC6151571.
21. Hinton GE, Zemel RS. Autoencoders, minimum description length and Helmholtz free energy. Adv Neural Inf Proces Syst. 1994;6:3–10.
22. Brechtmann F, Mertes C, Matusevičiūtė A, Yépez VA, Avsec Ž, Herzog M, Bader DM, Prokisch H, Gagneur J. OUTRIDER: a statistical method for detecting aberrantly expressed genes in RNA sequencing data. Am J Hum Genet. 2018;103(6):907–17. https://doi.org/10.1016/j.ajhg.2018.10.025. Epub 2018 Nov 29. PMID: 30503520; PMCID: PMC6288422.
23. Goodfellow IJ, Pouget-Abadie J, Mirza M, et al. Generative adversarial nets. Adv Neural Inf Proces Syst. 2014;27:2672–80.

Precision Medicine and Computational Cytology

11

Abstract

Precision medicine uses data of a person's genomic profile, proteins, environment and lifestyle to prevent to diagnose and to treat the disease.

Traditional pathology heavily depends on the tumour typing, differentiation and grading. In contrast, the precision medicine emphasizes on unique molecular and phenotypic characteristics of individual patients. Computational Cytology (pathology) with the help of artificial intelligence (AI) plays a pivotal role in the interpretation of clinical, whole slide imaging (WSI) of histopathology and cytology, biomarkers along with molecular data. The key components of precision medicine include genomic profiling, big data and bioinformatics, electronic health records, biomarkers, and preventive and public health data. AI can play an important role in precision medicine by cancer screening, cancer diagnosis, molecular data analysis, treatment planning and predicting prognosis. This chapter discusses the role of Computational Cytology and AI in personalized medicine.

Keywords

Precision medicine · Computational cytology artificial intelligence · Cancer screening · Cancer diagnosis · Molecular data analysis · Treatment planning

11.1 Introduction

Personalized medicine made a new era in health science where the diagnosis and treatment of the individual patient are tailored depending on their genomic profile. Traditional pathology heavily depends on the tumour typing, differentiation and grading. In contrast, personalized medicine emphasizes on unique molecular and phenotypic characteristics of individual patients. Computational

P. Dey, *Computational Cytology*, https://doi.org/10.1007/978-981-95-3272-8_11

Cytology (pathology) with the help of artificial intelligence (AI) plays a pivotal role in the interpretation of clinical, whole slide imaging (WSI) of histopathology and cytology, biomarkers along with molecular data. With the progress of science and technology, there are huge accumulations of data including proteomic, RNA expression and molecular genomic. Computational Cytology (CCyt) can do multimodal data fusion and help in personalized medicine. In the current chapter, the role of Computational Cytology and AI in personalized medicine has been described.

11.2 What Is Precision Medicine?

According to the National Cancer Institute [1], precision medicine is defined as "A form of medicine that uses information about a person's genes, proteins, environment, and lifestyle to prevent, diagnose, or treat disease." Precision medicine includes individual-patient data, all laboratory investigations, radiology imaging data and genomic data. In fact, precision medicine rapidly includes "multi-omics" data such as proteomics, epigenomics, pharmacomics, metabolomics. The integration of these datasets helps in disease prevention, precise diagnosis, targeted therapy, overall management and prediction of prognosis in individual patients.

Example Suppose an elderly patient presented with the diagnosis of advanced non-small cell lung carcinoma. The tumour shows TTF1 positivity and p40 negativity, indicating adenocarcinoma. The tumour cells show EGFR mutations.

Advise EGFR tyrosine kinase inhibitors (TKIs) like erlotinib as first-line therapy.

Personalised medicine term is often used interchangeably with precision medicine. In fact, the term "personalised medicine" is an older terminology and it should be replaced with "precision medicine".

11.3 Key Components of Precision Medicine

The key Components of Precision Medicine are described below (Fig. 11.1):

1. *Genomics and Molecular Profiling*: It includes whole genome sequences, single nucleotide polymorphisms (SNPs), structural variations (insertions, deletions) and epigenetic markers.
2. *Big Data and Bioinformatics*: Big data encompasses the integration of a vast amount of data regarding clinical features, socio-economic data, biochemical and laboratory investigations and molecular assays. Big data includes "omics" such as proteomics, epigenomics, pharmacomics, metabolomics, microbiomics. The big data is described by five "V": volume, velocity, variety, veracity and value. Volume refers to the huge complex data. Velocity indicates the speed of new data generation. Variety means the different types of data (structured/

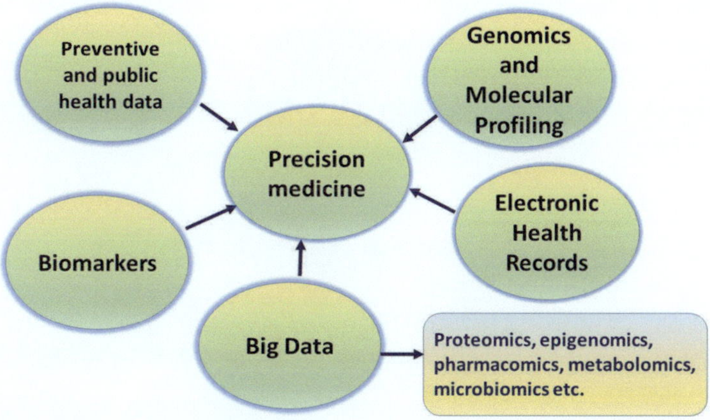

Fig. 11.1 Schematic diagram showing the essential components of precision medicine

unstructured data). Veracity indicates the accuracy and relevance of data. Value means the clinical need for the data.

3. *Electronic Health Records (EHRs)*: EHRs provide the detailed history of the patient.
4. *Biomarkers*: Various biomarkers are used for diagnosis, treatment and to predict the treatment response.
5. *Preventive and public health data.*

Figure 11.1 shows the essential components of precision medicine.

AI and Big Data The big data is described by five "V": volume, velocity, variety, veracity and value (Fig. 11.2). Volume refers to the huge complex data. Velocity indicates the speed of new data generation. Variety means the different types of data (structured/unstructured data). Veracity indicates the accuracy and relevance of data. Value means the clinical need for the data. In recent years, massive data (volume) has been generated at high speed (velocity). The large dataset is generated from the application of advanced technologies and different high-throughput platforms in tumour samples. The genomic profile data is generated by next-generation sequencing, RNA sequencing, single-cell RNA sequencing, DNA methylation profiles, proteomics and more. These datasets are publicly available in different domains. The Cancer Genome Atlas (TCGA) is one of the popular sites that consists of comprehensive tumour profiles including histopathology images, radiology images, genomic and epigenomic data [2].

The International Cancer Genome Consortium (ICGA) compiled the somatic mutations of various cancers [3]. The easy availability of the dataset provides a ready reference and one can utilize the data in precision medicine. The datasets are difficult to handle manually due to the high volume and complexity. Moreover, the

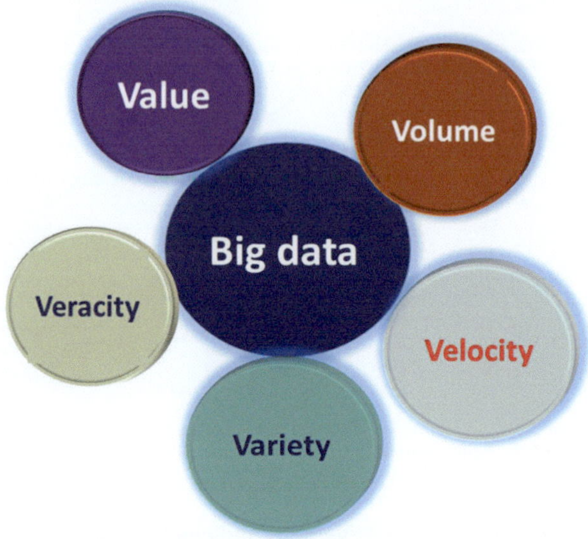

Fig. 11.2 The five "V" of big data

integration of different modalities is not possible manually. AI model may help in various ways by interpreting huge data and also by the fusion of multimodal datasets.

11.4 AI in Precision Medicine

Figure 11.3 shows the applications of AI in precision medicine.

11.4.1 Cancer Screening and Early Detection

It has been mentioned in the earlier chapter that the role of A- based cancer screening in cervical and urine smears. Various studies applied CNN-based models in cervical smears with high sensitivity and specificity (more than 90%) [4–6].

The AI-based screening of cervical smear is fast, less time-consuming, consistent and accurate. CNN has been used by various studies to detect malignant urothelial cells in smears from voided urine samples. The sensitivity and specificity of different studies ranged from 60% to 79.5%. However, the specificity of the AI model is 84.5–100% [7–9].

Liquid biopsy: Currently, liquid biopsy is a potential tool to detect early cancers. The study of circulating tumour DNA (ctDNA) and cell-free DNA (cfDNA) provides important information on cancer-specific genetic and epigenetic mutations [10].

Hoadley KA et al. [11] used the TCGA dataset of 10,000 samples of 33 different types of cancers. They analysed data on exome sequencing, DNA methylation, copy

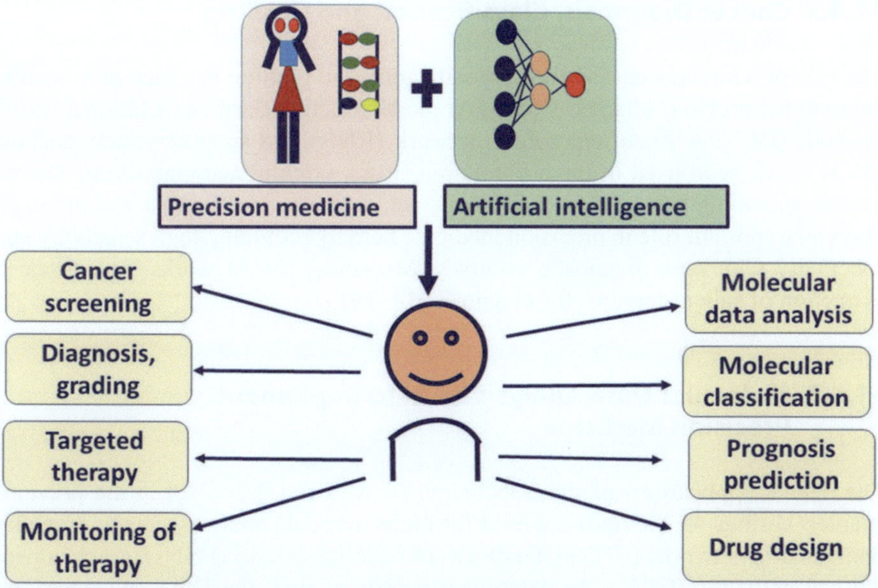

Fig. 11.3 The applications of AI in precision medicine

number in tumour DNA along with mRNA and miRNA expression levels and reverse-phase protein arrays. Interestingly, distinct DNA-methylation patterns in certain cancers were noted. The authors claimed that the pattern of methylation is helpful to predict the type of tumour cells.

In a prospective study, Cohen JD et al. [12] applied a novel blood test called the CancerSeek platform to detect cancer cells in 1005 patients. The test combined assays for genetic alterations and protein biomarkers. It was claimed that the test detected the cancer cells along with the cell of origin. The sensitivity of the test ranged from 69% to 98% and the specificity was 99%.

Chabon JJ et al. [13] made an AI model that can predict the cancer likelihood in the plasma of lung (Lung-CLiP) carcinoma from mutation analysis of cfDNA of blood sample. The model showed high predictive performance (AUC 0.98).

As the data accumulation increases in high speed, it is expected that a deep convolutional neural network (DCNN) model will be used extensively in liquid biopsy to analyse mutational changes and other protein biomarkers to identify cancer cells and also the cell of origin.

The major challenges in early detection of cancer by liquid biopsy are:

1. Limited shedding of ctDNA in the initial stage of cancer,
2. Only a few mutational changes are pathognomonic for a specific type of cancer,
3. Driver gene mutation may occur in aged persons.

11.4.2 Cancer Diagnosis, Classification and Grading

The role of AI in cancer diagnosis, classification and grading has been discussed in detail in the previous chapter. Various AI models such as deep convolutional neural network (DCNN), Recurrent neural network (RNN) and support vector machine (SVM) have been used in the accurate diagnosis, grading and classifying various cancers including breast, lung, colon, prostate, colorectal carcinomas and more. AI plays an important role in precision medicine here by providing high sensitivity and specificity with high diagnostic accuracy. Moreover, the AI works by automated extraction of salient features for diagnosis [14–19].

11.4.3 Molecular Data Analysis by AI to Implement Precision Medicine

The details applications of these techniques have been described in the previous chapter. Various AI Methods are used for molecular data analysis such as convolutional neural networks (CNNs), feedforward neural networks (FNNs), graph convolutional networks (GCN). As mentioned before, at first, the DNA sequences are encoded in 1D image and the CNN scans the image to find the local patterns. CNN is a powerful tool that automatically captures the important features. It also identifies the spatial relationship of the atoms. The applications of AI in molecular interpretations are listed below (Fig. 11.4):

- *Variant detection*: There are various toolkits available that can analyse the short reads. The Genome Analysis Toolkit (GATK) is a software package that can identify single-nucleotide variants (SNVs), insertions/deletions and many other genomic variations [20]. GATK is efficient and robust in analysing NGS data. Unlike traditional methods, a deep neural network interprets the sequencing data as an image and identifies different genetic variations with exceptional performance. DeepVariant is a type of deep neural network that can read the NGS data efficiently. Poplin R et al. [21] developed a DCNN called DeepVariant (Inception-V2 architecture) that helps to detect variants from aligned NGS reads. At first, the NGS read is aligned to a reference genome. The read and the reference data are encoded as an image and run into the DeepVariant model and the variant call is emitted. DeepVariant model showed greater accuracy and consistency across a variety.

  Abdelwahab O et al. [22] compared conventional and AI-based variant calling tools (BCFTools, GATK4, Platypus, DNAscope and DeepVariant). They showed that AI-based studies are far superior to conventional techniques in accuracy to detect SNV and insertion/deletions (INDELs).

  Oxford Nanopore Technologies (ONT) developed a portable real-time DNA sequencer that generates ultra-long reads. Bestcaling, a neural network-based tool, is able to transform the raw electrical signal to a nucleotide sequence. DeepVariant can be used for long-read variant calling [23].

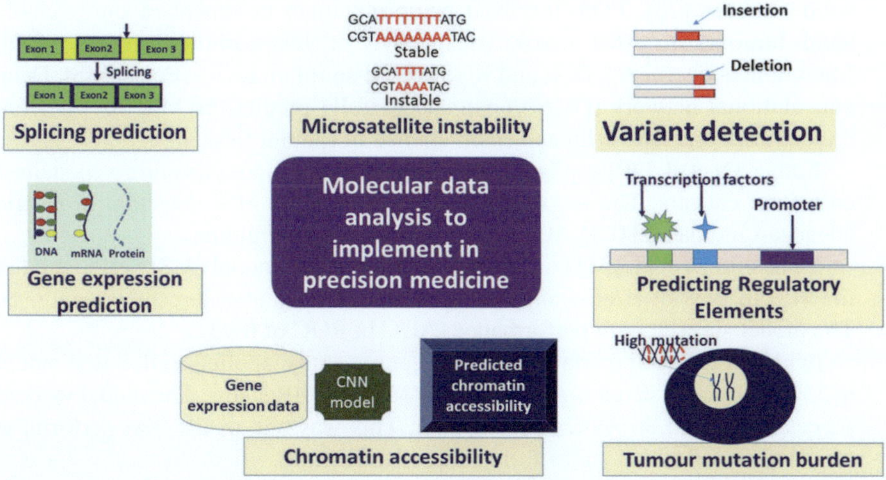

Fig. 11.4 Molecular data analysis to implement precision medicine

- *Predicting Regulatory Elements*: CNN can successfully identify the gene regulatory elements such as enhancers, promoters, and silencers. DeepSEA model can predict the transcription factor (TF) sites and DNA accessibility from genomic sequence and the model learns regulatory sequence code from genomic sequence [24].
- *Gene expression prediction*: CNN model can predict the transcription of RNA from the gene. Agarwal V et al. [25] developed a CNN model that uses simply the genomic sequence to predict mRNA expression levels. The model noted that the presence of CpG dinucleotides proximal to the promoter is one of the prime factor that strongly predicts transcriptional activity.
- *Splicing prediction*: Agathe JM et al. [26] applied SpliceAI deep learning splicing prediction algorithm to predict the splicing sites. The software provides graphical output. So it allows fast and precise interpretation.
- *Chromatin accessibility*: CNN model can predict the chromatin accessibility of a DNA chain. The CNN-based software FactorNet can predict the cell-type-specific transcription factor binding [27].
- *Microsatellite instability*: Microsatellites are short sequences (1–6 base pairs) of DNA situated both in non-coding and coding regions of DNA. These are error-prone regions during DNA replication. Microsatellite instability (MSI) indicates the change in the number and size of microsatellite sequences that are different from germ line DNA. In healthy people, DNA mismatch repair (MMR) proteins (MLHI, PMS2, MSH2, and MSH6) correct the mutational errors. High microsatellite instability (MSI-H) means frequent changes of MSI in different loci. Whereas, in low microsatellite instability (MSI-L), MSI occurs at low frequency. MSI-H is seen in colonic carcinoma and endometrioid carcinoma of the uterus. MSI-L is seen in prostate, gastrointestinal, and pancreatic carcinoma, and many

solid tumours [28]. FDA-approved pembrolizumab treatment of unresectable solid tumours in MSI cases, irrespective of histopathological type [29]. Immunohistochemistry, PCR and NGS are the common tests to detect MSI. Deep convolutional network (DCNN) can successfully predict the MSI simply from the digitized haematoxylin and eosin-stained of tumour tissue.

Kather JN et al. [30] applied CNN in digitized haematoxylin and eosin-stained colorectal cancers. The model showed 0.81AUCs for MSI detection in gastric adenocarcinoma and 0.84 AUC in colorectal adenocarcinoma.

Yamashita R et al. [31] built a deep learning based model (MSINet) to predict the MSI in WSI of H&E-stained images of 100 cases of colorectal carcinomas. The model showed high performance (AUC in ROC of 0·931).

Echle A et al. [32] in the largest multicentric study, applied a DL based model in 8500 colorectal carcinomas to identify MSI/dMMR status. The model worked successfully with an AUC of ROC 0.96. This was one of the best-performing model to classify MSI status from simple H&E slides.

- *Tumour mutation burden (TMB)*: Tumour mutation burden (TMB) means the total number of mutations in the cancer cells per megabase of DNA [33]. If the TMB is more than 20 mutations per megabase of DNA, then it is considered a high TMB. In June 2020, the FDA approved pembrolizumab therapy with unresectable or metastatic solid tumours with high TMB [34].

  TMB is normally estimated by gene-targeted sequencing with the help of NGS which is costly. Jain MS et al. [35] made a machine learning algorithm (Image 2TMB) which is able to predict TMB from the H&E-stained images of lung adenocarcinomas. The model had an AUC of 0.92 with an average precision of 0.89.

  Wang L et al. [36] applied a set of deep learning model (Resnet50, Googlenet, Inception v3, Alexnet, Squeezenet, Densenet) to predict TMB from digitized images of 644 gastrointestinal carcinomas. The images were downloaded from the open-access public domains. The model showed AUC 0.75–0.82.

  Shimada Y et al. [37] applied a CNN model (Inception V3) to predict TMB from the H&E-stained images of 278 cases of colorectal carcinomas. The model showed an AUC of 0.91.

11.4.4 Molecular Classification of Cancer

Currently, we classify cancers in different organs on the basis of histopathology or cytopathology. Microscopic images of the tumour tissue along with immunohistochemistry plays an important role in the classification of cancer. However, the current classification of cancers may not always be homogenous. In contrast, molecular classification of cancer reflects the treatment and management protocol and also the prognosis of the tumour. In 2001, Sørlie T et al. [38] first did molecular classification of breast carcinoma based on gene expression patterns.

Subsequently, molecular classification was done in colorectal and ovarian carcinomas [39, 40].

Deep learning technique has added advantages over the standard computational techniques (random forests, support vector machines and others) as it learns from the whole transcriptome. Gao F et al. [41] applied a novel deep learning-based framework (DeepCC) to do molecular subtyping of colon and breast cancers. It was noted that the DeepCC model had higher sensitivity, specificity and accuracy compared to standard computational techniques such as random forests (RF), support vector machine (SVM) and gradient boosting machine (GBM).

Deep learning can extract important features from the vast transcriptomic data and moreover, it is flexible and can incorporate previously acquired biological information to improve accuracy. Deep learning techniques have been successfully implemented to do molecular classification of lung and bladder carcinomas [42, 43].

11.4.5 Treatment Planning

AI can be used in chemotherapy planning for individual patients. Sundar R et al. [44] applied a random forest machine-learning model to select the patients of gastric carcinoma who may benefit from paclitaxel. The study included a total of 499 gastric carcinoma patients. A total of 19 genes were studied. A random forest model generated two groups: Pac-sensitive and Pac-resistant. Pac-sensitive patients had significant disease-free survival compared to Pac-resistant patients (66% vs. 40%). So, using a machine learning model, the authors identified a gene signature which predicted paclitaxel survival benefit in gastric carcinoma.

Kleppe A et al. [45] made a clinical decision support system based on DoMore-v1-CRC and pathological staging markers of stage II or III colorectal cancers. They identified the carcinoma with a favourable prognosis and so helped in avoiding unnecessary adjuvant chemotherapy.

Crispin-Ortuzar M et al. [46] made a machine learning model based on gene expression data and predicted the efficacy of platinum-based therapy on high-grade serous ovarian carcinoma with 80% accuracy. The AI model helped to avoid unnecessary treatment and toxicity.

11.4.6 Prognosis Prediction

Prediction of the prognosis of cancer is an essential part of management as it helps in the decision to avoid unnecessary aggressive treatment protocol. Cox proportional hazard regression model (Cox-PH) is the most common method of survival prediction [47]. It is a multivariate linear regression model that correlates survival and other prognostic variables.

It was noted that the genes displaying the linear relationship follow different biological processes than those of the non-linear relationship. Genes displaying a linear relationship were overall associated with substantially different biological processes than genes displaying a nonlinear relationship. Solvang HK et al. [48]

showed that Cox-PH is unable to handle the complex non-linear relationship of genomic data.

Deep learning model is non-linear and can provide better survival prediction from the complex molecular interactions [49]. Cox-net is the hybrid system that incorporates the Cox regression model into a neural network and shows better accuracy [50]. Table 11.1 highlights the different studies on prognostic prediction.

Chereda H et al. [52] developed a graph convolutional neural network based on gene expression profiles of a large breast cancer dataset to predict metastasis in individual patients. Chaudhary K et al. [56] made a DL-based model by integrating RNA sequencing (RNA-Seq), miRNA sequencing (miRNA-Seq) and methylation data of 360 hepatocellular carcinoma cases to predict survival. The model was robust and worked well in multiple cohorts.

The prognosis of the tumour depends on multiple data such as tumour typing, differentiation, mitotic activities [58], immune cells infiltration [59] and various other factors. Deep learning model can directly extract the essential features to predict the prognostic outcome. CNN model has been trained of H&E-stained images of colorectal, liver or renal cell carcinomas to predict the prognosis of colorectal, liver or renal cell carcinomas [55, 57].

Multimodal fusion of WSIs of carcinomas along with "omics data" may provide better prognostic prediction and also suggest personalized treatment profile. Hao J et al. [54] applied a deep learning model (PAGE-Net) to do multimodal data fusion of histopathological images and genomic data. The model provided better survival predictions. He B et al. [51] built a novel multimodal deep learning fusion model on 84 colorectal cancers (CRC). The model integrated WSI of H&E-stained images, clinical data, whole exome sequencing data and mRNA data to predict the 5-year survival of CRC patients. The multimodal compact bi-linear pooling method was used for data fusion. The model is promising to predict prognosis. However, the sample size was too small, and there was limited follow-up data. Moreover, the model was not tested on any cohort group.

11.4.7 Monitoring Therapy of the Patient

During the therapy of the patient, it is important to assess whether the ongoing therapy is effective or not. If the ongoing therapy is not effective, then the clinicians may have to change the therapy. Traditionally the cancer monitoring is done by assessing the shrinkage of the tumour tissue in a pathology sample or by radiology image and to check the appearance of the new tumour.

Table 11.2 highlights various studies on monitoring of cancer therapy by AI.

Dercle L et al. [64] used a machine learning algorithm on CT scans of non-small cell lung cancers to predict the response to chemotherapy.

Liquid biopsy is a non-invasive technique that can dynamically monitor treatment efficacy and detect resistance to therapy (Fig. 11.5). Circulating tumour DNA (ctDNA) dynamics are helpful in treatment response. Li et al. made a mathematical model of ctDNA kinetics and have shown that the ctDNA kinetics is helpful to

Table 11.1 Prognostic prediction by deep learning models

Tumour	Author	Year	Number of cases	AI model	Key findings	Comments
Colorectal cancers	He B [51],	2025	84	Multimodal deep learning fusion model	Predicted 5 year survival by integrating WSI of H & E stained images, clinical data, whole exome sequencing data, and mRNA data	Integration of clinical data and genomic data reinforced the histopathology based survival prediction
Breast	Chereda [52]	2021	12,179 genes in 969 patients	Graph convolutional neural network	Predicted distant metastasis based on gene expression data structured	Highly useful for prediction
Hepatocellular Carcinoma	Saillard C [53]	2020	A discovery set of194 cases and an independent validation set of 328 cases	Deep learning model	Predicted survival of patients from WSI of histopathology sections	A successful model that can bypass human interference
Glioblastoma Multiforme	Hao J [54]	2020	5404 genes of 447 GBM patients	Deep learning model (PAGE-Net)	Predicted survival by combining the histopathological images and genomic data	The study identified genetic and histopathological patterns responsible for survival difference
Renal Cell Carcinoma	Tabibu S [55]	2019	Exact number not mentioned	Convolutional neural networks (pre-trained Resnet 18 and Resnet 34)	Predicted survival of renal cell carcinomas from the digitized images	The number of cases are not mentioned
Hepatocellular carcinoma	Chaudhary K [56]	2018	360	DL-based model	Predict survival by integrating RNA sequencing, miRNA sequencing, and methylation data to	Multi-cohort robust study
Colorectal cancer	Bychkov D [57]	2018	420	Deep learning (convolutional and recurrent architectures)	Predicted survival of the patients on digitized H & E -stained tumour tissue Microarray samples	The performance of AI model (AUC 0.69) was better than visual microscopic impression (AUC 0.58)

Table 11.2 Monitoring therapy by a deep learning model

Tumour	Author	Year	Number of cases	AI model	Key findings	Comments
Melanoma	Widman AJ [60]	2024	48	Machine learning technology (MRD-EDGE)	Extremely low concentration of ctDNA was detected	Effective technology to detect extremely low concentration of ctDNA
Cancer type not mentioned	Li A, Lou E [61]	2024	Not mentioned	Mathematical model	Circulating tumour DNA (ctDNA) dynamics helped to predict the treatment response	ctDNA dynamic was helpful to predict tumour response
Four cancer types: Colon, breast, liver, ovary	Zhu [62]	2023	213 cancer cases	Ultrafast deep learning-based technique (Fragle)	Quantified ctDNA in plasma sample of the cancer patients to predict therapeutic response	Fragle is fast, and accurate method for ctDNA quantification
Lung carcinomas	Esfahani MS [63]	2022	329 blood samples (201 cancer and 87 healthy)	Epigenetic expression inference from cell free DNA-sequencing (EPIC-seq) by using machine learning technology	Detected therapeutic response by using EPIC-seq in serial blood samples of lung carcinomas	High potential in diagnosis and prognosis assessment
Non-small cell lung cancers	Dercle L [64]	2020	264	Machine learning algorithm	Predicted the response of chemotherapy based on radiomics signatures on CT scan images	Radiomics signatures successfully predicted tumour sensitivity to treatment

assess the therapeutic response of the tumour [61]. Deep learning models detect a quick drop in ctDNA levels during early cycles of chemotherapy. Zhu G et al. developed an ultrafast deep learning-based technique (Fragle) which can quantify ctDNA in plasma samples of cancer patients. The dynamic quantification can help in the treatment response of the patients [62].

ctDNA in the plasma of cancer patients is present in extremely low concentration. Widman AJ et al. [60] introduced a machine learning technology

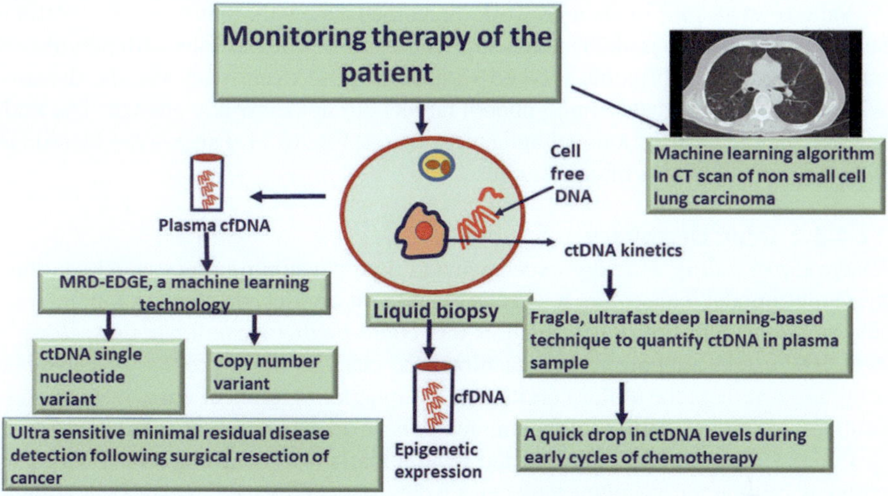

Fig. 11.5 Monitoring the therapy of the patient

(MRD-EDGE), that can simultaneously detect ctDNA single-nucleotide variant (SNV) and copy number variant (CNV) to enhance ctDNA detection. The technique is useful in the detection of therapeutic response and also to detect minimal residual disease.

Esfahani et al. [63] developed Epigenetic expression inference from cell-free DNA-sequencing (EPIC-seq) that uses machine learning technology to sequence the transcription start sites of cell-free DNA (cfDNA). They applied EPIC-seq in serial blood samples of lung carcinomas treated with PDL1 and correlated with clinical response. The authors highlighted that EPIC-seq can be used for monitoring the therapy of patients.

11.4.8 Targeted Therapy and Drug Discovery

Targeted therapy is one of the most promising areas in Cancer precision medicine [65]. AI is promising to identify the potential molecular target, drug generation and drug delivery. AI model integrates different "omics" data to develop target-oriented drugs. Medi K et al. [66] in a meta-analysis study tried to identify the potential therapeutic targets of cervical cancer by the integration of gene expression profiles with biomolecular networks.

Cantini L et al. generated a multi-network-based workflow to integrate different layers of genomic information including (1) Transcription Factor (TF) co-targeting network, (2) microRNA co-targeting network, (3) Protein–Protein Interaction (PPI) network and (4) gene co-expression network [67]. Then they applied a machine learning algorithm to discover the driver genes and noted that certain oncogenes are promising targets for pancreatic cancer.

Valle IF et al. [68] made a network medicine framework that showed a relationship between disease proteins and polyphenol targets. The diseases with polyphenol targets proximal to proteins showed significant gene expression and the diseases whose proteins are distal to polyphenol targets did not show any change. The finding may be the basis of a novel anticancer target. Figure 11.6 shows the identification of potential targets of cancer cells.

11.4.8.1 Drug Discovery

Discovery of a drug is a very expensive and time-consuming process. AI can integrate multimodal datasets such as gene expression profiles, protein–protein interaction and epigenetics to derive features that could predict a candidate drug. Tong Z et al. [69] used a support vector machine (one-class SVM) to predict the candidate drug target in hepatocellular carcinomas by integrating clinical data, gene expression profiles and protein–protein interaction networks.

López-Cortés A et al. [70] reported several markers as drug targets in breast carcinomas by integrating numerous cancer databases. Gilvary C et al. [71] applied ECLIPSE, a machine learning model using DepMap data to predict cancer specific drug targets by integrating genomic and essential genes in specific cancer cell lines. The model is useful to develop newer drugs against cancer.

11.4.8.2 Drug Design

De novo drug designs create novel chemical entities from the atomic building blocks that have no previous relationship. So, de novo means that the novel molecular structure can be generated without any starting template. There are several advantages of de novo drug designing. The compound has high potential for target-specific character in a cost and time-effective way. The de novo drug deigning needs only the information of the target receptors or its active binders (ligand) [72]. The 3D structures of the receptors are available by X-ray crystallography, NMR, or electron

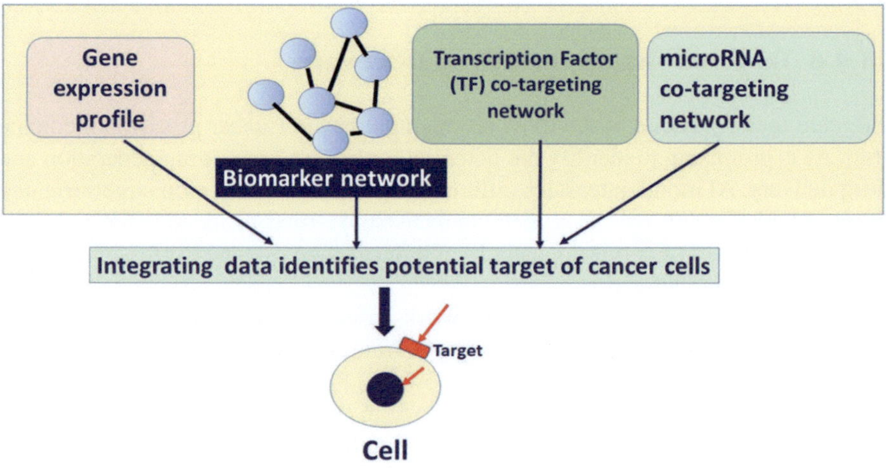

Fig. 11.6 Schematic diagram showing how to identify potential target of cancer cell

microscopy [73]. So the two major de novo drug designing approaches are structure-based and ligand-based design.

The rapidly increasing volume of complex data requires the use of deep learning models in drug designing. Various deep learning models are used in drug designing that include recurrent neural networks, convolutional neural networks, generative adversarial networks, autoencoders and graph convolutional networks. Graph convolutional networks give better molecular generation as it does not need computational conversion of the chemical molecules [74]. Deep reinforcement learning is a popular AI model. It amalgamates artificial neural networks with reinforcement learning. It is effective in drug designing as the model can handle the complex data and can provide feedback. Olivecrona et al. [75] have applied a deep reinforcement learning model to de novo design the compounds that were active against the dopamine receptor type 2.

11.5 Challenges and Limitations

AI has indisputable potential in precision medicine. However, AI faces several challenges in its implementation in health care.

Data Inconsistency The variability of data is a major challenge of AI. There is wide intra- and inter-laboratory variation of data regarding the quality of WSI of H&E-stained images of histopathology and also cytology. The intensity of immunostaining is also a major challenge. The transcriptomic data and even the list of "human genes" are variable. The multiple authorities publish their own findings. So the source and version of the genetic model should be mentioned.

Real-world Application of Data The electronic health record (EHR) data of different hospitals are often inconsistent and incomplete. This dataset needs preprocessing before use in AI. The outliers should be taken care of and if needed, should be removed. EHR consists of histopathology/cytopathology diagnosis, various laboratory reports and history of medications. The accuracy of these data is necessary for a successful AI model.

Data Safety AI deals with clinical history, genomics and social data. There is a great need of safety regarding data storage, management and sharing. The data should not be stolen or misused for commercial purposes. As the data is often private to the patient so it is needed to maintain privacy.

Rigorous Testing and Validation The rigorous testing and validation of AI model is an essential component of a safe and accurate AI model in the clinical world. The dataset should be huge and diverse. Moreover, it should represent the real-world scenario. The AI model should be monitored continuously to note any degradation of its performance. In addition, bias detection regarding gender, race, socioeconomic condition, method of data acquisition, etc., should be avoided.

Black Box Problems of AI Model The hidden layer of an artificial neural network is known as a black box. Any complex decision is made by this black box. We do not have any control over this black box. When we use a large number of parameters, we do not know the exact decision and AI model also does not provide any logic to make its final decision.

11.6 Conclusions

Deep learning is a promising technology in the field of precision medicine. It helps in early cancer detection, accurate identification and classification of cancer, molecular interpretation, targeting therapy, prediction of prognosis, and drug development. Overall, deep learning revolutionizes health care facilities. In addition, by integrating clinical data, imaging and genomics along with "multi-omics", deep learning gives us new insights into various disease mechanisms. There are several challenges and limitations in the implementation of deep learning in a clinical setting that includes consistent good quality data, unbiased data, and real-world data. The success of AI depends on rigorous validation, integrating innovative techniques and commitment of medical ethics.

References

1. https://www.cancer.gov/publications/dictionaries/cancer-terms/def/precision-medicine
2. Ding L, Bailey MH, Porta-Pardo E et al. Cancer Genome Atlas Research Network. Perspective on oncogenic processes at the end of the beginning of cancer genomics. Cell. 2018;173(2):305–320.e10. https://doi.org/10.1016/j.cell.2018.03.033. PMID: 29625049; PMCID: PMC5916814.
3. ICGC/TCGA Pan-Cancer Analysis of Whole Genomes Consortium. Pan-cancer analysis of whole genomes. Nature. 2020;578(7793):82–93. https://doi.org/10.1038/s41586-020-1969-6. Epub 2020 Feb 5. Erratum in: Nature. 2023 Feb;614(7948):E39. doi: 10.1038/s41586-022-05598-w. PMID: 32025007; PMCID: PMC7025898.
4. Rahaman MM, Li C, Yao Y, Kulwa F, Wu X, Li X, Wang Q. DeepCervix: a deep learning-based framework for the classification of cervical cells using hybrid deep feature fusion techniques. Comput Biol Med. 2021;136:104649.
5. Wang CW, Liou YA, Lin YJ, Chang CC, Chu PH, Lee YC, Wang CH, Chao TK. Artificial intelligence-assisted fast screening cervical high grade squamous intraepithelial lesion and squamous cell carcinoma diagnosis and treatment planning. Sci Rep. 2021;11(1):16244.
6. Holmström O, Linder N, Kaingu H, Mbuuko N, Mbete J, Kinyua F, Törnquist S, Muinde M, Krogerus L, Lundin M, Diwan V, Lundin J. Point-of-care digital cytology with artificial intelligence for cervical cancer screening in a resource-limited setting. JAMA Netw Open. 2021;4(3):e211740.
7. Lebret T, Paoletti X, Pignot G, et al. Artificial intelligence to improve cytology performance in urothelial carcinoma diagnosis: results from validation phase of the French, multicenter, prospective VISIOCYT1 trial. World J Urol. 2023;41(9):2381–8.
8. Zhang Z, Fu X, Liu J, Huang Z, Liu N, Fang F, Rao J. Developing a machine learning algorithm for identifying abnormal urothelial cells: a feasibility study. Acta Cytol. 2021;65(4):335–41. https://doi.org/10.1159/000510474. Epub 2020 Oct 6

9. Vaickus LJ, Suriawinata AA, Wei JW, Liu X. Automating the Paris system for urine cytopathology-a hybrid deep-learning and morphometric approach. Cancer Cytopathol. 2019;127(2):98–115. https://doi.org/10.1002/cncy.22099. Epub 2019 Jan 31
10. Bettegowda C, Sausen M, Leary RJ, et al. Detection of circulating tumor DNA in early- and late-stage human malignancies. Sci Transl Med. 2014;6(224):224ra24. https://doi.org/10.1126/scitranslmed.3007094. PMID: 24553385; PMCID: PMC4017867
11. Hoadley KA, Yau C, Hinoue T, et al. Cell-of-origin patterns dominate the molecular classification of 10,000 tumors from 33 types of cancer. Cell. 2018;173(2):291–304.e6. https://doi.org/10.1016/j.cell.2018.03.022. PMID: 29625048; PMCID: PMC5957518.
12. Cohen JD, Li L, Wang Y. Detection and localization of surgically resectable cancers with a multi-analyte blood test. Science. 2018;359(6378):926–30. https://doi.org/10.1126/science.aar3247. Epub 2018 Jan 18. PMID: 29348365; PMCID: PMC6080308.
13. Chabon JJ, Hamilton EG, Kurtz DM, et al. Integrating genomic features for non-invasive early lung cancer detection. Nature. 2020;580(7802):245–51. https://doi.org/10.1038/s41586-020-2140-0. Epub 2020 Mar 25. PMID: 32269342; PMCID: PMC8230734.
14. El Agouri H, Azizi M, El Attar H, El Khannoussi M, Ibrahimi A, Kabbaj R, et al. Assessment of deep learning algorithms to predict histopathological diagnosis of breast cancer: first Moroccan prospective study on a private dataset. BMC Res Notes. 2022;15(1):66.
15. Kanavati F, Toyokawa G, Momosaki S, Rambeau M, Kozuma Y, Shoji F, Yamazaki K, Takeo S, Iizuka O, Tsuneki M. Weakly-supervised learning for lung carcinoma classification using deep learning. Sci Rep. 2020;10(1):9297.
16. Kosaraju S, Park J, Lee H, Yang JW, Kang M. Deep learning-based framework for slide-based histopathological image analysis. Sci Rep. 2022;12:19075.
17. Chen CL, Chen CC, Yu WH, Chen SH, Chang YC, Hsu TI, Hsiao M, Yeh CY, Chen CY. An annotation-free whole-slide training approach to pathological classification of lung cancer types using deep learning. Nat Commun. 2021;12(1):1193.
18. Huang W, Randhawa R, Jain P, Iczkowski KA, Hu R, Hubbard S, Eickhoff J, Basu H, Roy R. Development and validation of an artificial intelligence-powered platform for prostate cancer grading and quantification. JAMA Netw Open. 2021;4(11):e2132554. https://doi.org/10.1001/jamanetworkopen.2021.32554. PMID: 34730818; PMCID: PMC8567112.
19. Dabass M, Vashisth S, Vig R. A convolution neural network with multi-level convolutional and attention learning for classification of cancer grades and tissue structures in colon histopathological images. Comput Biol Med. 2022;147:105680. https://doi.org/10.1016/j.compbiomed.2022.105680. Epub 2022 Jun 2.
20. McKenna A, Hanna M, Banks E, et al. The genome analysis toolkit: a MapReduce framework for analyzing next-generation DNA sequencing data. Genome Res. 2010;20(9):1297–303. https://doi.org/10.1101/gr.107524.110. Epub 2010 Jul 19. PMID: 20644199; PMCID: PMC2928508.
21. Poplin R, Chang PC, Alexander D, Schwartz S, Colthurst T, Ku A, et al. A universal SNP and small-indel variant caller using deep neural networks. Nat Biotechnol. 2018;36:983–7.
22. Abdelwahab O, Belzile F, Torkamaneh D. Performance analysis of conventional and AI-based variant callers using short and long reads. BMC Bioinformatics. 2023;24(1):472. https://doi.org/10.1186/s12859-023-05596-3. PMID: 38097928; PMCID: PMC10720095.
23. Wick RR, Judd LM, Holt KE. Performance of neural network basecalling tools for Oxford Nanopore sequencing. Genome Biol. 2019;20(1):129. https://doi.org/10.1186/s13059-019-1727-y. PMID: 31234903; PMCID: PMC6591954.
24. Zhou J, Troyanskaya OG. Predicting effects of noncoding variants with deep learning-based sequence model. Nat Methods. 2015;12:931–4. https://doi.org/10.1038/nmeth.3547.
25. Agarwal V, Shendure J. Predicting mRNA abundance directly from genomic sequence using deep convolutional neural networks. Cell Rep. 2020;31(7):107663. https://doi.org/10.1016/j.celrep.2020.107663.
26. de Sainte Agathe JM, Filser M, Isidor B, Besnard T, Gueguen P, Perrin A, Van Goethem C, Verebi C, Masingue M, Rendu J, Cossée M, Bergougnoux A, Frobert L, Buratti J, Lejeune É, Le Guern É, Pasquier F, Clot F, Kalatzis V, Roux AF, Cogné B, Baux D. SpliceAI-visual: a free

online tool to improve SpliceAI splicing variant interpretation. Hum Genomics. 2023;17(1):7. https://doi.org/10.1186/s40246-023-00451-1. PMID: 36765386; PMCID: PMC9912651.
27. Quang D, Xie X. FactorNet: a deep learning framework for predicting cell type specific transcription factor binding from nucleotide-resolution sequential data. Methods. 2019;166:40–7. https://doi.org/10.1016/j.ymeth.2019.03.020. Epub 2019 Mar 26. PMID: 30922998; PMCID: PMC6708499.
28. Middha S, Zhang L, Nafa K, et al. Reliable pan-cancer microsatellite instability assessment by using targeted next-generation sequencing data. Published online 3 Oct 2017.
29. Marcus L, Lemery SJ, Keegan P, et al. FDA approval summary: pembrolizumab for the treatment of microsatellite instability-high solid tumors. Clin Cancer Res. 2019;25(13):3753–8.
30. Kather JN, Pearson AT, Halama N, et al. Deep learning can predict microsatellite instability directly from histology in gastrointestinal cancer. Nat Med. 2019;25(7):1054–6. https://doi.org/10.1038/s41591-019-0462-y. Epub 2019 Jun 3
31. Yamashita R, Long J, Longacre T, Peng L, Berry G, Martin B, Higgins J, Rubin DL, Shen J. Deep learning model for the prediction of microsatellite instability in colorectal cancer: a diagnostic study. Lancet Oncol. 2021;22(1):132–41. https://doi.org/10.1016/S1470-2045(20)30535-0.).
32. Echle A, Grabsch HI, Quirke P, et al. Clinical-grade detection of microsatellite instability in colorectal tumors by deep learning. Gastroenterology. 2020;159(4):1406–1416.e11.
33. Dey P. In: Dey P, editor. Chapter 5: Pancancer biomarker in recent advances in pathology. New Delhi: Jaypee Brothers Medical Publishers Pvt Ltd; 2024.
34. https://www.fda.gov/drugs/drug-approvals-and-databases/fda-approves-pembrolizumab-adults-and-children-tmb-h-solid-tumors
35. Jain MS, Massoud TF. Predicting tumour mutational burden from histopathological images using multiscale deep learning. Nat Mach Intell. 2020;2:356–62.
36. Wang L, Jiao Y, Qiao Y, Zeng N, Yu R. A novel approach combined transfer learning and deep learning to predict TMB from histology image. Pattern Recogn Lett. 2020;135:244–8. https://doi.org/10.1016/j.patrec.2020.04.008.
37. Shimada Y, Okuda S, Watanabe Y, Tajima Y, Nagahashi M, Ichikawa H, Nakano M, Sakata J, Takii Y, Kawasaki T, Homma KI, Kamori T, Oki E, Ling Y, Takeuchi S, Wakai T. Histopathological characteristics and artificial intelligence for predicting tumor mutational burden-high colorectal cancer. J Gastroenterol. 2021;56(6):547–59. https://doi.org/10.1007/s00535-021-01789-w. Epub 2021 Apr 28.
38. Sørlie T, Perou CM, Tibshirani R, Aas T, Geisler S, Johnsen H, Hastie T, Eisen MB, van de Rijn M, Jeffrey SS, Thorsen T, Quist H, Matese JC, Brown PO, Botstein D, Lønning PE, Børresen-Dale AL. Gene expression patterns of breast carcinomas distinguish tumor subclasses with clinical implications. Proc Natl Acad Sci USA. 2001;98(19):10869–74. https://doi.org/10.1073/pnas.191367098. PMID: 11553815; PMCID: PMC58566.
39. Komor MA, Bosch LJ, Bounova G, Bolijn AS, Delis-van Diemen PM, Rausch C, et al. Consensus molecular subtype classification of colorectal adenomas: CMS classification of colorectal adenomas. J Pathol. 2018;246:266–76. https://doi.org/10.1002/path.5129.
40. Tothill RW, Tinker AV, George J, Brown R, Fox SB, Lade S, Johnson DS, Trivett MK, Etemadmoghadam D, Locandro B, Traficante N, Fereday S, Hung JA, Chiew YE, Haviv I, Australian Ovarian Cancer Study Group, Gertig D, de Fazio A, Bowtell DDL. Novel molecular subtypes of serous and endometrioid ovarian cancer linked to clinical outcome. Clin Cancer Res. 2008;14(16):5198–208. https://doi.org/10.1158/1078-0432.CCR-08-0196.
41. Gao F, Wang W, Tan M, Zhu L, Zhang Y, Fessler E, Vermeulen L, Wang X. DeepCC: a novel deep learning-based framework for cancer molecular subtype classification. Oncogene. 2019;8(9):44. https://doi.org/10.1038/s41389-019-0157-8. PMID: 31420533; PMCID: PMC6697729.
42. Hu F, Zhou Y, Wang Q, Yang Z, Shi Y, Chi Q. Gene expression classification of lung adenocarcinoma into molecular subtypes. IEEE/ACM Trans Comput Biol Bioinform. 2020;17:1187–97.

43. Woerl A-C, Eckstein M, Geiger J, Wagner DC, Daher T, Stenzel P, et al. Deep learning predicts molecular subtype of muscle-invasive bladder cancer from conventional histopathological slides. Eur Urol. 2020;78:256–64. https://doi.org/10.1016/j.eururo.2020.04.023.
44. Sundar R, Barr Kumarakulasinghe N, Huak Chan Y, et al. Machine-learning model derived gene signature predictive of paclitaxel survival benefit in gastric cancer: results from the randomised phase III SAMIT trial. Gut. 2022;71(4):676–85. https://doi.org/10.1136/gutjnl-2021-324060. Epub 2021 May 12. PMID: 33980610; PMCID: PMC8921574.
45. Kleppe A, Skrede OJ, De Raedt S, et al. A clinical decision support system optimising adjuvant chemotherapy for colorectal cancers by integrating deep learning and pathological staging markers: a development and validation study. Lancet Oncol. 2022;23(9):1221–32. https://doi.org/10.1016/S1470-2045(22)00391-6. Epub 2022 Aug 11.
46. Crispin-Ortuzar M, Woitek R, Reinius MAV, et al. Integrated radiogenomics models predict response to neoadjuvant chemotherapy in high grade serous ovarian cancer. Nat Commun. 2023;14(1):6756. https://doi.org/10.1038/s41467-023-41820-7. PMID: 37875466; PMCID: PMC10598212.
47. Cox DR. Regression models and life-tables (with discussion). J R Stat Soc Ser B Methodol. 1972;34(2):187–220.
48. Solvang HK, Lingjærde OC, Frigessi A, Børresen-Dale AL, Kristensen VN. Linear and non-linear dependencies between copy number aberrations and mRNA expression reveal distinct molecular pathways in breast cancer. BMC Bioinformatics. 2011;12:197.
49. Huang Z, Johnson TS, Han Z. Deep learning-based cancer survival prognosis from RNA-seq data: approaches and evaluations. BMC Med Genet. 2020;13(Suppl 5):41. https://doi.org/10.1186/s12920-020-0686-1. PMID: 32241264; PMCID: PMC7118823.
50. Ching T, Zhu X, Garmire LX. Cox-nnet: an artificial neural network method for prognosis prediction of high-throughput omics data. PLoS Comput Biol. 2018;14(4):e1006076. https://doi.org/10.1371/journal.pcbi.1006076. PMID: 29634719; PMCID: PMC5909924.
51. He B, Wang L, Zhou W, Liu H, Wang Y, Lv K, He K. A fusion model to predict the survival of colorectal cancer based on histopathological image and gene mutation. Sci Rep. 2025;15(1):9677. https://doi.org/10.1038/s41598-025-91420-2. PMID: 40113813; PMCID: PMC11926114.
52. Chereda H, Bleckmann A, Menck K, et al. Explaining decisions of graph convolutional neural networks: patient-specific molecular subnetworks responsible for metastasis prediction in breast cancer. Genome Med. 2021;13(1):42. https://doi.org/10.1186/s13073-021-00845-7. PMID: 33706810; PMCID: PMC7953710.
53. Saillard C, Schmauch B, Laifa O, Moarii M, Toldo S, Zaslavskiy M, Pronier E, Laurent A, Amaddeo G, Regnault H, Sommacale D, Ziol M, Pawlotsky JM, Mulé S, Luciani A, Wainrib G, Clozel T, Courtiol P, Calderaro J. Predicting survival after hepatocellular carcinoma resection using deep learning on histological slides. Hepatology. 2020;72(6):2000–13. https://doi.org/10.1002/hep.31207.
54. Hao J, Kosaraju SC, Tsaku NZ, Song DH, Kang M. PAGE-Net: interpretable and integrative deep learning for survival analysis using histopathological images and genomic data. Pac Symp Biocomput. 2020;25:355–66.
55. Tabibu S, Vinod PK, Jawahar CV. Pan-renal cell carcinoma classification and survival prediction from histopathology images using deep learning. Sci Rep. 2019;9(1):10509. https://doi.org/10.1038/s41598-019-46718-3. PMID: 31324828; PMCID: PMC6642160.
56. Chaudhary K, Poirion OB, Lu L, Garmire LX. Deep learning-based multi-omics integration robustly predicts survival in liver cancer. Clin Cancer Res. 2018;24:1248–59. https://doi.org/10.1158/1078-0432.CCR-17-0853.
57. Bychkov D, Linder N, Turkki R, Nordling S, Kovanen PE, Verrill C, Walliander M, Lundin M, Haglund C, Lundin J. Deep learning based tissue analysis predicts outcome in colorectal cancer. Sci Rep. 2018;8(1):3395. https://doi.org/10.1038/s41598-018-21758-3. PMID: 29467373; PMCID: PMC5821847.

58. Wang H, et al. Mitosis detection in breast cancer pathology images by combining handcrafted and convolutional neural network features. J Med Imaging (Bellingham). 2014;1:34003. https://doi.org/10.1117/1.JMI.1.3.034003.
59. Turkki R, Linder N, Kovanen P, Pellinen T, Lundin J. Antibody-supervised deep learning for quantification of tumor-infiltrating immune cells in hematoxylin and eosin stained breast cancer samples. J Pathol Inform. 2016;7:38. https://doi.org/10.4103/2153-3539.189703.
60. Widman AJ, Shah M, Frydendahl A, et al. Ultrasensitive plasma-based monitoring of tumor burden using machine-learning-guided signal enrichment. Nat Med. 2024;30(6):1655–66. https://doi.org/10.1038/s41591-024-03040-4. Epub 2024 Jun 14. PMID: 38877116; PMCID: PMC7616143.
61. Li A, Lou E, Leder K, Foo J. Early ctDNA kinetics as a dynamic biomarker of cancer treatment response. bioRxiv [Preprint]. 2024 Jul 3:2024.07.01.601508. doi: 10.1101/2024.07.01.601508. Update in: JCO Clin Cancer Inform. 2025 Mar;9:e2400160. doi: 10.1200/CCI-24-00160. PMID: 39005329; PMCID: PMC11244961.
62. Zhu G, Rahman CR, Getty V et al. Fragle: universal ctDNA quantification using deep learning of 2 fragmentomic profiles. BioRxiv 20 Sept 2023.
63. Esfahani MS, Hamilton EG, Mehrmohamadi M, et al. Inferring gene expression from cell-free DNA fragmentation profiles. Nat Biotechnol. 2022;40(4):585–97. https://doi.org/10.1038/s41587-022-01222-4. Epub 2022 Mar 31. PMID: 35361996; PMCID: PMC9337986.
64. Dercle L, Fronheiser M, Lu L, Du S, Hayes W, Leung DK, et al. Identification of non-small cell lung cancer sensitive to systemic cancer therapies using radiomics. Clin Cancer Res. 2020;26:2151–62.
65. You Y, Lai X, Pan Y, Zheng H, Vera J, Liu S, et al. Artificial intelligence in cancer target identification and drug discovery. Signal Transduct Target Ther. 2022;7(1):156. https://doi.org/10.1038/s41392-022-00994-0.
66. Medi K, Kazim YA, Craig M. Potential biomarkers and therapeutic targets in cervical cancer: insights from the meta-analysis of transcriptomics data within network biomedicine perspective. PLoS One. 2018;13:e0200717. https://doi.org/10.1371/journal.pone.0200717.
67. Cantini L, Medico E, Fortunato S, Caselle M. Detection of gene communities in multi-networks reveals cancer drivers. Sci Rep. 2015;5:17386. https://doi.org/10.1038/srep17386.
68. do Valle IF, et al. Network medicine framework shows that proximity of polyphenol targets and disease proteins predicts therapeutic effects of polyphenols. Nat Food. 2021;2:143–55. https://doi.org/10.1038/s43016-021-00243-7.
69. Tong Z, Zhou Y, Wang J. Identifying potential drug targets in hepatocellular carcinoma based on network analysis and one-class support vector machine. Sci Rep. 2019;9(1):10442.
70. López-Cortés A, Paz-Y-Miño C, Cabrera-Andrade A, Barigye SJ, Munteanu CR, González-Díaz H, Pazos A, Pérez-Castillo Y, Tejera E. Gene prioritization, communality analysis, networking and metabolic integrated pathway to better understand breast cancer pathogenesis. Sci Rep. 2018;8(1):16679. https://doi.org/10.1038/s41598-018-35149-1. PMID: 30420728; PMCID: PMC6232116
71. Gilvary C, Madhukar NS, Gayvert K, Foronda M, Perez A, Leslie CS, et al. A machine learning approach predicts essential genes and pharmacological targets in cancer. bioRxiv 692277. https://doi.org/10.1101/692277.
72. Nicolaou CA, Kannas C, Loizidou E. Multi-objective optimization methods in De novo drug design. Mini-Rev Med Chem. 2012;12:979–87. https://doi.org/10.2174/138955712802762284.
73. Burley SK, Berman HM, Bhikadiya C, Bi C, Chen L, Di Costanzo L, Christie C, Dalenberg K, Duarte JM, Dutta S, et al. RCSB protein data bank: biological macromolecular structures enabling research and education in fundamental biology, biomedicine, biotechnology and energy. Nucleic Acids Res. 2019;47:D464–74.
74. Mouchlis VD, Afantitis A, Serra A, Fratello M, Papadiamantis AG, Aidinis V, Lynch I, Greco D, Melagraki G. Advances in de novo drug design: from conventional to machine learning methods. Int J Mol Sci. 2021;22(4):1676.
75. Olivecrona M, Blaschke T, Engkvist O, Chen H. Molecular de-novo design through deep reinforcement learning. J Cheminform. 2017;9(1):48. https://doi.org/10.1186/s13321-017-0235-x. PMID: 29086083; PMCID: PMC5583141.

Part IV

Advanced Topics and Emerging Trends

12 Natural Language Processing and Its Role in Computational Cytology

Abstract

Natural language processing (NLP) deals with the interaction of computer and human language. Algorithmic model of NLP helps the computer to understand the human language, interpret it and then generates the response. It can handle both the written and oral form of language and can translate oral language into written form and vice versa. In health care & medical applications, NLP can extract structured data such as in a particular tumour it can extract information on tumour types, grades, morphological details, prognostic factors. The NLP typically uses deep learning particularly recurrent neural network. There are several challenges to implement NLP in routine practice in cytology such as unstructured data, complexity of data and privacy concerns. The current chapter discusses the basic principles and applications of NLP in computational cytology.

Keywords

Natural language processing · Deep learning · Language translation · Cytology reporting

12.1 Introduction

Natural language processing (NLP) is a part of artificial intelligence (AI) that deals with the interaction of computer and human language. Algorithmic model of NLP helps the computer to understand the human language, interpret it and then generate the response. NLP can deal both the written and oral form of language and can translate oral language into written form and vice versa. The NLP typically uses deep learning particularly recurrent neural network. There is a great prospect of NLP in the field of pathology/cytology [1].

P. Dey, *Computational Cytology*, https://doi.org/10.1007/978-981-95-3272-8_12

12.2 Importance of Natural Language Processing

Natural language processing is important for various reasons (Fig. 12.1):

1. *NLP facilitated human and computer communication*: It helps the virtual assistant to communicate with the human and provides instant response. In this way NLP diminishes the human workload.
2. *Information Extraction & Summarization*: NLP extracts information from large volume of text and process it in the accessible format.

   Example: The doctor wants the different treatment protocols of a particular cancer. Here, NLP provides the extract of all the published treatment protocol.
3. *Sentiment Analysis*: NLP analyses the sentiment of the text data. In medical report it can analyse the good or bad prognostic disease, successful treatment protocol etc.

   Example: CT scan detects majority of lung carcinoma but it has radiation hazards. NLP interprets the effectivity of CT scan in the detection of carcinoma of lung, but concerns about the health hazard of the technique.
4. *Healthcare & Medical Applications*: NLP is helpful in the medical diagnosis, and analysing the research work.

   Example: "A 60-year patient with back pain having 70% plasma cells in the bone marrow". Here, NLP answered:

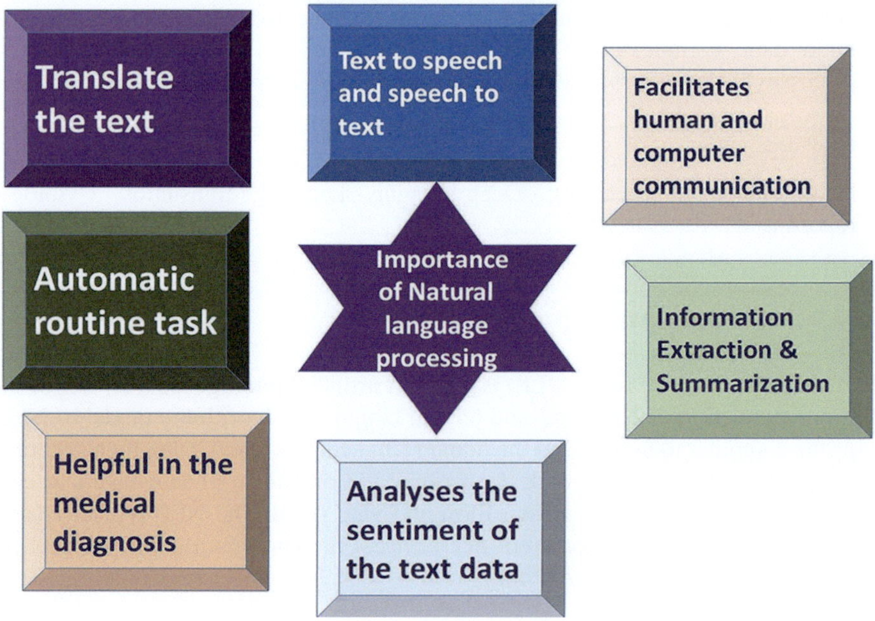

Fig. 12.1 Importance of natural language processing

Code

```
!pip install spacy scikit-learn
!python -m spacy download en_core_web_sm
import spacy
import re
# Load spaCy language model
nlp = spacy.load("en_core_web_sm")
# Sample clinical text
text = "A 60-year patient with back pain having 70% plasma cells in the bone marrow"
# Run NLP pipeline
doc = nlp(text)
# Extract named entities, POS and custom keywords
print("Entities:")
for ent in doc.ents:
    print(f"{ent.text} - {ent.label_}")
# Rule-based extraction
def extract_medical_info(text):
    age = re.findall(r'(\d+)-year', text)
    symptoms = re.findall(r'with (.+?) having', text)
    plasma_cells = re.findall(r'(\d+)% plasma cells', text)
    info = {
        "Age": int(age[0]) if age else None,
        "Symptom": symptoms[0] if symptoms else None,
       "Plasma Cell %": int(plasma_cells[0]) if plasma_cells else None
    }
    # Simple medical condition guess
    if info["Plasma Cell %"] and info["Plasma Cell %"] > 60:
        info["Possible Diagnosis"] = "Multiple Myeloma"
    else:
        info["Possible Diagnosis"] = "Unknown"
    return info
# Run function
info = extract_medical_info(text)
# Display extracted information
print("\nExtracted Info:")
for key, value in info.items():
    print(f"{key}: {value}")
```

Extracted Info and response:
Age: 60.
Symptom: back pain.
Plasma Cell %: 70.
Possible Diagnosis: Multiple Myeloma.

5. *Automatic routine task*: NLP performs many automatic routine tasks such as identifying spams in email, detecting frauds etc.
6. *Translation*: NLP can translate the text from one language to the other language.

   translate from English to Spanish by NLP "I love this planet earth. It is my mother."

   NLP Response: "Amo este planeta tierra, es mi madre".

   Code:

```
!pip install transformers sentencepiece
from transformers import MarianMTModel, MarianTokenizer
# Load the English to Spanish translation model
model_name = 'Helsinki-NLP/opus-mt-en-es'
tokenizer = MarianTokenizer.from_pretrained(model_name)
model = MarianMTModel.from_pretrained(model_name)
# Input text
text = "I love this planet earth. It is my mother."
# Tokenize input and translate
tokens = tokenizer(text, return_tensors="pt", padding=True, truncation=True)
translated = model.generate(**tokens)
# Decode output
translated_text = tokenizer.decode(translated[0], skip_special_tokens=True)
print("Translated Text:", translated_text)
```

7. *Text to speech and speech to text*: NLP can convert text data to speech and vice versa.

12.3 Principles of Natural Language Processing

The key principles of Natural Language Processing are following:

- *Sentence segmentation*: The model breaks the paragraph into sentences.
- *Tokenization*: It splits the sentence into words or tokens.
  Example: Pranab played football.
  Input: " Pranab played football"
  Tokens: ["Pranab ", " played ", " football "]
- *Lowercasing*: All the uppercases are converted to lowercases.
  New Delhi is the capital of India.
  Lowercasing Example: new delhi is the capital of india

- *Stop word Removal*: All the stop words (common words that do not have any meaning} are removed such as "the", "a", "an" etc.
  Example: The newspaper mentioned the violent earthquake in Tibet.
  newspaper mentioned violent earthquake Tibet
- *Punctuation Removal*: All the punctuations are removed.
  Example: Immunochemistry report: HER2: 3+, Ki67: 65%.
  Example: Immunochemistry report HER2 3+, Ki67 65%
- *Stemming*: Converts the words into their root form.
  Example: "walking", "swimming", "easily".
  After stemming: "walk", "swim", "easily"
- *Lemmatization*: It is almost same as stemming, but the root words bear some meaning.
  Example: "bathing", "flies", "running", "better", "ate".
  After lemmatization: "bath"," fly", "run", "good", "eat"
- *Part-of-Speech (POS) Tagging*: POS assigns the grammatical category of word within the sentence.
  Example: "Ramesh likes good fish".
  Ramesh: Noun.
  likes: verb.
  good: adjective.
  fish: pronoun
- *Named Entity Recognition (NER)*: NER identifies the named entity such as person's name, company, location, date etc.
  Example: Mrinal joined in Starlink in 2024.
  Mrinal = Person.
  Starlink = Company.
  2024 = Date
- *Syntax Parsing (Dependency Parsing)*: It analyses the grammatical structures of the sentence.
  Example: I love music.
  I = subject.
  Love = verb.
  Music = object
- *Semantic Analysis*: It means understanding the meaning of the word in the sentence.
  Example: The manager became red by seeing the product.
  Here "red" means angry.
- *Sentiment Analysis*: It means understanding the exact vibes of the expression.
  Example:
  The teacher feels *down* seeing the student's progress report: negative.
  The captain feels *great* after conquering the enemy's checkpoint: Positive.

12.4 Techniques in NLP

Several techniques are used in NLP in the pathology practice [2].

These are mentioned below:

1. *Rule-Based Approaches*: In rule-based approach manually created rules are used to process the human language. The rules are made by the linguistic and domain experts based on pattern matching, and strict pre-defined language rule.

   The components of Rule-Based Approaches:

   (a) *Lexicons*: It is a predefined vocabulary related with certain data such as.
   Word forms: walk: walks, walking, walk.
   Different entities of the name: name of person, organization, country.
   Part of speech (POS): Noun, pronoun, verb, adjective

   (b) *Grammar Rules*: It deals with grammatical rules.
   Parsing Rules: It determines the structure of a sentence such as subject-verb-object format.
   POS tagging rule**:** The set criteria to determine the verb, noun etc. such as word ends with "ing" is a verb.

   (c) *Pattern Matching*: It is used to determine the specific words, phrase or the construction of the sentence.
   Example: Medical diagnosis: If a patient has weakness, polyuria, and high blood sugar level then the patient has diabetes mellitus.
   Spam detection: If an e-mail contains "*Get the lottery prize*" and "*click the link*"

   (d) *Named Entity Recognition (NER)*: NER identifies the name, location, organization, date etc.
   Example: On July 2008, Pranab Dey became Professor in PGIMER.
   NER extraction will be in this Table 12.1.

   (e) *Knowledge Base & Ontology*: In Knowledge Base & Ontology, there is a store of facts regarding words, organization, relationships etc.

Advantages:

- Rule-Based Approach has high interpretability.
- It works well in medical coding.

Disadvantages:

- Introduction of any rule needs manual addition.
- It cannot manage linguistic variations.

Table 12.1 Named entity recognition

Entity	Category
July 2008	Date
Pranab Dey	Person
Professor	Title
PGIMER	Organizations (ORG)

2. *Statistical NLP*: Statistical NLP does not follow any rule based predefined laws. It mainly gives attention on the frequency of word, co-occurrence, and statistical patterns.

Example:

Incorrect sentence: Leena goes too school.

Correct sentence: Leena goes to school.

The model knows from the frequency of the word after "go" that 'too" is incorrect and it should be "to".

Advantages:

- It is efficient in the ambiguous cases.
- In case of enough data, Statistical NLP can adapt in different languages.

Disadvantages:

- It needs huge dataset to work.

3. *Machine Learning based Approaches*: It uses following algorithms:
   Support Vector Machines (SVM): Classification of medical report.
   Naïve Bayes: Detecting spam.
   Decision Trees & Random Forests: Feature based tasks.

Advantages:

- It can quickly adapt the new data and works well over time.
- It adopts better than rule based approaches.

Disadvantages:

- It requires labelled data.
- Manually designed features are needed.

4. *Deep Learning in NLP*: Modern NLP uses deep learning based algorithm [3].
   (a) *Recurrent Neural Networks* (RNNs): RNN is used for sequence based data processing. RNN can do text generation and NER. It often faces problem of vanishing gradient.
   (b) *Long Short-Term Memory* (LSTM): LSTM is a specialized form of RNN. It does not have vanishing gradient problem. LSTM manages long-term dependency learning [4].
   (c) *Gated Recurrent Unit* (GRU): GRU is a simplified form of LSTM and is computationally efficient as it deals with fewer parameters. GRU uses only reset and update gates.
   (d) *Convolutional Neural Networks* (CNNs) for NLP: CNN uses filters that capture the various features of text. It is efficient in classification of text and sentiment analysis.
   (e) *Transformer Models*: It is a revolutionary NLP model which uses self – attention mechanism. It is efficient as it does parallel processing of words.

The various transformer models are used such as Bidirectional Encoder Representations from Transformers (BERT), Generative Pre-Trained Transformer (GPT), Text-To-Text Transfer Transformer (T5).

Advantages:
- It can handle complex NLP with high accuracy.
- It can do multiple tasks.

Disadvantages:
- Huge dataset is required.
- Full interpretability is lacking due to “black box effect”.

The Table 12.2 compares the different NLP models.

Table 12.2 Comparison of different Natural Language Processing models

	Rule-Based NLP	Statistical NLP	Machine Learning NLP	Deep Learning NLP
Definition	Uses manually created already defined linguistic rules and patterns.	Uses statistic based probabilistic models in language	Uses machine learning algorithms to learn from text dataset	Applies deep neural networks in text dataset
Data dependency	Predetermined rules on the dataset	Huge dataset is needed to make probabilistic model	Labelled dataset needed	Huge dataset for training
Interpretability	High	Moderate	Moderate	Low due to Black-box effect
Accuracy	Low to moderate	Moderate	High	Very high
Scalability	Poor and manual update of rules is needed	Better	Good and it retraining helps in learning from new data	Excellent
Handling ambiguity	Poor	Moderate	Good	Excellent and it has the ability to understand deep contextual meaning
Common applications	Grammar correction.	Spelling check, Named Entity Recognition (NER).	Sentiment analysis and text classification	Automatic summarization, speech-to-text.
Training time	No training needed	Faster than machine learning.	Medium	High

12.5 Applications of Natural Language Processing (NLP) in Cytology/Pathology

The various applications of NLP are described below (Fig. 12.2).

1. Automated Structured Extraction of Diagnostic entities
   The pathology reports usually contain descriptive text data. NLP can help in following ways:
   - NLP can extract structured data such as in a particular tumour it can extract information on tumour types, grades, morphological details, prognostic factors etc. [5, 6]
   - It can help in the cancer registry by standardizing the terminologies.

Example: NLP algorithms can extract data from The Bethesda system reporting for thyroid cytopathology (TBSRTC) reports and can make a standardized data models for better clinical insights.

2. Enhancing Summarization of Cytopathology Report
   Pathologists generate complex reports and clinicians need the summary of the cytopathology report. NLP can:
   - Summarize the report by highlighting the salient diagnostic and prognostic points.
   - Generate structured reports that may be helpful to take clinical action.

Example: An NLP-based tool can automatically summarize lung cancer pathology reports, emphasizing tumour type, size, and receptor status.

3. Integration with Digital Cytology
   NLP may take important role by integrating the digital imaging particularly whole slide imaging (WSI) with the patient's metadata such as clinical information, textual cytology report, and laboratory reports.

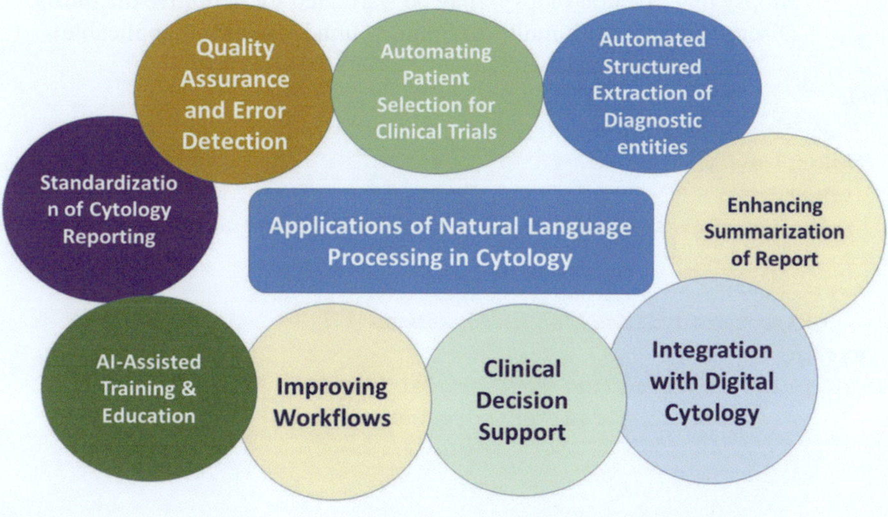

Fig. 12.2 The various applications of natural language processing in cytology

Example: In pleural effusion sample, NLP can match the reports describing "atypical cells suspicious for malignancy" with AI analysed digital image.

4. Clinical Decision Support (CDS) for Cytology Diagnoses
   NLP can help Clinical Decision Support (CDS) for the cytology diagnosis by:
   - Suggesting differential diagnosis based on the description of textural cytology report.
   - Providing cross-reference.
   - Giving clinical guidelines.
   - NLP based AI system can suggest immunocytochemistry, and further molecular tests.

Example:

Original Statement in cytology: A 57 Year Female, pleural effusion fluid reported as "Atypical cells suspicious for malignancy".

Comments by NLP:

Patient Information:

Age: 57

Gender: Female

Specimen Information:

Type: Pleural Effusion Fluid

Diagnosis Details:

Atypical Cells Present: True

Suspicious for Malignancy: True

Clinical Decision Support Recommendations:

- **High suspicion of malignancy.**
- Recommend further workup:

  Clinical correlation with patient history and imaging.

  Consider repeat cytology with cell block for ancillary studies (e.g., immunohistochemistry).

  Biopsy (e.g., pleural biopsy) may be warranted for definitive diagnosis.

  Discuss findings with multi-disciplinary tumour board (if applicable).

Code

```
import spacy
import re
# Load a pre-trained English NLP model (you might need to download it: python -m spacy
download en_core_web_sm)
try:
    nlp = spacy.load("en_core_web_sm")
except OSError:
    print("Downloading spaCy model 'en_core_web_sm'...")
    spacy.cli.download("en_core_web_sm")
```

```
    nlp = spacy.load("en_core_web_sm")
def analyze_cytology_report(report_text):
    """
    Analyzes a cytology report to extract key information and provide
    clinical decision support.
    """
    doc = nlp(report_text)
    patient_info = {
        "age": None,
        "gender": None
    }
    specimen_info = {
        "type": None
        }
    diagnosis_info = {
        "text": report_text,
        "malignancy_suspicion": False,
        "atypical_cells": False
    }
    decision_support_recommendations = []
    # --- 1. Extract Patient Demographics (Rule-based/Pattern Matching) ---
    age_match = re.search(r'(\d+)\s*Year', report_text, re.IGNORECASE)
    if age_match:
        patient_info["age"] = int(age_match.group(1))
    if re.search(r'Female', report_text, re.IGNORECASE):
        patient_info["gender"] = "Female"
    elif re.search(r'Male', report_text, re.IGNORECASE):
        patient_info["gender"] = "Male"
    # --- 2. Extract Specimen Type (Keyword Matching/NER) ---
    # spaCy's NER might identify "fluid" as a product, but we can refine
    if "pleural effusion fluid" in report_text.lower() or "pleural effusion" in report_text.lower():
        specimen_info["type"] = "Pleural Effusion Fluid"
    else:
        # Broader search for common fluid types if "pleural effusion" isn't present
        fluid_keywords = ["fluid", "effusion", "ascitic fluid", "peritoneal
fluid", "pericardial fluid", "CSF"]
        for token in doc:
            if token.text.lower() in fluid_keywords:
                specimen_info["type"] = token.text
                break
# --- 3. Analyze Diagnosis/Impression (Keyword/Phrase Matching) ---
    if re.search(r'atypical cells', report_text, re.IGNORECASE):
        diagnosis_info["atypical_cells"] = True
    if re.search(r'suspicious for malignancy', report_text, re.IGNORECASE) or \
```

```
         re.search(r'malignancy suspected', report_text, re.IGNORECASE) or \
         re.search(r'positive for malignancy', report_text, re.IGNORECASE):
            diagnosis_info["malignancy_suspicion"] = True
    # --- 4. Clinical Decision Support Logic ---
    if diagnosis_info["atypical_cells"] and diagnosis_info["malignancy_suspicion"]:
        recommendations = [
            "**High suspicion of malignancy.**",
            "Recommend further workup:",
            "- Clinical correlation with patient history and imaging.",
            "- Consider repeat cytology with cell block for ancillary studies (e.g., immunohistochemistry).",
            "- Biopsy (e.g., pleural biopsy) may be warranted for definitive diagnosis.",
            "- Discuss findings with multi-disciplinary tumor board (if applicable)."
        ]
        decision_support_recommendations.extend(recommendations)
    elif diagnosis_info["atypical_cells"] and not diagnosis_info["malignancy_suspicion"]:
        recommendations = [
            "**Atypical cells of uncertain significance.**",
            "Recommend:",
            "- Clinical correlation.",
            "- Consider follow-up cytology or further investigation if clinically indicated."
        ]
        decision_support_recommendations.extend(recommendations)
    else:
        decision_support_recommendations.append("Diagnosis does not indicate atypical cells or suspicion for malignancy based on current rules.")
    return {
        "patient_info": patient_info,
        "specimen_info": specimen_info,
        "diagnosis_info": diagnosis_info,
        "decision_support_recommendations": decision_support_recommendations
    }
# --- Example Usage ---
cytology_statement = "A 57 Year Female, pleural effusion fluid reported as \"Atypical cells suspicious for malignancy\""
analysis_results = analyze_cytology_report(cytology_statement)
print("--- Cytology Report Analysis ---")
print(f"Original Statement: {analysis_results['diagnosis_info']['text']}")
print("\nPatient Information:")
print(f"  Age: {analysis_results['patient_info']['age']}")
print(f"  Gender: {analysis_results['patient_info']['gender']}")
print("\nSpecimen Information:")
print(f"  Type: {analysis_results['specimen_info']['type']}")
print("\nDiagnosis Details:")
```

```
print(f"  Atypical Cells Present: {analysis_results['diagnosis_info']['atypical_cells']}")
print(f"  Suspicious for Malignancy: {analysis_results['diagnosis_info']['malignancy_suspicion']}")
print("\nClinical Decision Support Recommendations:")
for rec in analysis_results['decision_support_recommendations']:
    print(f"- {rec}")
# --- Another Example ---
print("\n--- Another Example: Atypical cells of uncertain significance ---")
another_statement = "A 62 Year Male, ascitic fluid reported as
\"Atypical glandular cells, favor reactive\""
another_analysis = analyze_cytology_report(another_statement)
print(f"Original Statement: {another_analysis['diagnosis_info']['text']}")
print("\nDecision Support:")
for rec in another_analysis['decision_support_recommendations']:
    print(f"- {rec}")
```

5. Improving Workflows of Pap Smear Screening
   NLP helps cervical cancer screening by:
   - Automated categorization of Bethesda report on cervical cytology.
   - Suggesting follow up and further investigations.
   - Prioritizing high-risk cases.

Example: NLP can detect phrases like "Atypical glandular cells favours neoplasia" in reports and flag cases for urgent management.

6. Standardization of Cytology Reporting
   NLP helps in the standardization of the cytology report across the different institutions by the following ways:
   - Textural cytology descriptions are converted into standard terminologies.
   - It may help in research and collaborative study by improving the consistency of data.
7. Quality Assurance and Error Detection in Cytology
   - NLP helps in detecting discrepancies and inconsistencies in cytology reports.
   - It may identify the missing critical information in the report.
   - It can highlight the proper follow-up recommendations in the cytology report.

   Example: NLP can flag a report on FNAC of thyroid with the diagnosis "Atypia of undetermined significance" without mentioning the further recommendations of repeat FNAC or other investigations.

8. Automating Patient Selection for Clinical Trials
   NLP takes important role for the selection of patients for clinical trial and research. The cases fulfilling the key criteria are identified by textural data analysis. In addition, information on biomarkers of the patients are also extracted for the trial of precision medicine.

   Example: In a research project, NLP can extract the data of EGFR positive adenocarcinoma of lung with the prognosis after specific therapy.

9. AI-Assisted Training & Education for Cytologists
   NLP assisted educational tool helps the students to understand the terminologies, and classification of diseases. AI can teach case-based learning to the students by analysing the cytology reports with the help of NLP.
   Example:
   An NLP model can help the students to understand Paris classification of urine cytology case by case.

12.6 Challenges in Application of NLP in Cytology

Complexity of Medical Language: Cytology reports often contain abbreviations, variable terminologies and jargon. It is a challenge to NLP to extract the real information from this complex text of medical report.

Data availability: A successful NLP needs high-quality annotated dataset for the training.

Unstructured data: The most cytology reports are unstructured and therefore difficult to standardize.

Computational Complexity: The deep-learning based NLP needs huge computational resources.

Integration with Healthcare Systems: NLP must be incorporated into laboratory information system (LIS) and other digital pathology platforms.

12.7 Conclusions

NLP is a very important part of computational cytology. It extracts necessary data from the text and summarize the cytology report. NLP helps in standardization of the report, improving cancer diagnosis and giving essential recommendations for the management of the patient. There are several challenges to implement NLP in routine practice in cytology such as unstructured data, complexity of data and privacy concerns. However, in future it is expected that NLP will overcome all these challenges and will be an essential tool in the cancer diagnosis, treatment and research.

References

1. López-Úbeda P, Martín-Noguerol T, Aneiros-Fernández J, Luna A. Natural language processing in pathology: current trends and future insights. Am J Pathol. 2022;192(11):1486–95.
2. Burger G, Abu-Hanna A, de Keizer N, Cornet R. Natural language processing in pathology: a scoping review. J Clin Pathol. 2016;69:949:jclinpath-2016-203872.
3. Minaee S, Kalchbrenner N, Cambria E, Nikzad N, Chenaghlu M, and Gao J. Deep learning based text classification: a comprehensive review. arXiv preprint arXiv:2004.03705. 2020.
4. Zhou C, Sun C, Liu Z, Lau F, A C-LSTM neural network for text classification. arXiv preprint arXiv:1511.08630. 2015.

5. Kim BJ, Merchant M, Zheng C, Thomas AA, Contreras R, Jacobsen SJ, Chien GW. A natural language processing program effectively extracts key pathologic findings from radical prostatectomy reports. J Endourol. 2014;28(12):1474–8.
6. Nguyen Wenker T, Natarajan Y, Caskey K, Novoa F, Mansour N, Pham HA, Hou JK, El-Serag HB, Thrift AP. Using natural language processing to automatically identify dysplasia in pathology reports for patients with Barrett's esophagus. Clin Gastroenterol Hepatol. 2023;21(5):1198–204.

13 Multimodal Data Fusion by Combining Imaging, Clinical and Molecular Data

Abstract

The rapid development in health care and research is responsible for the data explosion from diverse modalities such as clinical data, imaging data and molecular data. It is necessary to extract salient features from these multimodal datasets. Multimodal data fusion is the process that integrates the data acquired from different modalities to improve the diagnostic accuracy, management, and implementing personalized medicine. In addition, multimodal data fusion provides a complete understanding of the system. The level of data fusion may be in the early, intermediate and late stages. Autoencoders, Multi-Channel Neural Networks and Generative Adversarial Networks are used for data fusion. The present chapter discusses the technique of multimodal data fusion, challenges and its application in cytology.

Keywords

Multimodal data fusion · Autoencoders · Multi-channel neural networks · Generative adversarial networks

13.1 Introduction

The rapid development in health care and research leads to the accumulation of data from diverse modalities such as clinical data, imaging data and molecular data. Multimodal data fusion is the process that integrates the data acquired from different modalities to improve the diagnostic accuracy, management, and implementing personalized medicine. In addition, it provides a complete understanding of the system. The present chapter discusses the technique of multimodal data fusion, challenges and its application in cytology.

P. Dey, *Computational Cytology*, https://doi.org/10.1007/978-981-95-3272-8_13

13.2 Types of Data Modalities

- *Imaging Data*: It includes whole slide imaging of cytology or histopathology images, radiological images and other functional images.
- *Clinical Data*: Clinical data is mostly text data. It consists of data from the hospital information system (HIS), laboratory information system (LIS) and other necessary data related to the patient.
- *Molecular Data*: Molecular data includes next-generation sequencing data, proteomics and microbiome data.
- *Audio data*: speech, sounds
- *Sensor data*: temperature, various physiological signals

13.3 Level of Data Fusion

The level of data fusion may be in the early, intermediate and late levels.

13.3.1 Early Level Fusion

In early level fusion, the raw data derived from various modalities are fused at the input level before feature extraction (Fig. 13.1).

Example WSI image data of cytology is combined with the molecular data before feature extraction.

- *Advantages*:
  - The information of each modality is maximally preserved.
  - Potential to demonstrate rich correlations across different data modalities.
- *Challenges*:
  - Alignment of data is a problem.
  - As raw data is not modified much so there remains high dimensionality and data redundancy.

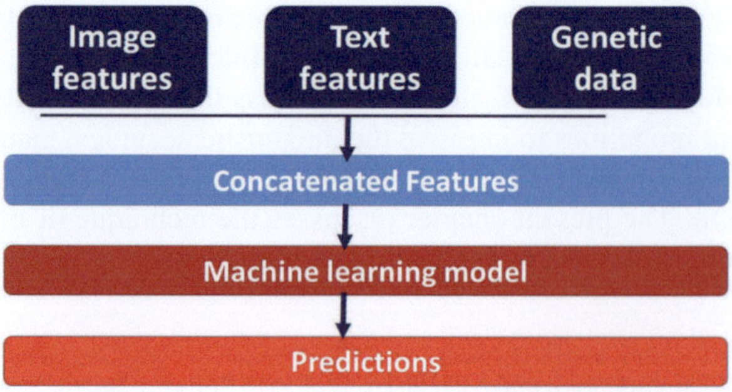

Fig. 13.1 Early fusion of data

13.3.2 Intermediate Fusion (Representation-Level Fusion)

In intermediate fusion, each modality of data is processed separately and the features are extracted. The data is then fused for analysis.

Examples The salient features are extracted from the WSI of a cytology smear. The molecular genomic data is also extracted by deep learning. Then the features of two modalities of data are combined and analysed.

- *Advantages*:
  - It reduces the complexity of raw data as the modality-specific features are extracted.
- *Challenges*:
  - In intermediate fusion, it needs proper feature extraction and reduction of dimension.
  - It may require intense computation.

13.3.3 Late Fusion (Decision-Level Fusion)

In late fusion, the individual data modalities are processed and analysed separately. After that, the individual model outputs, are derived initially, then all the outputs are further combined to make a final decision (Fig. 13.2).

Example The WSI of cytology smear and molecular genomic data are processed separately. The outputs are recorded for both WSI data, and molecular data. Then, finally both the outputs are combined to reach a final decision.

- *Advantages*:
  - No raw data fusion is needed
  - Robust to missing data

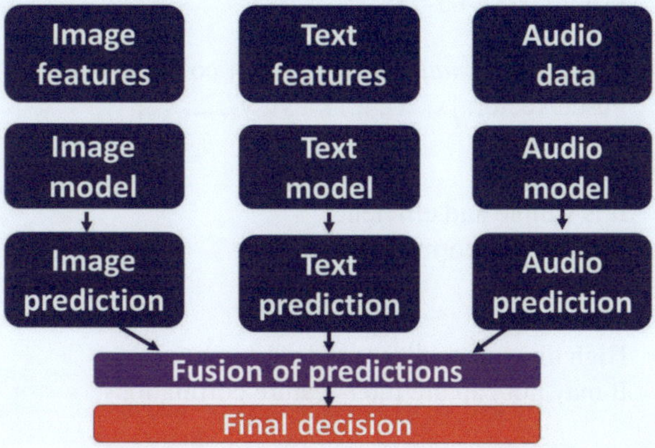

Fig. 13.2 Late level fusion

Table 13.1 Comparison of different levels of fusion

Level of fusion	Principle	Advantage	Algorithms used
Early	Raw data is fused	Information of each modality is maximally maintained	Concatenation-Based Fusion, Autoencoders, Multi-Channel Neural Networks, Generative Adversarial Networks
Intermediate	At first, features are extracted	Reduces the complexity of raw data	Deep Canonical Correlation Analysis, Graphical Neural Networks, Tensor Fusion Networks
Late	The fusion is done at the decision level	No raw data fusion is needed	Ensemble Learning, Meta-Learners

- *Challenges*:
  - Overall, less synergy between the different modalities of data

Table 13.1 compares the different levels of fusion.

13.4 Techniques for Multimodal Data Fusion

13.4.1 Early Fusion Technique

In the case of early fusion techniques, the raw data is combined from the multiple modalities before the feature extraction.

13.4.1.1 Concatenation-Based Fusion

Here, the raw data from the multiple sources are combined together into a single specific axis.

If you have two or more feature vectors:

- Feature vector x: $[x_1, x_2, ..., x_n]$
- Feature vector y: $[y_1, y_2, ..., y_m]$

Then *concatenation-based fusion* combines them as:
Fused vector: $[x_1, x_2, ..., x_n, y_1, y_2, ..., y_m]$

Advantages

- It is simple and efficient
- No loss of information

Disadvantages

- High dimensionality may lead to overfitting
- It may not capture inter-feature correlations.

13.4.1.2 Multi-Channel Neural Networks

In multi-channel neural networks, each channel focuses on one modality of data. Each channel is processed individually and finally the results are combined together to have the final prediction.

The Architecture Overview is shown in Fig. 13.3.

Advantages

- Spatial relationship of the different modalities of the data is retained.
- One can add more channels or different types of data.

Challenges

- It is computationally costly as we use multiple channels of data.
- Careful synchronization of inputs is needed.

13.4.1.3 Autoencoders (AEs)

Autoencoders is an unsupervised neural network. It encodes the input data into a compressed reorientation which is also called as latent space.

So it works as

- *Encoder*: Encodes input data into a latent vector.
- *Decoder*: Reconstructs the original input from the latent vector.

Architecture The architecture of the Autoencoder is highlighted in Fig. 13.4.

Advantages

- Learns compact, meaningful multimodal features.
- Missing data is successfully handled.
- Useful for downstream tasks like classification or generation.

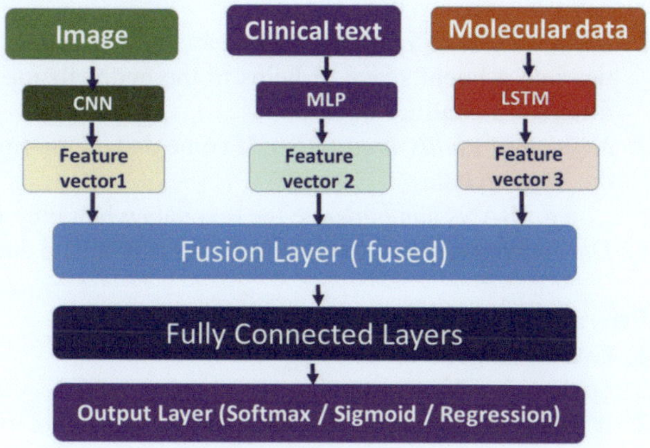

Fig. 13.3 Multi-channel neural networks

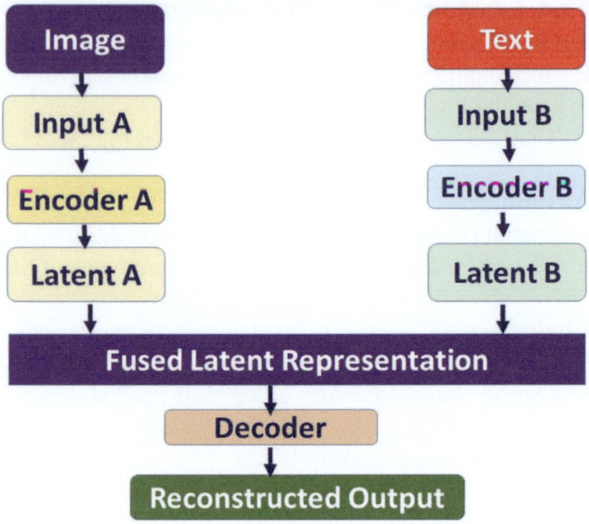

Fig. 13.4 The architecture of an Autoencoder

13.4.1.4 Generative Adversarial Networks (GANs)

GANs may help in multimodal data fusion in various ways.

1. *Cross-Modal Generation*: GANs can generate one data modality from another.

Example
- Text to image: If text data is provided, it can generate a practical image (Fig. 13.5).
- Image to text data (Fig. 13.6): It can generate text data from the images.
- MRI to CT scan: It can translate the radiological imaging.
- Image to sound: GANs can generate sound from an image or vice versa.

2. *Representation Learning*: GANs can learn to map different types of data modalities into a latent space. It helps in the better fusion of data and comparison of different modalities of data.
3. *Missing Modality Imputation*: If some data is missing, then GANs can generate the missing data.
   e.g., GANs can generate the text data when only image data is available.
4. *Data Augmentation*: GANs can artificially create data to enhance training.

Pros and Cons
1. GANs can generate missing data modalities.
2. GANs are difficult to train.
3. It is very difficult to assess the quality of data fusion.

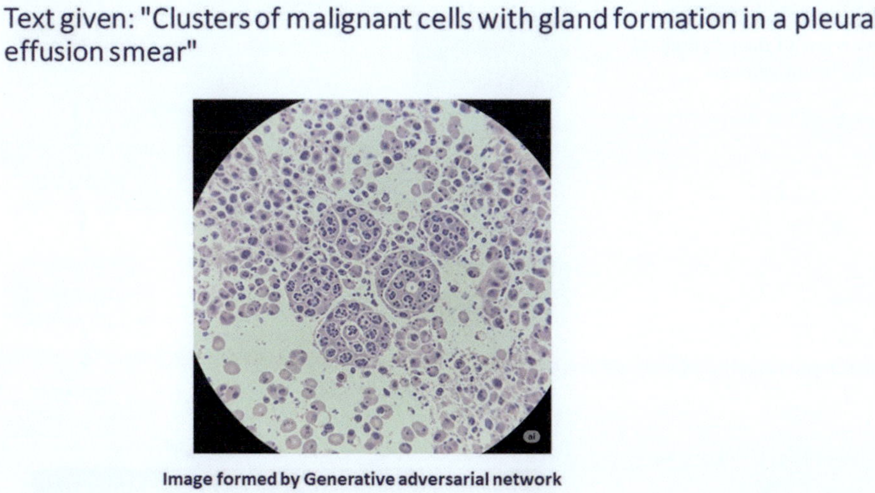

Fig. 13.5 Text to image. The image is formed by the given text

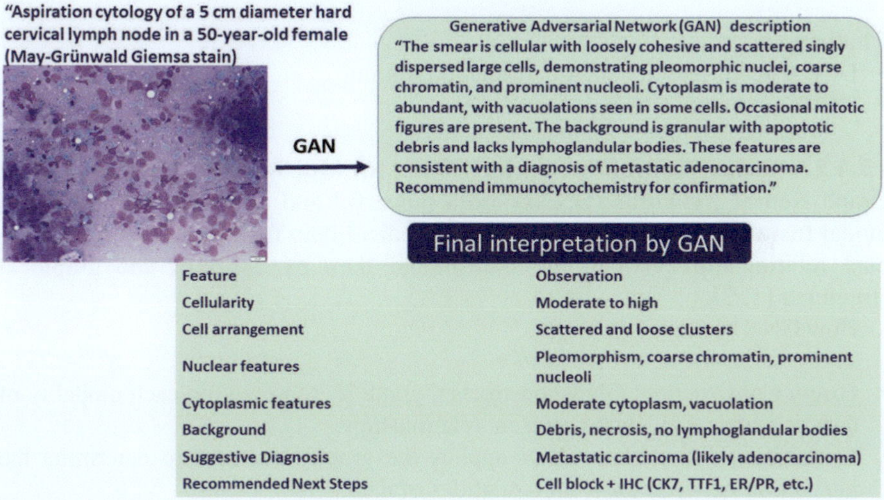

Fig. 13.6 Image to text data: Complete text data with interpretation is provided by GAN

13.4.2 Intermediate Fusion

These are techniques used in intermediate fusion:

- *Deep Canonical Correlation Analysis (DCCA)*: DCCA is commonly used for intermediate fusion. DCCA processes individual data modalities separately in deep networks in a shared latent space by maximizing correlation between them.

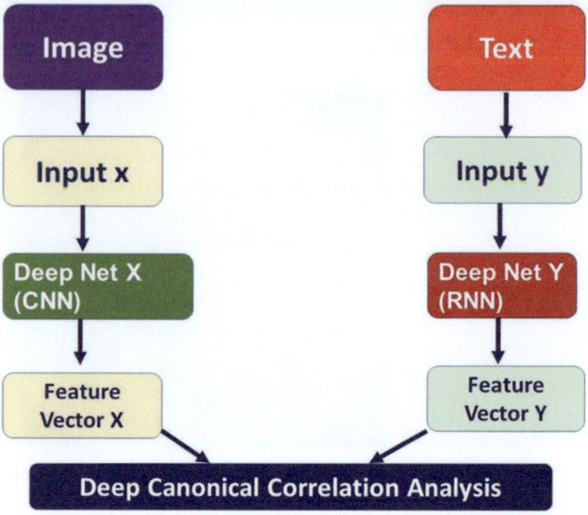

Fig. 13.7 Architectural overview of deep canonical correlation analysis

An architectural overview of DCCA is shown in Fig. 13.7.

Challenges

- DCCA needs paired data for correlation training.
- DCCA is sensitive to hyperparameters.

13.4.2.1 Graph Neural Networks (GNNs) for Multimodal Fusion

Graph Neural Networks (GNNs) are a powerful and effective tool for multimodal fusion. It is especially useful for medical data fusion to determine complex relationship between the multimodal data by applying the graphical structures [1, 2].

How GNN works

- *Graph Construction*: GNN constructs a graph by representing each modality of data as a node and edges represent relationships.
- *Information Interaction:* GNN applies the graph structures to determine the interaction between different modalities of data.
- *Intra-modal Context*: GNN captures contextual information between each modalities of data.
- *Inter-modal Complementary Information*: GNN helps to determine the complementary information between different modalities of data.

Advantage GNN is very good for structured, interconnected data.

13.4.2.2 Tensor Fusion Networks (TFN)

Tensor Fusion Networks (TFN) is a powerful tool for multimodal data fusion.

It works by (Fig. 13.8):

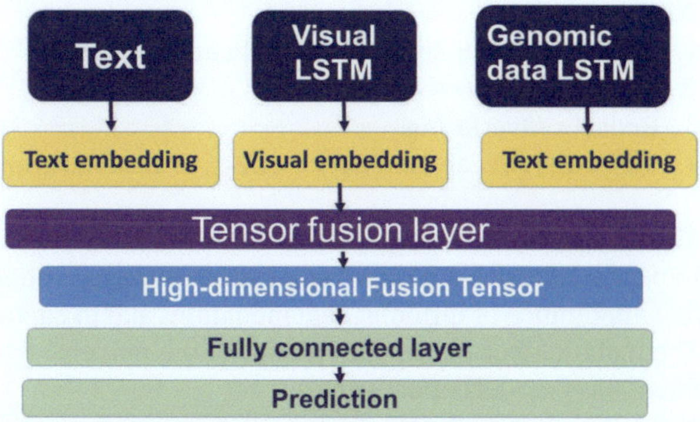

Fig. 13.8 Tensor flow multimodal data fusion (LSTM Long Short-Term Memory)

1. *Tensor Fusion Layer formation*: TFN generates a multimodal tensor that interacts with all the data modalities. The 3D tensors identify all possible interactions between the data modalities.
2. *Fully Connected Layers*: After generating the fusion tensor, one or more fully connected layers are formed to create the final predictions.

Example TFN can be applied to generate meaningful interaction between radiology, genomics and pathology.

Advantages of TFN

- *Multimodal interaction modelling*: TFN maintains high-order correlations between different data modalities.
- *Flexible*: TFN can work with any number of modalities.

13.4.3 Late Fusion (Decision-Level Fusion) Techniques

In the late fusion technique, the different modalities of the data are trained individually and finally integrated to predict. The following techniques are used in late fusion:

13.4.3.1 Ensemble Learning

Ensemble Learning combines predictions from multiple modalities of data by using majority voting, weighted averaging or meta-learning [3].

Common ensemble methods are:

- Bagging
- Boosting
- Stacking: Here, the initial model's output is combined by another model.
- Voting

Application In healthcare, ensemble learning is applied to combine clinical data, images (WSI/ CT scan/MRI) or other data for diagnosis.

Advantage

1. Improved Accuracy: It provides better prediction
2. Simple and effective
3. Reduces Overfitting
4. Versatility**:** It can be used for effective classification

13.4.3.2 Neural Network-Based Meta-Learners

In neural Network-Based Meta-Learners, a meta-model is applied to learn the relative importance of different data modalities and to capture cross-modal interactions. The meta-learner means the "model of the models" that learns to combine the different base models effectively.

How it works

1. *Train base models*: Individual data modalities are trained.
2. *Extract outputs*: The output from each data modality is extracted.
3. *The output data is incorporated into a neural network meta-learner*: Meta-learner learns to combine the features for the final prediction.
4. *End-to-end fine-tuning*: At times, fine-tuning of the base models and the meta-learner may be needed.

Advantages

1. *Captures complex relationships* between different data modalities.
2. *Better performance*: It is efficient in classification.
3. *Adaptive weighting*: the network learns the importance of the particular modality in a particular situation.

13.4.3.3 Applications of Multimodal Data Fusion

Healthcare

- *Diagnosis*: Multimodal data fusion combines WSI, radiological images (MRI/CT scan), clinical data and genetic data to reach a comprehensive diagnosis.
- *Patient Monitoring*: The combination of electronic health records and real-time vitals may have an immense role in patient monitoring.

Autonomous Systems

- *Self-driving Cars*: Integrating radar, cameras, GPS, and vehicle sensors help in automatic self-driving car to work.
- *Robotics*: Combining tactile, vision, and auditory data for robotics.

Others

- *Sentiment Analysis*: Combining and analysing facial expressions, audio, and textual content to assess sentiment.
- *Biometric Systems*: Multimodal data fusion combines fingerprint, face recognition, and voice recognition to identify the person.

13.4.3.4 Challenges in Multimodal Fusion

- *Data Alignment and Synchronization*: In the early fusion level, alignment of data and synchronization are great challenges.
- *Missing or Incomplete Data Modalities*: In real world, the data may often be incomplete or missing.
- *Data Modality dominance*: At times, the particular modality of data may be of higher volume and of high quality. This data modality may dominate leading to data imbalance.

13.5 Conclusions

Multimodal data fusion is a challenging area of artificial intelligence. By incorporating the multimodal data, a more sensitive system can be generated that will be able to diagnose reasonably and accurately along with proper management of the patient and prognostic assessment. Multimodal data fusion is not simply combining different modalities of data but creating a holistic perception of the machine. We expect that in the future it will take a great role in computational cytology.

References

1. D'Souza NS, Wang H, Giovannini A, Foncubierta-Rodriguez A, Beck KL, Boyko O, Syeda-Mahmood TF. Fusing modalities by multiplexed graph neural networks for outcome prediction from medical data and beyond. Med Image Anal. 2024;93:103064. https://doi.org/10.1016/j.media.2023.103064. Epub 2023 Dec 27.
2. Xing T, Dou Y, Chen X, et al. An adaptive multi-graph neural network with multimodal feature fusion learning for MDD detection. Sci Rep. 2024;14:28400. https://doi.org/10.1038/s41598-024-79981-0.
3. Ding W, Wu S, Nugent C. A multimodal fusion enabled ensemble approach for human activity recognition in smart homes. Health Informatics J. 2023;29(2) https://doi.org/10.1177/14604582231171927.

14 Applications of Quantum Computation in Artificial Neural Network: Opportunities and Challenges

Abstract

Quantum neural network is one of the advanced technologies in the field of artificial intelligence and machine learning. The quantum nature of the network provides many added advantages of the network such as high speed of learning, handling complex topology of the network and optimization of the hyperparameters.

In this chapter, the basic concepts, application in pathology, advantages, and challenges of the quantum neural network are discussed.

Keywords

Quantum physics · Neural network · Deep learning · Artificial neural network · Quantum computing

14.1 Introduction

Recently, machine learning technology has been an emerging field in medical systems, including pathology. Machine learning includes artificial neural networks and deep learning [1, 2]. Deep learning deals with images and huge data that need high speed and many advanced computational capabilities. This is particularly true for the histopathology sections that deal with whole slide imaging with huge data. Moreover, molecular technique including the data of next-generation sequencing, clinical data and other ancillary data demands high-speed learning technique of an artificial neural network. Quantum computing is the most promising area of computer science that applies the technology of quantum physics and has immense capability to solve many complex problems that cannot be solved by traditional computers. Quantum computing applies the various properties of the quantum dynamics, such as superposition, quantum entanglement and

P. Dey, *Computational Cytology*, https://doi.org/10.1007/978-981-95-3272-8_14

interference [3]. The amalgamation of technology of quantum computation and machine learning is innovative and can produce an extremely powerful quantum machine learning (QML) technology [4]. Quantum artificial neural network (QNN) is a part of QML. The major works in this field are in progress. In the present paper, the basic concepts of quantum deep learning, its achievements and challenges are discussed.

14.2 The Unique Characteristics of Quantum Dynamics

Quantum dynamics has certain interesting characteristics:

- Quantum superposition: Quantum superposition is one of the basic principles of quantum dynamics. It means that the quantum system can remain in multiple states till you measure it.
- Quantum entanglement: Quantum entanglement is a strange phenomenon that says if two entangled subatomic particles are separated by a large distance (even by billions of light-years), the identification of one particle describes the state of the other particle.
- Quantum tunnelling: Quantum tunnelling is a peculiar mechanical phenomenon when a particle can cross a potential energy barrier.

14.3 How Quantum Computing Differs from Traditional Computing

The traditional computer uses bits. The bit is the basic unit of information. The bit may be 0 or 1 (off or on). At any one point in time, the bit may be either of these phases, 0 or 1. However, in quantum computation, we use quantum bits or qubits, the basic unit of the quantum computer (Fig. 14.1). Unlike the traditional bit, the qubit [5] may be in 0, 1 or in the coherent superposition state of both 0 and 1. In a classical computer, n number of bits represents only one value between 0 and 2^{n-1}. Whereas in the qubit, the n number of values represents 2^n values at the same time. When multiple qubits are used in the computer, they are connected by quantum entanglement. The identification of the first qubit immediately identifies the second qubit. Table 14.1 highlights the differences between the traditional bits and qubits.

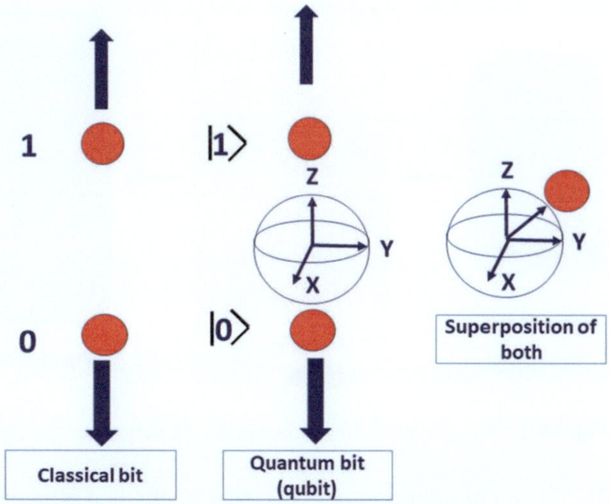

Fig. 14.1 The schematic diagram showing the characteristics of a classical bit and a quantum bit (Qubit)

Table 14.1 Qubit versus ordinary traditional bit

Features	Bit	Qubit
Computer	The traditional computer uses bit	The quantum computer uses qubit
Work function	The traditional computer uses bit by logical gates such as AND, OR, etc	The quantum computer uses a qubit in quantum logic.
State	At any point in time, the bit may be either 0 or 1	At any point in time, the bit may be 0, 1 or a superimposition of these bits.
Speed of work	Bits work slowly	Qubits work very fast
Circuit behaviour	The circuit behaviour of the bit follows the laws of classical physics	The circuit behaviour of the qubit follows the laws of quantum physics

14.4 Various Models of the Quantum Neural Network

A. *Parametrized quantum circuits (PQCs)*: PQC is a hybrid quantum and classical algorithm which is composed of a set of parametrized qubit gates with noise, and the parameters are tuned to solve the desired task. PQC maintains the power of quantum supremacy or quantum advantages [6]. The variational quantum algorithm (VQA) is a type of PQC-dependent protocol. Here, the classical data is translated into a quantum state known as quantum embedding. Unlike classical artificial neural networks, VQA uses quantum entanglement as an activation function. The VQA operates in three stages (Fig. 14.2): (A) Data encoding: Here, the classical or quantum data is loaded into the quantum circuit with the help of a quantum operation. (B) Variational Ansatz: This consists of multiple layers of repeated applications of the operation. (C) Measurement: The qubit is measured to get the relevant information [7].

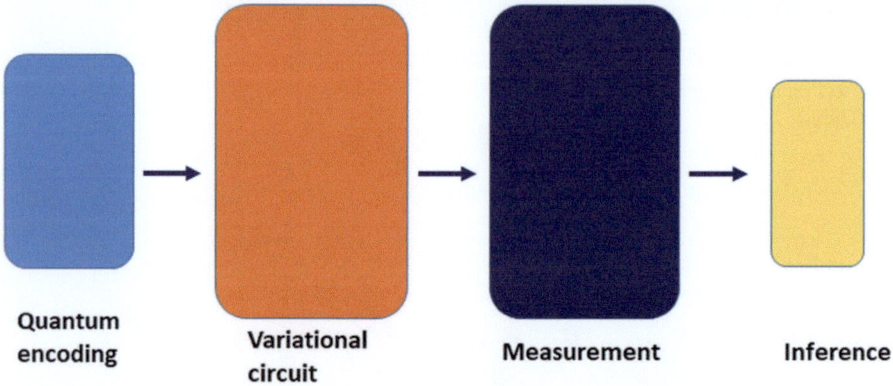

Fig. 14.2 The schematic diagram showing the variational quantum algorithm

B. *Quantum neural network (QNN)*: QNN is a type of parametrized quantum circuit. Figure 14.3a and b describe the simple ANN and QNN. In the case of QNN, the classical data is encoded into qubits. The qubit state is then processed through multiple parametrized layers. Finally, the qubits are measured and interpreted. QNN has the major advantage of speed and performance over the ordinary ANN [8].
C. *Quantum convolutional neural network (QCNN)*: In QCNN, the repeated convolutional and pooling layers are done in the quantum circuits [9].

   At first like QNN, the classical input data is encoded into a qubit state. The repeated convolution and pooling operations are done in the quantum circuit till we get a sufficiently small-sized feature map. Finally, the outcome of the system is obtained by measuring the desired small number of qubit states (Fig. 14.4). Till now, the QCNN has not proved as a better performing network than the classical CNN. However, it is expected that QCNN will show better performance if we do it in a completely quantum environment with natural qubit data.
D. *Quantum Kernel methods*: In the quantum kernel method (QKM), the input data is mapped into a higher-dimensional vector space. The QKM finally computes the kernel functions by applying the quantum computer. By mapping the data into higher-dimensional space, it is possible to do the classification which is ordinarily impossible to do by the low-dimensional representation of data. The QKM is very expressive as the dimension of the kernel data is infinite [10].

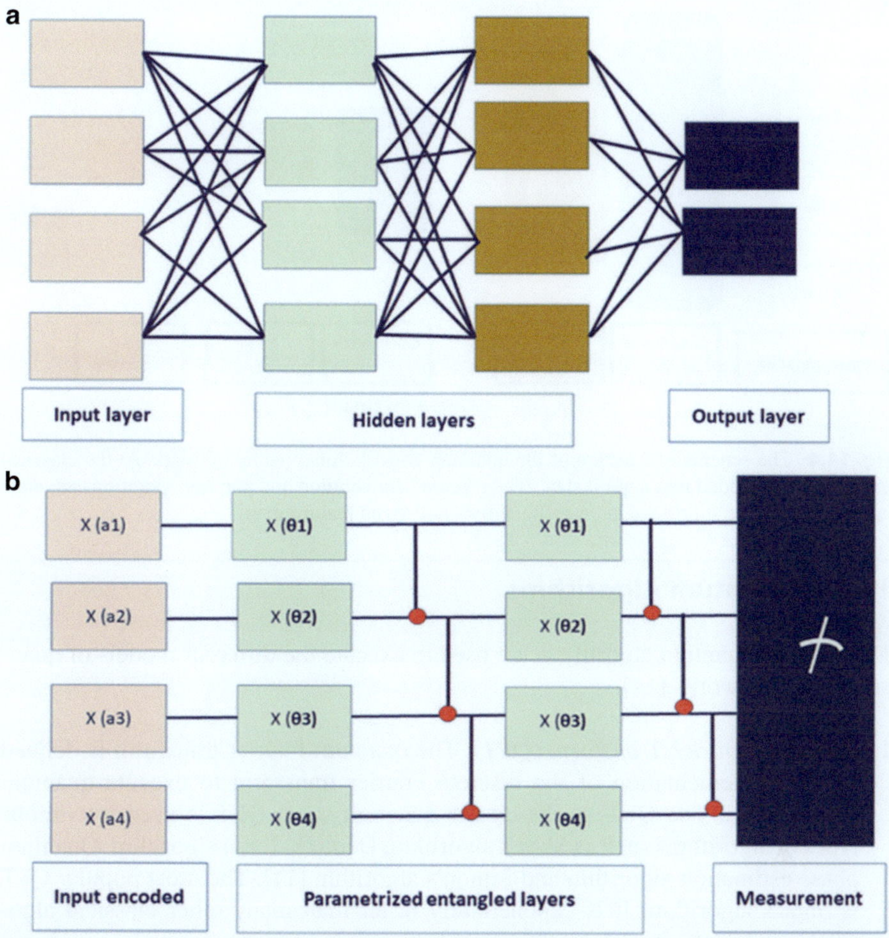

Fig. 14.3 (**a**) Traditional artificial neural network is composed of an input layer, a hidden layer and an output layer. (**b**) The quantum neural network is almost similar to that of traditional artificial neural networks. The input data is encoded into a qubit. The qubit state is processed through multiple parametrized layers, and finally, the qubits are measured and interpreted.

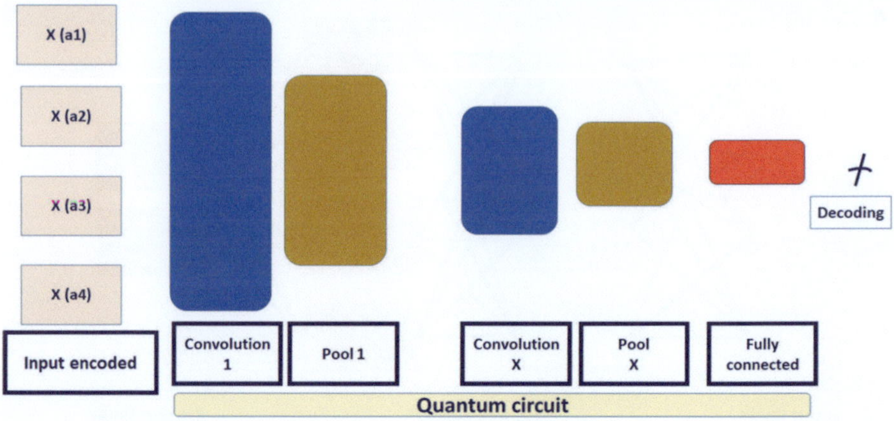

Fig. 14.4 The schematic diagram of the quantum convolutional neural network. At the classical input, data is encoded into a qubit state. The repeated convolution and pooling operations are done in the quantum circuit till we get a sufficiently small-sized feature map

14.5 Quantum Algorithms

The various Quantum algorithms are used to execute the different models of quantum neural networks [11].

1. *Quantum Fourier Transform (QFT)*: The quantum Fourier transform is defined as the implementation of the discrete Fourier transform to execute quantum computation. The QFT works on the quantum state. QFT is used by various types of algorithms such as Shor's algorithm, Deutsch-Jozsa algorithm, Quantum phase estimation algorithm and Simon's algorithm [11]. The most popular QFT is Shor's algorithm. It is exponentially faster than many other classical algorithms and is effective for polynomial time problems [12].
2. *Amplitude amplification algorithm*: It mainly deals with the amplitude and frequency of the quantum state. Grover's algorithm is the most commonly used amplitude amplification algorithm which is equally fast as Shor's algorithm [13].
3. *Quantum walks algorithm*: It is just like the classical random walk. The quantum walks algorithm is highly suitable to speed up the black box challenges [14]. The commonly used quantum walk algorithms are complete knot invariants and quantum simulation.
4. *Hybrid algorithm*: The Hybrid algorithm combines both quantum and classical algorithms. It is designed to take the benefits of "the best of both worlds". The commonly used hybrid algorithms are QADA and variational quantum eigensolver [15, 16].

5. *Bounded-error quantum polynomial time (BQP)*: BQP algorithm runs in polynomial time. The commonly used BQP algorithms are quantum simulation, solving linear systems of equations and computing knot invariants [17].

14.6 Advantages of the Quantum Neural Network

Quantum computer is supposed to be superior to their classical counterpart which is popularly known as quantum supremacy [18].

(a) *High-speed training time*: QNN has the quantum properties such as quantum coherence, superimposition and quantum entanglement. So, it can process data at high speed which cannot be done by a classical computer.
(b) *Handling complex topology*: The QNN has the immense capability to handle the complex topology of the deep learning network which may not be possible for the traditional computer. In addition, the quantum associative memory algorithm may help to store the data exponentially.
(c) *Automated optimization of the hyperparameters*: QNN has the potential to automatically adjust various hyperparameters such as the rate of learning, number of hidden layers, and number of iterations. Quantum entanglement or non-locality, the crucial characteristics of the QNN, help in the auto adjustment of the hyperparameters.
(d) *Manipulation of the tensor*: The other unique advantage of QNN is to handle the complex matrix and tensor in a very high speed [19]. Tensors are the fundamental pieces that help to build up the quantum state and quantum entanglement helps to adhere these pieces.
(e) *Quantum tunnelling effect*: The ordinary ANN uses gradient descent to reach the optimization of the neural network. However, QNN applies the quantum tunnelling phenomenon to achieve the true objective goal (Fig. 14.5) [20].

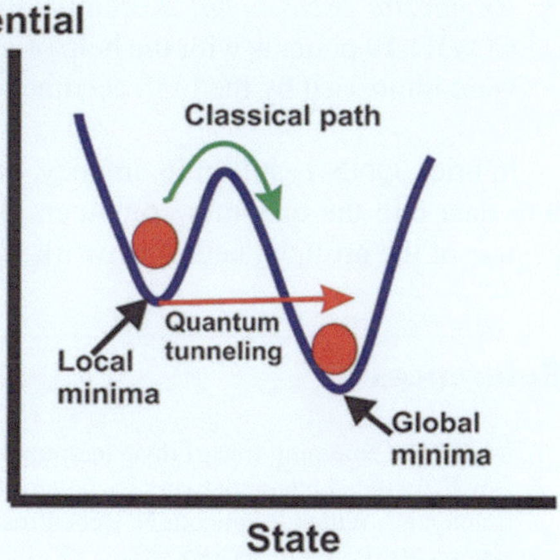

Fig. 14.5 The quantum tunneling effect bypasses the classical gradient

14.7 Limitations of Quantum Neural Network

Quantum data set In the QNN, commonly, the classical data is encoded into a quantum data set which means the classical bits are converted into qubits. However, till now, it is not clear how to perfectly encode the classical data set into the quantum bits [21]. The quantum data may be more promising than the classical data encoded into quantum bits [22].

Barren plateau Barren plateau indicates the vanishing gradient of the quantum landscape with an increasing number of qubits. This is the major challenge of the QNN. The possible reasons for barren plateau include global cost functions [23], high noise [24] and large entanglements. The barren plateau can be avoided by layer-by-layer training, pre-training and local cost function [25].

14.8 Applications of Quantum Neural Network in Pathology

Currently, there are a limited number of publications in this emerging field.

1. *Disease identification*: Hybrid Quantum machine learning is used in the histopathology section of skin to detect early skin cancer [26].
2. *Disease classification*: Jain S et al. first used quantum machine learning (QML)with the help of a quantum Boltzmann machine to distinguish adenocarcinoma and squamous cell carcinoma of the lung based on the gene expression data of 104 lung cancer patients [27]. In another study, the QML technique was applied to classify several types of cancer (brain, breast, kidney, lung, liver and colorectal cancers) based on the molecular data from Cancer Genome Atlas [28]. Iliyasu AM et al. applied QML to identify dysplastic cells in cervical lesions [29]. They considered the technique crucial for cervical cancer detection.
3. *Prognostic assessment*: Recently, El-shafeiy et al. predicted the outcome of COVID-19 patients with the help of a quantum neural network [30]. The authors were impressed by the high accuracy and effectiveness of QNN.

In brief, QNN is still in its infancy. In the future, we need to have natural quantum data into the quantum computer. Quantum computation is a completely new avenue of the artificial neural network with immense potential.

References

1. Dey P. The emerging role of deep learning in cytology. Cytopathology. 2021;32(2):154–60.
2. Dey P. Artificial neural network in diagnostic cytology. Cytojournal. 2022;19:27.
3. Biamonte J, Wittek P, Pancotti N, Rebentrost P, Wiebe N, Lloyd S. Quantum machine learning. Nature. 2017;549(7671):195–202.

4. Cerezo M, Verdon G, Huang HY, et al. Challenges and opportunities in quantum machine learning. Nat Comput Sci. 2022;2:567–76.
5. Tzyy-Chyang L, Gwo-Ruey Y, Juang J-C. Quantum-based algorithm for optimizing artificial neural networks. IEEE Trans Neural Netw Learn Syst. 2013;8:1266–78.
6. Farhi E, Harrow AW. Quantum supremacy through the quantum approximate optimization algorithm. arXiv preprint arXiv:2016. https://doi.org/10.48550/arXiv.1602.07674.
7. Biamonte J. Universal variational quantum computation. Phys Rev A. 2021;103:L030401.
8. Oh S, Choi J, Kim J-K, Kim J. Quantum convolutional neural network for resource-efficient image classification: a quantum random access memory (QRAM) approach. In: Proceedings of the IEEE International Conference on Information Networking (ICOIN); 2021. p. 50–2.
9. Cong I, Choi S, Lukin MD. Quantum convolutional neural networks. Nat Phys. 2019;15:1273–8.
10. Havlíček V. Supervised learning with quantum-enhanced feature spaces. Nature. 2019;567:209–12.
11. García DP, Cruz-Benito J, García-Peñalvo FJ. Systematic literature review: quantum machine learning and its applications; 2022. https://doi.org/10.48550/arXiv.2201.04093.
12. Shor PW. Algorithms for quantum computation: discrete logarithms and factoring. In: Proceedings of the 35th Annual Symposium on Foundations of Computer Science; 1994. p. 124–34.
13. Lin J, Ye M, Zhu JW, Li XP. Machine learning assisted quantum adiabatic algorithm design. Acta Phys Sin. 2021;70(14):140306.
14. Childs AM. Universal computation by quantum walk. Phys Rev Lett. 2009;102(18):180501.
15. Farhi E, Goldstone J, Gutmann S. A quantum approximate optimization algorithm; 2014. https://doi.org/10.48550/arXiv.1411.4028.
16. Ryabinkin IG, Genin SN, Izmaylov AF. Constrained variational quantum eigensolver: quantum computer search engine in the Fock space. J Chem Theor Comput. 2018;15(1):249–55.
17. Aaronson S. BQP and the polynomial hierarchy. In: Proceedings of the 43rd ACM Symposium on Theory of Computing. (STOC); 2010. p. 141–50.
18. Harrow AW, Montanaro A. Quantum computational supremacy. Nature. 2017;549(7671):203–9.
19. Das S, Khatri S, Dowling JP. Robust quantum network architectures and topologies for entanglement distribution. Phys Rev A. 97(1):012335.
20. Ohzeki M, Okada S, Terabe M, et al. Optimization of neural networks via finite-value quantum fluctuations. Sci Rep. 2018;8:9950.
21. Havlíček V, Córcoles AD, Temme K, Harrow AW, Kandala A, Chow JM, Gambetta JM. Supervised learning with quantum-enhanced feature spaces. Nature. 2019;7747:209–12.
22. Huang HY, Broughton M, Cotler J, Chen S, Li J, Mohseni M, Neven H, Babbush R, Kueng R, Preskill J, McClean JR. Quantum advantage in learning from experiments. Science. 2022;6598:1182–6.
23. Cerezo M, Sone A, Volkoff T, Cincio L, Coles PJ. Cost function dependent barren plateaus in shallow parametrized quantum circuits. Nat Commun. 2021;12(1):1791.
24. Wang S, Fontana E, Cerezo M, Sharma K, Sone A, Cincio L, Coles PJ. Noise-induced barren plateaus in variational quantum algorithms. Nat Commun. 2021;12(1):6961.
25. Grant E, Wossnig L, Ostaszewski M, Benedetti M. An initialization strategy for addressing barren plateaus in parametrized quantum circuits. Quantum. 2019;3:214.
26. Iyer V, Ganti B, Hima Vyshnavi AM, Krishnan Namboori PK, Iyer S. Hybrid quantum computing based early detection of skin cancer. J Interdiscip. 2020;23(2):347–55.
27. Jain S, Ziauddin J, Leonchyk P, Yenkanchi S, Geraci J. Quantum and classical machine learning for the classi_cation of non-small-cell lung cancer patients. Social Netw Appl Sci. 2020;2(6):1–10.
28. Li RY, Gujja S, Bajaj SR, Gamel OE, Cilfone N, Gulcher JR, Lidar DA, Chittenden TW. Quantum processor-inspired machine learning in the biomedical sciences. Patterns (N Y). 2021;2(6):100246.

29. Iliyasu AM, Fatichah C. A quantum hybrid PSO combined with fuzzy k-NN approach to feature selection and cell classification in cervical cancer detection. Sensors (Basel). 2017;17(12):2935.
30. El-shafeiy E, Ella Hassanien A, Sallam AKM, Abohany AA. Approach for training quantum neural network to predict severity of COVID-19 in patients. Comput Mater Contin. 2021;66(2):1745–55.

Advanced Techniques in Artificial Intelligence

15

Abstract

Over the last few years, there has been rapid progress in the field of artificial intelligence (AI). The various advanced techniques in AI have opened newer horizons in this field. These advanced technologies include multimodal foundation models, retrieval-augmented generation, diffusion models, neuro-symbolic AI, self-supervised learning, causal AI and causal inference and transfer learning. It is necessary to be acquainted with these newer techniques to implement them in an AI model. The present chapter discusses the basic principles and applications of various advanced AI technologies.

Keywords

Artificial intelligence · Multimodal foundation models · Retrieval-augmented generation · Diffusion models · Neuro-symbolic AI · Self-supervised learning · Causal AI and causal inference · Transfer learning

15.1 Introduction

Since the last few years, there has been rapid progress in the field of artificial intelligence. The various advanced techniques in AI have opened newer horizons in this field. It is necessary to be acquainted with these newer techniques to implement an AI model. In this present chapter, various advanced AI technologies have been described.

P. Dey, *Computational Cytology*, https://doi.org/10.1007/978-981-95-3272-8_15

15.1.1 Multimodal Foundation Models

The Multimodal Foundation Models (MFM) are pre-trained models that are trained to perform a wider range of tasks, such as text generation and text-to-image generation, etc. [1] (Fig. 15.1, Box 15.1).

In fact, technically, MFM is a type of transfer learning that makes MFM possible. The recent launch of large multimodal foundation models (LMFM) such as ChatGPT-4-Turbo by OpenAI and Gemini by Google have generated huge opportunities and challenges.

Key Characteristics

- Pre-trained: MFMs are self-supervised or unsupervised models.
- Scalable: MFMs use billions of parameters.
- General-purpose: The models are adaptable and can do multiple tasks.

Tasks of MFM

1. *Cross-Modal Understanding*: This means understanding the relationship between different modalities of data.
   (a) *Matching the image and text data*: It verifies whether the index image and the text data are matching or not.
      - Example: In a given microscopic image of metastatic carcinoma, text caption matches the image or not.
      - Model: Contrastive Language-Image Pretraining.
   (b) *Visual Question Answering (VQA)*: Here, the questions are asked based on a visual image.
      - Example: Microscopic image of a papillary carcinoma of the thyroid is shown and the question is asked "Please tell whether the microscopic picture has intranuclear inclusion or not?" (Fig. 15.2)
      - Model: GPT-4 with vision, Flamingo, BLIP

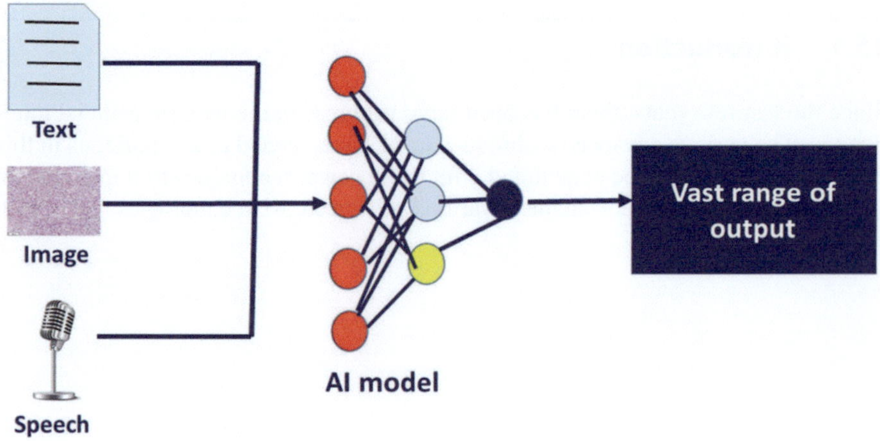

Fig. 15.1 Multimodal Foundation Model

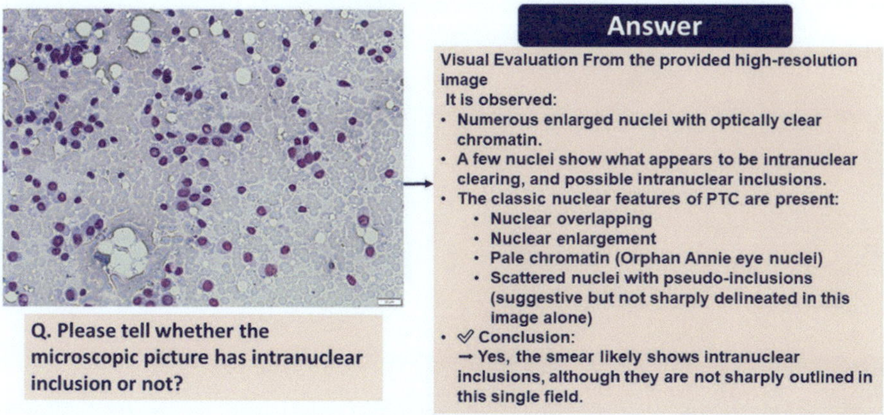

Fig. 15.2 Visual question answering: Please tell whether the microscopic picture has an intranuclear inclusion or not? The answer was given in the right part of the image

2. *Multimodal Generation*: This particular model generates the data content from one modality to another modality.
   (a) *Text-to-Image Generation*: In this task, from the given text description, an image is generated.
      - Example: "A lion is in the cage".
      - Models: DALL·E, Midjourney, Stable Diffusion
   (b) *Image Captioning*: In this task, a descriptive caption is generated from the given image (Fig. 15.3).
      - *Example*: Fig. 15.3 is a photograph of mine (Dr Pranab Dey). The caption was given by the Multimodal Foundation Models.
        Output: *Caption*:
        "A pathologist intently examines a slide under a microscope in a clinical laboratory, focusing on cellular details for diagnostic evaluation".
   (c) *Text-to-Audio/Audio-to-Text*: This task involves the generation of text to speech and speech to text.
      - *Models*: Whisper (OpenAI), GPT-4o (Omni), Bark (Suno)
   (d) *Text-to-Video/Video-to-Text*: The video is generated from the descriptive text data and vice versa.
      - *Models*: Sora (OpenAI), Make-A-Video (Meta)
3. *Multimodal Reasoning*: In this task, the information across the modalities is combined to do the complex reasoning.
   (a) *Diagram or Chart Interpretation*: The complex visual structure is provided and a question is asked.
      - *Example*: "Explain bar chart".
      - *Models*: GPT-4 with vision, Gemini
   (b) *Multimodal Arithmetic/Logic Tasks*: Both image and text data are provided to ask for reasoning.
      - *Example*: Microscopic image is given along with clinical data. Then the specific diagnosis is asked (Figs. 15.4 and 15.5).

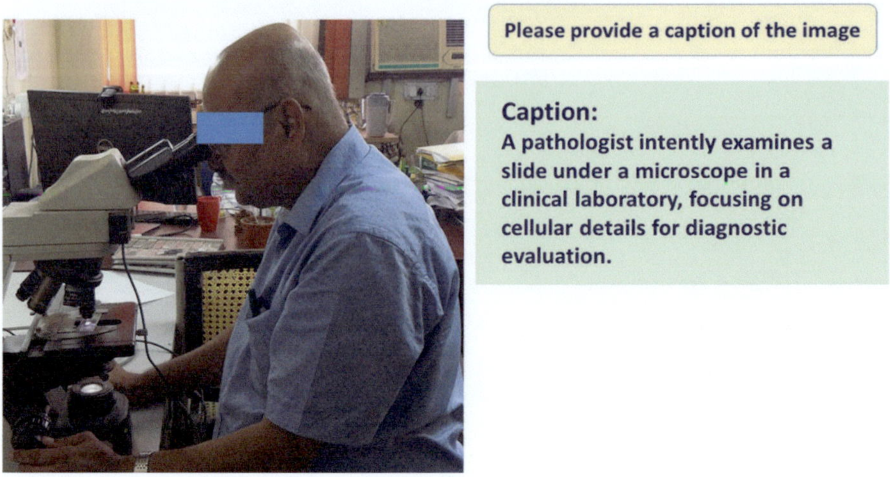

Fig. 15.3 Captioning of the image

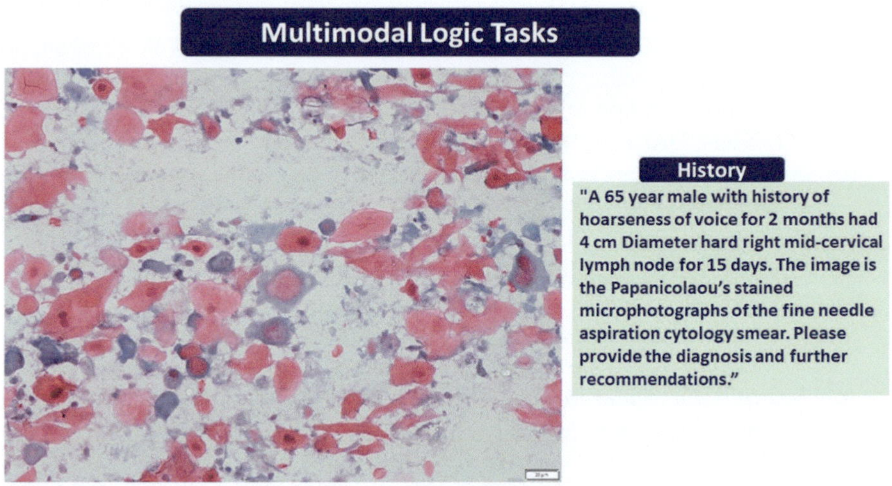

Fig. 15.4 Microscopic image and history are provided

4. *Interactive Tasks*: This task is mainly used in robotics.
   (a) *Instruction Following in Robotics*: It involves understanding voice or text instructions and performing a physical task.
   - *Example*: "Pick up the pen from the table."
   - *Models*: Gato, PaLM-E

Properties (Fig. 15.6)

- Scalable: MFM is versatile model and can be used in various purposes.

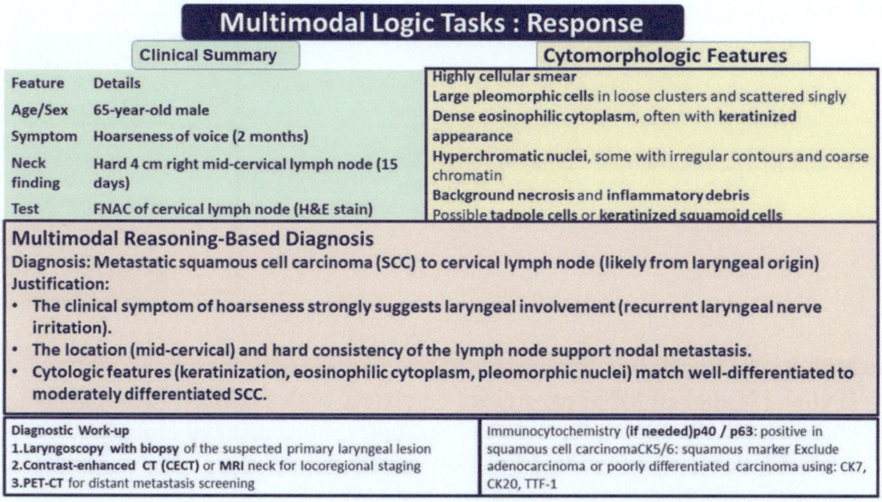

Fig. 15.5 Multimodal reasoning-based diagnosis and justification (unaltered)

Box 15.1 Multimodal Foundation Models (MFMs)

MFMs are pre-trained models and can do wider types of tasks such as text generation, text-to-image generation, etc.

Characteristics

- Pre-trained.
- Self-supervised or unsupervised models.
- Scalable: MFMs use billions of parameters.
- General-purpose: Adaptable and can do multiple tasks

Tasks of MFM

- *Cross-Modal Understanding*: MMF understands the relationship between different modalities of data.
- *Multimodal Generation*: It can generate the data content from one modality to another modality, e.g. text to image and vice versa.
- *Multimodal Reasoning*: Such as reasoning with the chart or diagram.
- *Interactive Tasks*: Such as ordering the robot to do a task.

Properties

- Scalable
- Multimodal Capability
- Cross-Modal Reasoning
- Emergent Capabilities: MFM can do certain unexpected work such as writing a poem by seeing the specific image.
- Transferability: It can do tasks that are not even trained.

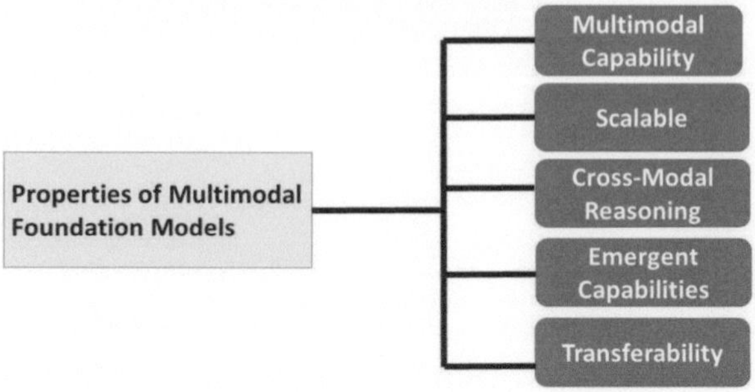

Fig. 15.6 Properties of Multimodal Foundation Models

- Multimodal Capability: It is capable of integrating multiple modules of data Cue H et al. [2] applied MFM pre-trained on diverse omics datasets (genomic, epigenomics, etc.) to expose the extremely complex molecular cell biology.
- Cross-Modal Reasoning: MFM can draw inferences between different modalities such as it can describe an image in text.
- Emergent Capabilities: MFM can do certain unexpected work such as writing a poem by seeing the specific image.
  Transferability: It may do tasks that are not even trained.

15.2 Retrieval-Augmented Generation (RAG)

RAG is an advanced technique in natural language processing (NLP). It links text models with external knowledge bases (e.g., search engines or databases) and retrieves relevant documents from external data sources (Fig. 15.7, Box 15.2).

RAG has two components:

- *Retrieval*: The retrieval system fetches relevant documents from the external knowledge system.
- *Generation*: A generator is a large language model that produces contextually relevant responses from retrieved data.

Advantages

- *Improved factual accuracy*: The retrieved facts are accurate.
- *Up-to-date knowledge*: RAG provides the dynamic current knowledge.
- *Smaller model footprint*: There is no need to store data internally as the model only retrieves data from the external source.

Example

- *User question*: *Question: "Do you need mastectomy in a 5 cm diameter carcinoma of right breast with liver metastasis?"*
- *RAG system*: It provides a detailed answer (Fig. 15.8).

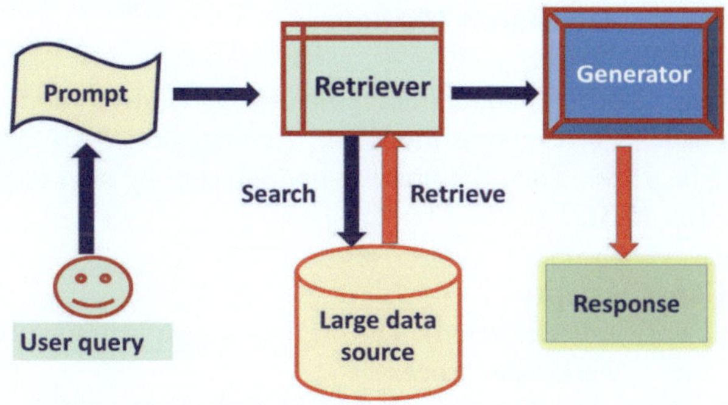

Fig. 15.7 Retrieval-Augmented Generation model

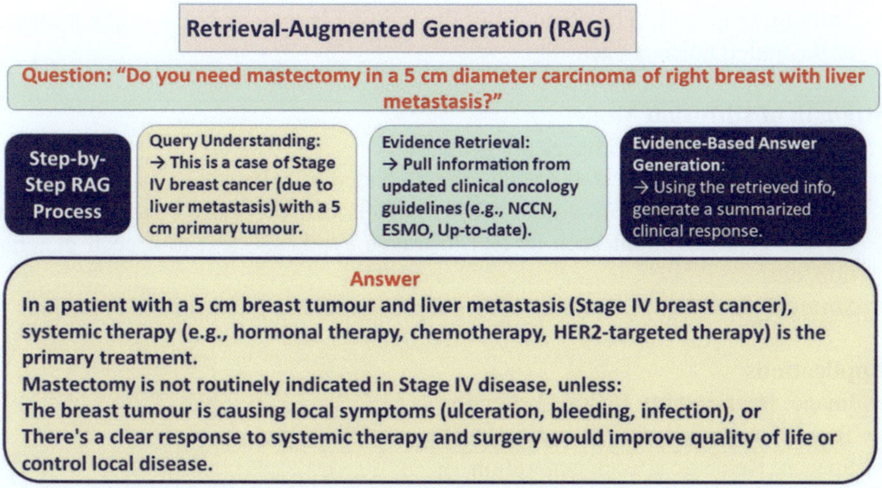

Fig. 15.8 Example of Retrieval-Augmented Generation

Box 15.2 Retrieval-Augmented Generation (RAG)

RAG links text models with external knowledge bases and retrieves relevant documents from external data sources.

Components

- *Retrieval*: It fetches relevant documents from the external knowledge system.
- *Generation*: It produces contextually relevant responses from retrieved data.

Advantages

- Improved factual accuracy
- Up-to-date knowledge
- Smaller model footprint: There is no need to store data internally as the model only retrieves data from the external source.

15.3 Diffusion Models

The diffusion models are powerful generative models to generate high-quality images by reversing the noise. At first, noise is imparted to the original image (Fig. 15.9). Then the noise is undone step by step to generate high-quality image (Box 15.3).

Core Concepts
- Forward (Diffusion): The original image is gradually corrupted by adding noise by a Markovian process.
- Reversing (Denoising): It is the process of training the artificial neural network by reversing the noise step by step to get back the image.
- Training Objective: The objective of the training is to recover the original image or the added noise at each step.

Strength of Diffusion Model
- *Quality*: High-quality images are generated
- *Stable*: The training is stable and has less chance of collapsing
- *Highly Flexible Conditioning*: Diffuse models can be easily conditioned with various types of input such as text-to-image synthesis, text-to-speech generation, etc.
- *Strong Theoretical Foundation*: The diffuse model has interpretable behaviour.

Applications
- Image: High-quality Image Generation
- Text to image generation: Image development from text
- Speech: Realistic speech generation
- Video: To generate a coherent video

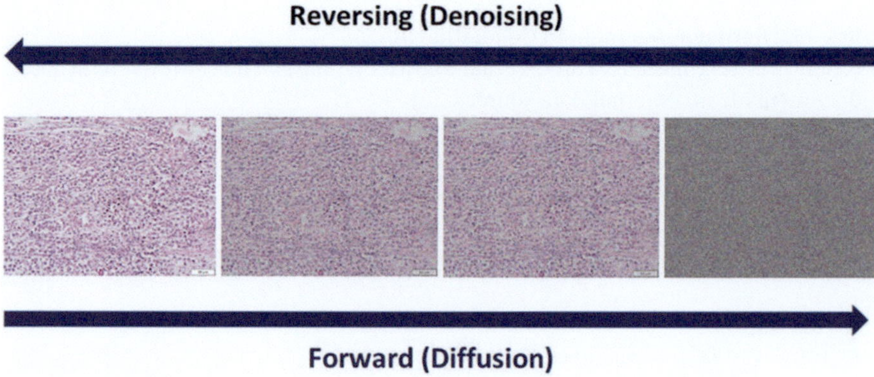

Fig. 15.9 Diffuse model showing image destruction by adding noise, followed by reversing to generate an image

Box 15.3 Diffusion Models

It generates high-quality images by reversing the noise. At first, noise is imparted to the original image and then the noise is undone step by step to generate high-quality image.

Core Concepts

- Forward (Diffusion): The original image is gradually corrupted.
- Reversing (Denoising): Reversing the noise step by step to get back the image with the help of an artificial neural network.
- Training Objective: The objective of the training is to get back the original image.

Strength of Diffusion Model

- *Quality*: High-quality images
- *Stable*: The training is stable
- Highly Flexible Conditioning
- *Strong Theoretical Foundation*: The diffuse model has interpretable behaviour

Applications

- Image: High-quality Image Generation
- Text to image generation: Image development from text
- Speech: Realistic speech generation
- Video: To generate a coherent video

15.4 Neuro-Symbolic AI

Neuro-Symbolic AI is the combination of neural networks with symbolic reasoning systems (Fig. 15.10). The symbolic reasoning system is based on logic and is interpretable. So the combination of a deep learning network and symbolic reasoning generates the powerful system that can reason like human (Box 15.4) [3].

The differences between deep learning and Neuro-Symbolic AI are highlighted in Table 15.1.

Advantages

- Generalization: It can do well in novel or unseen situations
- Hybrid Intelligence: It has neural perception and reasoning
- Interpretability: The decision can be interpreted and explained
- Data Efficiency: It can work well with scanty data

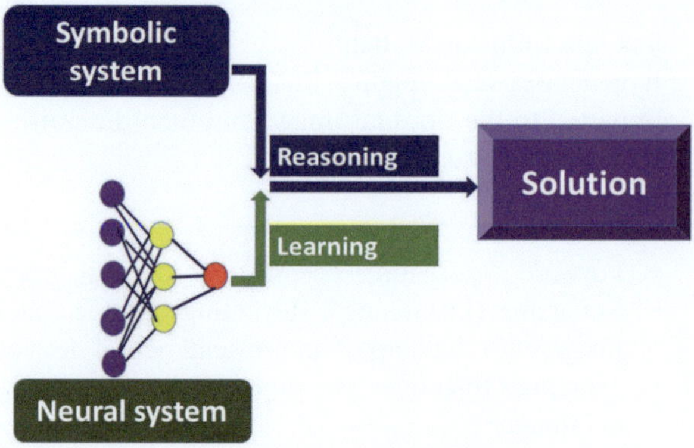

Fig. 15.10 Symbolic system provides reasoning and neural system gives pattern recognition

Table 15.1 The differences between deep learning and Neuro-Symbolic AI

Feature/Aspect	Deep learning	Neuro-Symbolic AI
Core Approach	Pattern recognition	Combination of Deep Learning and symbolic reasoning
Data Requisite	Huge amounts of labelled data	Less amount of data can be used by symbolic knowledge
Reasoning power	No ability for logical or abstract reasoning	Good logical reasoning power
Black box problem	Poor interpretability due to black-box problem	High interpretability as symbolic components can be interpreted and explained
Scalability	Highly scalable	Less scalable due to symbolic components
Knowledge Transfer	Weak	Strong
Examples of Systems	GPT, ResNet, BERT	DeepProbLog, IBM NS-CL, AlphaGeometry

Challenges

- *Scalability*: The symbolic systems are difficult to scale.
- *Differentiability*: Integration of discrete logical operations into neural pipelines is difficult.
- *Training Complexity*: It is difficult to design and optimize the combined models.

Applications

- Visual Question answering: The system can understand the image and can give an answer to any logical question related to the image.
- Scientific Discovery: Neural network proposes patterns and explains them.
- Mathematics & Code: The code generated by the neural network is corrected by a symbolic system.

Box 15.4 Neuro-Symbolic AI

Neuro-Symbolic AI is the combination of neural networks with symbolic reasoning systems.

Advantages

- Generalization: Do well in unseen situations
- Hybrid Intelligence: It has neural perception and reasoning
- Interpretability: The decision can be interpreted and explained
- Data Efficiency: It can work well with scanty data

Challenges

- *Scalability*: Difficult to scale
- *Differentiability*: Integration of discrete logical operations into neural pipelines is difficult
- *Training Complexity*: It is difficult to design and optimize the combined models

Applications

- Visual Question answering: It can give an answer to any logical question related to the image.
- Scientific Discovery: It proposes patterns and explains them.
- Mathematics & Code: The code generated by the neural network is corrected by a symbolic system.

15.5 Self-Supervised Learning

Self-Supervised Learning (SSL) is the machine learning technique where the model learns by unsupervised learning from the unlabelled data that conventionally needs supervised learning (Fig. 15.11). So, SSL is the bridge between supervised and unsupervised learning (Box 15.5) [4].

Importance of Self-Supervised Learning

- Labelled data is time-consuming and laborious
- Unlabelled data is abundant
- SSL can use the raw data to make AI scalable and efficient

Advantages of SSL

- Label efficiency: Efficient labelling of data and avoids a labelled dataset
- Generalization: Robust model
- Scalability: It can handle a huge amount of raw data
- Performance: It is equal to or better than supervised learning

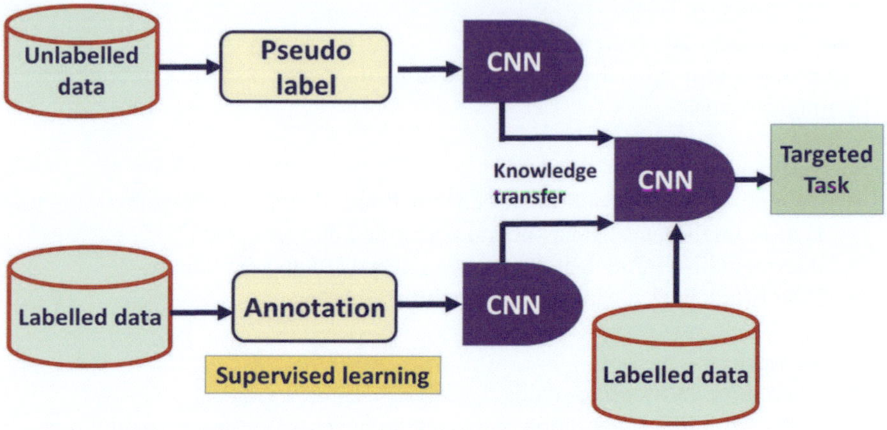

Fig. 15.11 Self-Supervised Learning (CNN convolutional neural network)

Limitations

- *Designing*: A good design is needed for good performance.
- *Computational cost*: Large SSL models are expensive.
- *Evaluation difficulty*: Difficult to assess the quality.

Box 15.5 Self-supervised learning (SSL)

Here, the model learns by unsupervised learning from the unlabelled data that conventionally needs supervised learning.

Importance of Self-Supervised Learning

- Labelled data is time-consuming and laborious
- Unlabelled data is abundant
- SSL can use the raw data to make AI scalable and efficient

Advantages of SSL

- Label efficient
- Generalization: Robust model
- Scalability: It can handle a huge amount of raw data
- Performance: Good

Limitations

- *Designing*: A good design is needed for good performance
- *Computational cost*: Expensive
- *Evaluation difficulty*: Difficult to assess the quality

15.6 Causal AI and Causal Inference

Causal AI is a type of AI that gives attention to cause–effect relationships within the data for precise prediction. It reveals the underlying mechanism of the outcome [5]. The causal inference identifies the cause-and-effect relationships from data. Causal AI classically employs the tool of causal inference. The traditional AI focuses on correlational relationships, whereas causal AI focuses on cause–effect relationships (Box 15.6).

15.6.1 Strength of Causal AI

- *Ability to explain*: Causal AI understands the cause of the decision taken by the model.
- *Fairness*: It avoids false correlations.
- *Robustness*: Causal AI is robust and works well in new environments.
- Decision Support: It helps in healthcare for improved decisions.

15.6.2 Building Causal AI

These are the steps to build causal AI (Fig. 15.12):

1. *Define the Problems and Objectives*: The problems should be identified first and tasks should also be defined.
2. *Collecting Observational Data*: Collect the observational data in large amounts as this is the cornerstone to build causal AI.

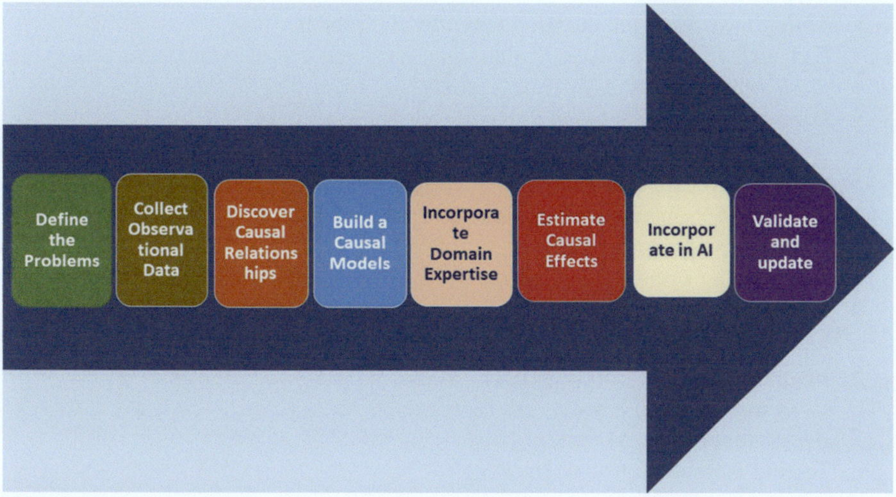

Fig. 15.12 Steps of causal AI

3. *Discovering Causal Relationships*: At first, identify the relevant variables. Apply a directed acyclic graph to analyse the pattern and identify the causal relationships between variables.
4. *Building Causal Models*: Make a structural causal model based on the identified relationships.
5. *Incorporating Domain Expertise*: It means to design, refine and validate the causal model with the help of knowledge gained from the subject matter experts (SME) such as physicians, engineers. The insights of SME are incorporated into the causal AI model.
6. *Estimating Causal Effects*: Estimate the causal effect by applying computational methods such as regression analysis or propensity score.
7. *Integrate with AI system*: Incorporate the causal model into reinforcement learning agents **or** decision support systems.
8. *Testing Interventions and Iterating*: Apply the causal AI and monitor the effects. Refine the models in the course of time to improve their accuracy and predictive power.

Applications

- Healthcare: To take important decision in treatment
- AI system: To take decision in dynamic environment
- Marketing: It may help to increase sell

Box 15.6 Causal AI and Causal Inference

Causal AI gives attention to cause–effect relationships within the data for precise prediction.

Strength of causal AI

- *Ability to explain* the decision taken by the model
- *Fairness*: It avoids false correlations.
- *Robustness*: Causal AI is robust
- *Decision Support*: It helps in healthcare for improved decisions

Steps to build Causal AI

1. Define the Problems and Objectives
2. Collecting Observational Data
3. Discovering Causal Relationships
4. Building Causal Models: Make a structural causal model based on the identified relationships
5. Incorporating Domain Expertise
6. Estimating Causal Effects
7. Integrate with the AI system
8. Testing Interventions and Iterating

(continued)

Box 15.6 (continued)

Applications

- To take an important decision in treatment
- To take a decision in a dynamic environment
- It may help to increase sell

15.7 Conclusions

In conclusions, the various innovative types of neural network models are generated in the last few years. These systems overcome various limitations of AI such as causal AI describes the reasoning, and thereby overcomes the black box problem. Self-supervised learning helps us to work with unlabelled data and saves time to label the data. Retrieval-Augmented Generation system can give direct answer of the questioning and also can help the differential diagnosis of the disease by retrieving large amount of data from the website. Multimodal Foundation Models can help us to generate one type of data to other type. All these newer AI systems are highly innovative. It is expected that incorporation of these newer AI systems will bring revolution in pathology/cytology.

References

1. Bommasani R, Hudson DA, Adeli E, Altman R, Arora S, von Arx S, Bernstein MS, Bohg J, Bosselut A, Brunskill E, et al. On the opportunities and risks of foundation models. arXiv preprint arXiv:2021. https://doi.org/10.48550/arXiv.2108.07258.
2. Cui H, Tejada-Lapuerta A, Brbić M, et al. Towards multimodal foundation models in molecular cell biology. Nature. 2025;640:623–33. https://doi.org/10.1038/s41586-025-08710-y.
3. Sarker MK, Zhou L, Eberhart A, Hitzler P. Neuro-symbolic artificial intelligence: current trends. AI Commun. 2021;34(3):197–209.
4. Raj A, Dutta S. A review on self-supervised learning. Int J New Technol Res. 2023;9(1):06–10.
5. Feuerriegel S, Frauen D, Melnychuk V, Schweisthal J, Hess K, Curth A, Bauer S, Kilbertus N, Kohane IS, van der Schaar M. Causal machine learning for predicting treatment outcomes. Nat Med. 2024;30(4):958–68. https://doi.org/10.1038/s41591-024-02902-1. Epub 2024 Apr 19.

16 Generative Adversarial Networks: Basic Concepts and Applications

Abstract

The Generative Adversarial Networks (GAN) is newer entity in deep learning networks with the unique power of data creation. It is probably the most innovative and dynamic machine learning technique. GAN consists of a generator (G) and a discriminator (D) that compete with each other and ultimately, a synthetic image is produced indistinguishable from the original one. There are many variants of GAN with unique features. The large number of synthetic images generated by GANs help to train the neural network. Moreover, GAN can make high-quality realistic images and can be used for different purposes. In this chapter, the basic concept and applications of GAN have been discussed.

Keywords

Generative adversarial networks · Synthetic data · Fake image · Generator · Discriminator

16.1 Introduction

The Generative Adversarial Network (GAN) is a relatively newer entity in deep learning networks with the unique power of data creation. Deep learning (DL) is mainly used as a discriminatory model that can discriminate between different objects such as a crow from a pigeon. Unlike DL, the generative model notes the underlying pattern and distribution of data and then generates new data to produce a synthetic/fake sample or image. This concept has produced a new techniques of Generative Adversarial Network (GAN) that help to generate synthetic images or videos mimicking the original one. Goodfellow IJ et al. [1] first introduced the concept of GAN in 2014. GAN is the combination of two neural networks: a generator

P. Dey, *Computational Cytology*, https://doi.org/10.1007/978-981-95-3272-8_16

(G) and a discriminator (D) that compete with each other and ultimately, a synthetic image is produced indistinguishable from the original one.

16.2 Key Concepts of GAN: Police Versus Counterfeiter

The key concept of GAN is just like a police officer and a counterfeiter. The counterfeiter makes fake currency and the police identify it. In the course of time, the counterfeiter makes the currency in such a way that it is indistinguishable from the original one and deceives the police.

In GAN, the story is about same as to generate synthetic data. There are two components of GAN: The generator (G) and the discriminator (D):

- Generator: The generator is like "counterfeiter"' that learns to create synthetic or fake data (image). The image looks so authentic that it resembles the real image and the discriminator cannot identify it as fake.
- Discriminator: The discriminator neural network is just like a policeman and tries to distinguish the fake data from the real data in the training set. It gives the output as the possibility of an image as real.

So, the generator and discriminator are the two competitors. The generator tries to deceive the discriminator by making synthetic or fake data. Whereas the discriminator tries to identify the fake data. At one point in time, the discriminator cannot recognize the fake data (Fig. 16.1).

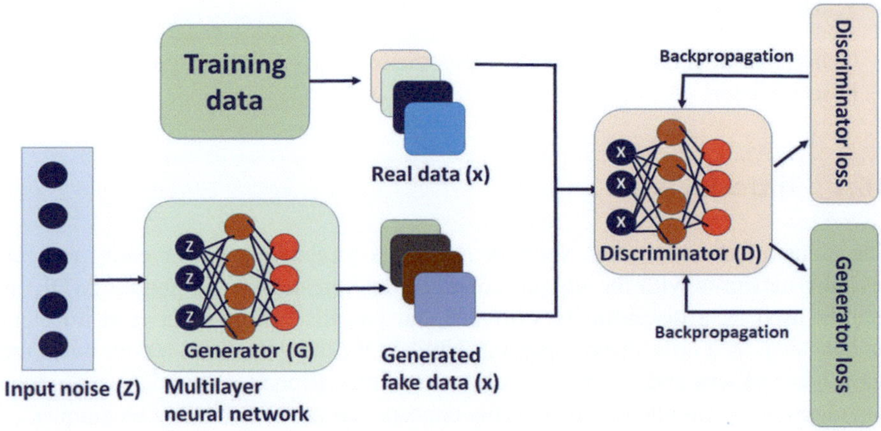

Fig. 16.1 Generative artificial network: It consists of a generator (G) and a discriminator (D). The generator generated fake data and the discriminator tries to discriminate the fake from the real data. Finally, the discriminator cannot distinguish between fake and the real data

16.3 Neural Network Architecture of GAN

Generative network (G): Here, a random noise vector called as "Z vector"' is used to generate a synthetic image. The noise vectors are usually more than 100 dimensions that provide the raw material to develop the synthetic images.

Input: Random Noise vectors

Output: The synthetic/fake image

The Discriminator Network (D): The discriminator network receives either training set data (image) or the synthetic data. The input data is processed by the convolutional neural network (CNN) and gives the output as the possibility of real image.

Input: Real or synthetic data.

Output: A binary scalar probability (0 for synthetic, 1 for real).

16.4 The Training Process of GAN

The training process of GAN is iterative by which both neural networks are updated. Here, the competition occurs between the Generative network and the Discriminator Network till the generative network wins the game and the adversarial network cannot distinguish synthetic or fake data from the real one.

These are the *steps of GAN*:

1. Define the problem: The problem is defined and based on which the architectural network of both generator (G) and discriminator (D) is designed.
2. Train the discriminator: At first, the discriminator is trained on real data or the original image on a training set made of only real images. In this training process, the discriminator knows how to distinguish a real image from the fake one.
3. Train the generator: With the help of inserting random noise in the input, the generator produces fake image. Now the output of the generator's data is given to the discriminator as input data.
4. Train the discriminator: The discriminator is trained on synthetic and real data. Now the discriminator is given training on both synthetic and real data, and it tries to identify the real one.
5. Generator training: The output of the discriminator is now fed in the generator so that the discriminator's ability to correct classification is minimized.
6. Alternative training: Alternative training of the generator and discriminator is going on. The generator continuously produces fake images to deceive the discriminator.
7. Loss function: The whole operating system applies the loss function to measure the difference between real and synthetic data. Commonly, Adam optimizer is used.
8. Evaluation: After training, the data produced by the generator is evaluated.

16.5 Strength of GAN

- *High-Quality Data Generation*: GAN can generate high-resolution and realistic image that looks like the true images. In cytology, it can generate realistic but fake images.
- *Powerful for Data Augmentation*: It can generate synthetic images so that the training set is balanced. So, in case of a low dataset (in rare tumours), GAN can help to increase training data.
- *Image-to-Image Translation*: GAN can do complex mapping between the domains such as haematoxylin and eosin stained images and immunohistochemistry images are developed from one to the other and vice versa (Fig. 16.2).
- *Generate Highly Diverse Outputs*: It can develop diverse variations of images such as to develop images of higher grade in cytology (Fig. 16.3).

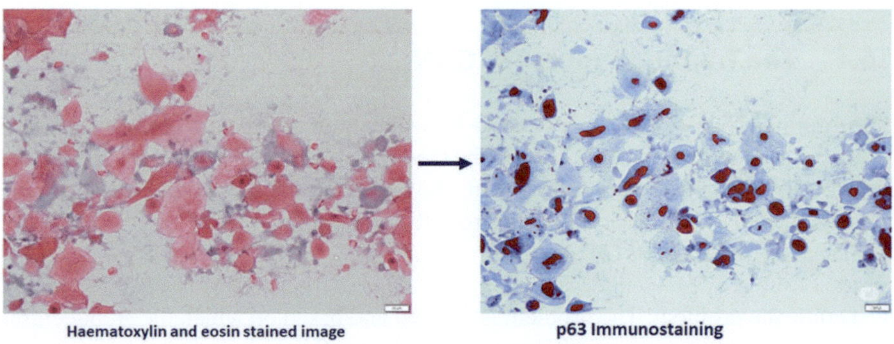

Fig. 16.2 Image-to-Image translation by generative adversarial network

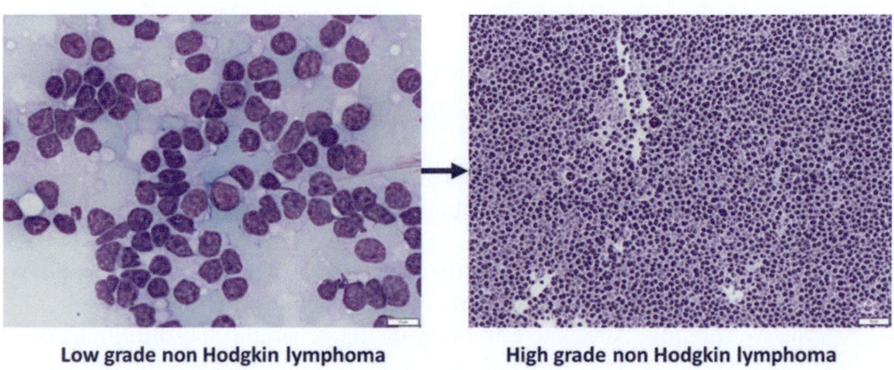

Fig. 16.3 Conversion of images of higher grade in cytology

16.6 Limitations in Training GANs

There are several limitations to training GANs:

- *Collapsing mode*: It may happen if the generator generates only a limited variety of samples. The generator observes that the discriminator is fooled by certain sets of images (data) and then it produces only those sets of data. The process affects the distribution of data.
- *Vanishing gradient*: If the discriminator is strong in the early part of training, then its output for a generated sample will be close to zero and loss function may not provide sufficient gradient for effective learning.
- *Difficult to evaluate*: The quality assessment of the generative output is difficult.
- *Unstable training*: The game of GAN may be unstable with completely divergence output and to have a stable equilibrium is difficult.

16.7 Advanced GAN Architectures

Several advanced variations of GAN have been developed to increase its performance.

1. *Deep Convolutional GAN (DCGAN)*: In DCGAN, the CNNs are applied both in the generator and discriminator networks to make the GAN more stable [2].

   Main innovation: In DCGAN, the fully connected layer is replaced by a CNN to get top-quality images.

   Applications:
   - Synthetic image: To generate synthetic cytology images.
   - Augmentation: To expand the limited dataset.
   - Simulations of virtual cells: The cells with different shapes and sizes are generated.
2. *Conditional GANs (cGANs)*: In cGANs, the generator is directed to generate a particular type of image. Both the generator and discriminator are conditioned by feeding of certain additional information. This additional information may be a text description, image or class labels (Fig. 16.4).

   Advantages of Conditional GANs:
   - Controlled generation: The main benefit of cGAN is to get a specific category of images.
   - Faster and stable training is possible in cGAN.
   - Higher quality and relevant images are produced.

   Applications
   - Image-to-image translation: One type of image domain can be transformed to another type of domain such as day can be changed to night.
   - Text-to-image synthesis: It can generate an image from the text description.

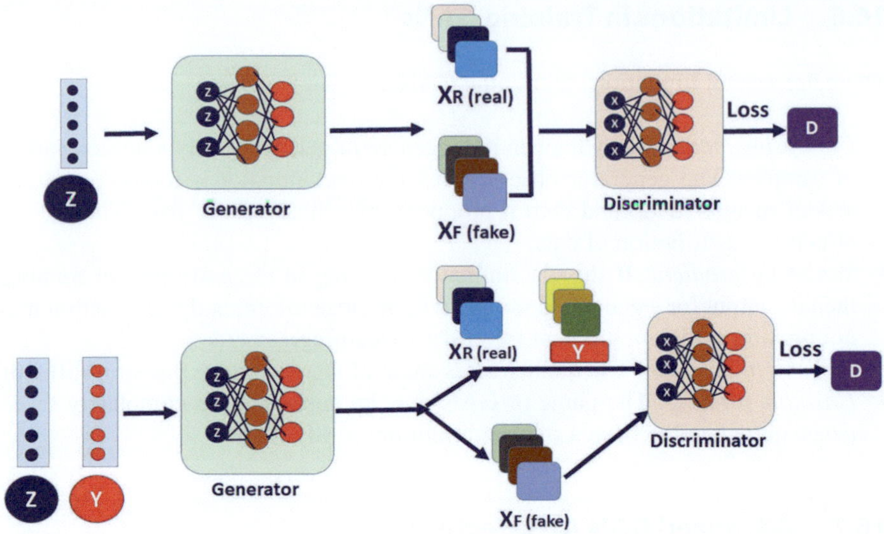

Fig. 16.4 Schematic diagram of cGAN

- Image editing: it can edit the images according to the operator's motive.
- Data Augmentation: To generate more synthetic data for training.
- Video generation.

3. *Wasserstein GAN (WGAN)*: In WGAN, the Wasserstein distance is applied as a loss function and the gradient remains stable. No problem of vanishing gradient is faced.
4. *Cycle-Consistent Generative Adversarial Network (CycleGAN)*: CycleGAN is an innovative program [3]. It is mainly used for "unpaired image-to-image translation" that means transforming one domain to another without any corresponding input–output pairs (e.g., converting crows to pigeons) (Fig. 16.5)

   Crucial concept: In CycleGAN, two generators and two discriminators along with cycle consistency loss are used.

   Two Generators:

   G:X Y (cat to rat)

   F:Y X (rat to cat)

   Two Discriminators:

   $\mathbf{D_Y}$: It distinguishes real versus fake images in domain Y.

   $\mathbf{D_X}$: It distinguishes real versus fake images in domain X.

   Main advantages

   - No need of paired data
   - Effective in translation of medical modality

5. *Style-Based Generative Adversarial Network (StyleGAN)*: Here a "style-based" generator architecture is applied to get exceptionally high-resolution and realistic images. In StyleGAN, instead of a random vector, a style-based vector is used [4].

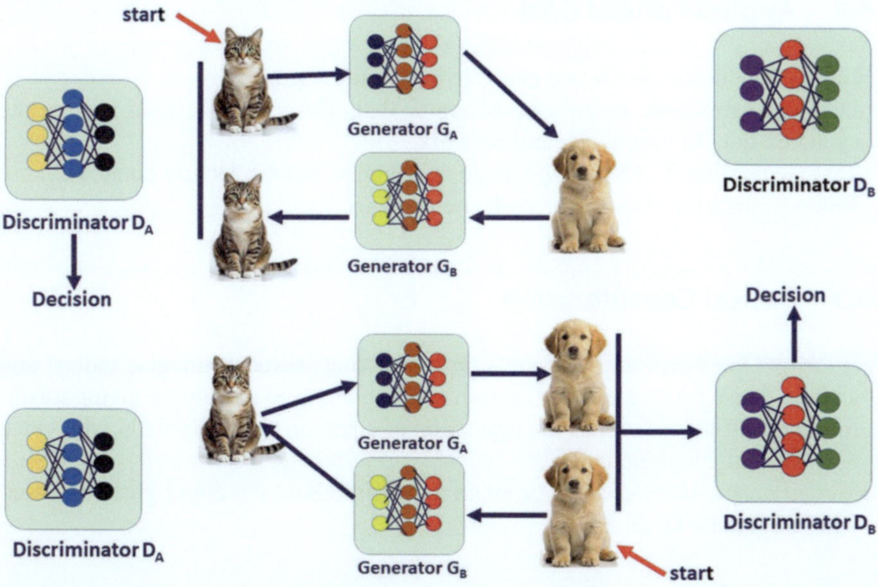

Fig. 16.5 Schematic diagram of cycleGAN

Key Concepts

- Style-Based Architecture: Instead of a random vector, a style-based vector is used.
- Adaptive Instance Normalization (AdaIN): AdaIN is used in each layer of the generator to develop the specific features such as the facial expression of a human being.

Advantages

- High-resolution images
- Innovative image generation

6. *Big Generative Adversarial Network (BigGAN)*: It is a class conditional GAN. BigGAN generates an image of a specific class such as a horse or tiger only. The scaling capacity of BigGAN is very high. Instead of a random noise vector, the generator receives a specific vector with class label [5].

   Strength of BigGAN

   - *Large batch size*: it deals with more than 2000 batch size.
   - *Large capacity of the model*: Both the generator and discriminator have millions of parameters.
   - *Class level*: Along with the vector, it includes the class label.
   - *Orthogonal Regularization*: The application of Orthogonal Regularization helps preventing overfitting.

16.8 Applications of GAN

- Image Generation: GAN can generate high-quality images.
- Data Augmentation: In the case of scarce data, GANs can be used to generate synthetic data to train the neural network.
- Text Generation: GANs can generate text such as poems, lecture notes, etc.
- Video Generation: GANs can make new videos.

16.9 Ethical Consideration

Deepfakes: Deepfakes are the synthetic media that includes images, videos and audios. These fake videos or images may be a threat to society by giving misinformation. It may also hurt the reputation of a person by manipulating the video or images in a malicious way.

Copyright and Authorship: The problem may arise about the copyright of the contents created by GAN.

16.10 Conclusions

The Generative Adversarial Network is a powerful deep learning program with vast potential. It can generate a large number of synthetic data (images). These synthetic data are helpful in the training process of CNN. The variants of GAN have many unique features, e.g. to transform one image to another category or to produce a specific type of image. These advanced software programs will be very helpful in pathology images. The GAN has many ethical problems as it can generate images or videos with intentionally wrong information to misguide people. The fake images created by GAN can cause defamation. In the future, GAN should be used judiciously with a good intention.

References

1. Goodfellow IJ, Pouget-Abadie J, Mirza M, et al. Generative adversarial networks. arXiv:1406.2661v1.
2. Radford A, Luke Metz L, Chintala S. Unsupervised representation learning with deep convolutional generative adversarial networks. arXiv:1511.06434v2.
3. Jun-Yan Zhu JY, Park T, Isola P, Efros AA. Unpaired image-to-image translation using cycle-consistent adversarial networks. arXiv:1703.10593v7.
4. Karras T, Laine S, Aila T. A style-based generator architecture for generative adversarial networks. arXiv:1812.04948v3.
5. Brock A, Donahue J, Simonyan K. Large scale GAN training for high fidelity natural image synthesis. arXiv:1809.11096v2.

Transfer Learning: Leveraging Pre-trained Knowledge for Efficient Models in Deep Learning

17

Abstract

Transfer learning (TL) is a powerful technique in machine learning. Here, a pre-trained model carrying experience with similar types of tasks is applied to improve the efficacy of the base model with similar tasks. In current days, TL is widely applied in disease classification, identification of malignant cells and natural language processing. It is a promising area with high potential. The domain shifts, negative transfer, and overfitting are the major challenges and limitations of TL. In future, TL will overcome its limitations and will be widely applied in pathology. The present chapter discusses the basic principles, strengths, limitations and applications of transfer learning.

Keywords

Transfer learning · VGG · ResNet · Inception · EfficientNet · MobileNetV2 · Xception

17.1 Introduction

Transfer learning (TL) is an important addition to machine learning. It uses a pre-trained model that works on a similar problem with a large dataset. The pre-trained model is applied to improve the efficacy of the base model especially with a limited dataset. In current days, TL is widely applied in disease classification, identification of malignant cells and natural language processing [1]. It is a promising area with high potential. The present chapter discusses the basic principles, strengths, limitations and applications of transfer learning.

P. Dey, *Computational Cytology*, https://doi.org/10.1007/978-981-95-3272-8_17

17.2 What Is Transfer Learning?

Definition Transfer Learning is defined as gaining knowledge from one pre-trained model and transferring the learned features to a smaller model that deals with the related problem (Fig. 17.1).

This is just like learning in detail on the badminton game and then using the knowledge in lawn tennis. The skills and different techniques of the badminton game may help the lawn tennis player to be efficient in lawn tennis game.

In Transfer learning, the knowledge acquired by training on one type of dataset is reused partially or completely to improve the performance of another model with a related task (Fig. 17.1) (Box 17.1). The parameters and their weight of the pre-trained model remain intact to help in the training.

Example In case of detection of metastatic breast carcinoma in the Sentinel lymph node [2], at first, the winner team trained the network in *Inception-v3* or *ResNet*, pre-trained on *ImageNet*. The model was fine-tuned to detect metastatic carcinoma of breast.

Strength of Transfer Learning (Box 17.1)

- *Knowledge Reusability*: A pre-trained ANN model transfers the captured generalized features and the knowledge is transferred to do a different but similar task.
- *Data Scarcity*: In real life, the collection of a huge dataset may be difficult.
- The TL reduces the need of a large dataset as the pre-trained ANN model already extracted the essential features.
- *Reduced training time*: TL avoids extensive re-training of the deep learning model.

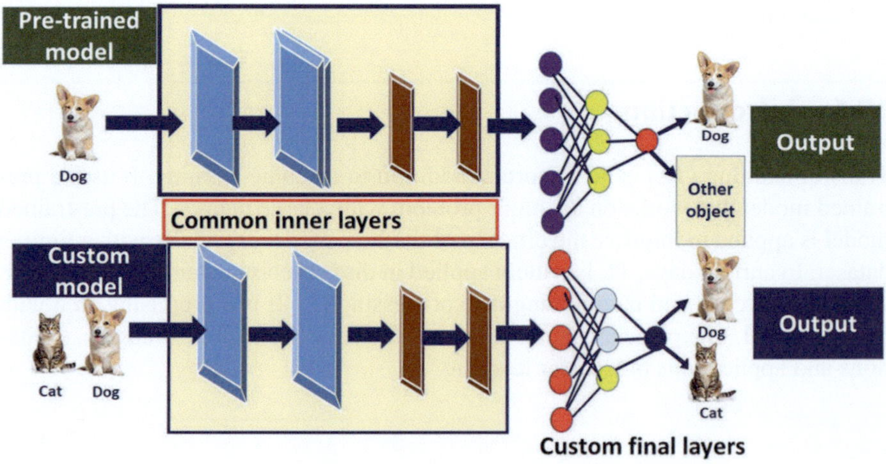

Fig. 17.1 Example of transfer learning model showing the pre-trained model (to identify dog) and custom model to apply the experience of the pre-trained model

- *Computational cost*: As the model is pre-trained so TL reduces training, avoiding computational cost.
- *Domain Adaptation*: TL can adjust the pre-trained deep learning model of one domain to work on another domain. Only fine-tuning may be needed to make it function in another domain.

Example To standardize Haematoxylin and eosin stain colour between source and target datasets.

When to Use Transfer Learning
- When there is limited labelled data.
- Reusing the previous knowledge of the network for performing related tasks.
- Rapid deployment of a new model using the pre-trained models.

The salient features of TL have been highlighted in Box 17.1.

Box 17.1: Transfer Learning Model

In Transfer learning, the knowledge acquired by training of one type of dataset is reused partially or completely to improve the performance of another model with a related task.

Strength of Transfer Learning
- Reduces the training time.
- Improve the performance of AI, particularly if the dataset is small
- It does not need much labelled data

Steps of Transfer Learning

1. *Select a Pre-Trained Model*
2. *Load: Import the pre-trained model with architecture and weights*
3. *Tune the Model for the New Task*
4. *Freeze the Base Layers*
5. *Train the New Top Layers*
6. *Fine-Tune the Model*
7. *Evaluate and Validate*
8. *Deploy the Model*: Implement the model in real real-world situation. Continuously monitor the model for performance

Types of Transfer Learning
- Inductive Transfer Learning
- Transductive Transfer Learning
- Unsupervised Transfer Learning

(continued)

Box 17.1 (continued)

When to Use Transfer Learning

- In case of limited labelled data
- Reusing the previous knowledge of the network for performing related tasks
- Rapid deployment of the new model

Applications

- Medical image classification
- Detection of object
- Natural language processing
- In the case of reinforcement learning

Limitations

- Domain shift
- Risk of Negative Transfer
- Overfitting
- Limited Interpretability and explainability

17.3 Types of Transfer Learning

A. *Inductive Transfer Learning*: Here, the source task and target tasks are different but related and labelled data is available for the target task.

   Example:

   Aim: to detect malignant cells in pleural effusion

   Source Domain: Breast histology images

   Source Task: Tumour detection

   Target Domain: Images of effusion cytology smear

   Target Task: To classify the effusion cytology as benign or malignant.

B. *Transductive Transfer Learning*: Here, the source and target tasks are almost similar but the domains are different. The source data are labelled but the target data are unlabelled.

   Example:

   Source: Labelled urine cytology smear for the detection of malignant cells.

   Target: Unlabelled pleural effusion cytology to detect malignant cells.

C. *Unsupervised Transfer Learning*: Here, no labelled data is available in both source and target domains. The knowledge of one domain is transferred to the other domain without any supervision.

   Example:

   Aim: We wish to identify malignant cells in pleural effusion (target domain) without any labelled data. However, we have a large dataset of unlabelled cervical Papanicolaou's smear.

   Source domain: Images of unlabelled cervical Papanicolaou's smear.

Table 17.1 The comparison of different types of transfer learning

Feature	Inductive transfer learning	Transductive transfer learning	Unsupervised transfer learning
Labelled data in source domain	Yes	Yes	No
Labelled data in target domain	Yes	No	No
Typical techniques	Fine-tuning	Domain adaptation	Autoencoders, self-supervised learning
Main aim	Improve performance on a new task using source knowledge	Adaptation of the model to a new domain with no target labels	Learn transferable representations without any supervision

Target domain: Images of pleural effusion cytology smear.
Source task: Self-supervised learning.
Target task: Identification of malignant cells.
Label: No labelled data in either domain.

Table 17.1 shows the comparison of different types of transfer learning

17.4 Core Concepts and Strategies in Transfer Learning

Pre-trained Models The pre-trained models are already trained for the general task on a very large dataset.

Examples: VGG, ResNet, Inception, EfficientNet, MobileNetV2, Xception.

Strength of These Models They are already trained on a large amount of data.

Feature Extraction The basic concept is using a pre-trained model as a feature extractor.

17.5 Steps of Transfer Learning

The steps of transfer learning are described below (Fig. 17.2):

Step 1: Selecting and Loading a Pre-trained Model A pre-trained model is loaded.

Available models: VGG, ResNet, Inception, EfficientNet, MobileNetV2, Xception.

Code

```
from tensorflow.keras.applications import ResNet50
base_model = ResNet50(weights='imagenet', include_top=False,
input_shape=(224, 224, 3))
```

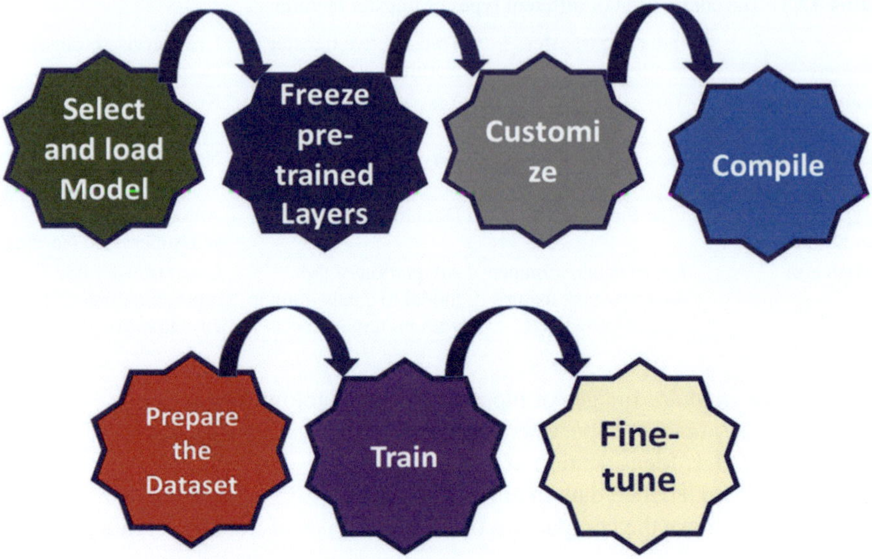

Fig. 17.2 Steps to build the transfer learning

Step 2: Freezing the Pre-trained Layers Weights of the layers are frozen so that they are not updated at the time of training.

Code

```
for layer in base_model.layers:
 layer.trainable = False
```

Step 3: Adding a Custom Classifier Head A new dense layer is attached which is suitable for the new task.

Code

```
from tensorflow.keras import layers, models
model = models.Sequential([
 base_model,
 layers.GlobalAveragePooling2D(),
 layers.Dense(128, activation='relu'),
 layers.Dropout(0.3),
layers.Dense(1, activation='sigmoid') # for binary classification
])
```

Step 4: Compiling the Model Appropriate optimizer and loss function are selected for the new task.

Code

```
model.compile(
 optimizer='adam',
 loss='binary_crossentropy',
 metrics=['accuracy']
)
```

Step 5: Preparing the Dataset The data is pre-processed according to the requirements of the base model.

Code

```
from tensorflow.keras.applications.resnet50 import preprocess_input
from tensorflow.keras.preprocessing.image import ImageDataGenerator

datagen = ImageDataGenerator(preprocessing_function=preprocess_input,
validation_split=0.2)

train_gen = datagen.flow_from_directory(
 'urine_cytology_data',
 target_size=(224, 224),
 batch_size=32,
 class_mode='binary',
 subset='training'
)

val_gen = datagen.flow_from_directory(
 'urine_cytology_data',
 target_size=(224, 224),
 batch_size=32,
 class_mode='binary',
 subset='validation'
)
```

Step 6: Train the Model In this stage, the base model weights remain frozen and only the new classifier head is updated.

Code

```
history = model.fit(train_gen, validation_data=val_gen, epochs=10)
```

Step 7 (Optional): Fine-Tuning Once the top layers have been trained, then the deeper layer can be unfrozen and fine-tuned.

Code

```
# Unfreeze last few layers for fine-tuning
for layer in base_model.layers[-30:]:
 layer.trainable = True

# Recompile with a lower learning rate
model.compile(
 optimizer=tf.keras.optimizers.Adam(1e-5),
 loss='binary_crossentropy',
 metrics=['accuracy']
)
# Continue training
model.fit(train_gen, validation_data=val_gen, epochs=5)
```

17.6 Selection Criteria of Models

The selection of the pre-trained models in transfer learning is very important for maximizing the performance, reducing the training time and resources. The following factors play key roles in the selection of the pre-trained models:

1. *Type of Task*
   The specific task of the target domain determines the selection of the pre-trained models.
   Image classification: ResNet, DenseNet, EfficientNet
   Object Detection: YOLO, Faster R-CNN
   Image Segmentation: U-Net, DeepLabV3+
   Natural language processing: BERT, GPT
2. *Domain Similarity* (source–target relationship):
   High similarity: If the task of the target is highly similar to the task of the pre-trained model of the source, then the result is expected to be good.

Example To classify the histopathological images of different tumours, ImageNet-pre-trained models such as ResNet and VGG are good to use.

Low Similarity If the source and target-specific tasks are totally dissimilar, then the transfer learning model may not be effective or it may need extensive fine-tuning.

3. *Size of the Target Dataset*
   Large dataset (more than 100k): If the size of the target dataset is large, then Fine-tuned deeper model such as ResNet-101 can be used.

Small dataset (less than 5k): In the case of small size of target dataset, a lightweight models such as MobileNet, EfficientNet-B0 can be used with freeze early layers.

4. *Computational Resources*

   High resources: Here, Vision Transformers, ResNet, EfficientNet-B7

   Low resource: MobileNet, SqueezeNet, EfficientNet-lite

5. *Model Size & Number of Parameters*:

   Larger Models: The large pre-trained model may have 100 million parameters and have higher accuracy. However, they need more computational resources (more memory, training time, etc.)

   Example: ResNet-152, ViT-L, BigGAN, Swin-L

   Smaller Models: The smaller models have only few million parameters and they are good choice for low resourceful situations. However, these pre-trained models may be less accurate.

   Example: MobileNet, SqueezeNet

   Figure 17.3 shows the selection criteria of different transfer learning models.

The comparison of different transfer models is highlighted in Table 17.2.

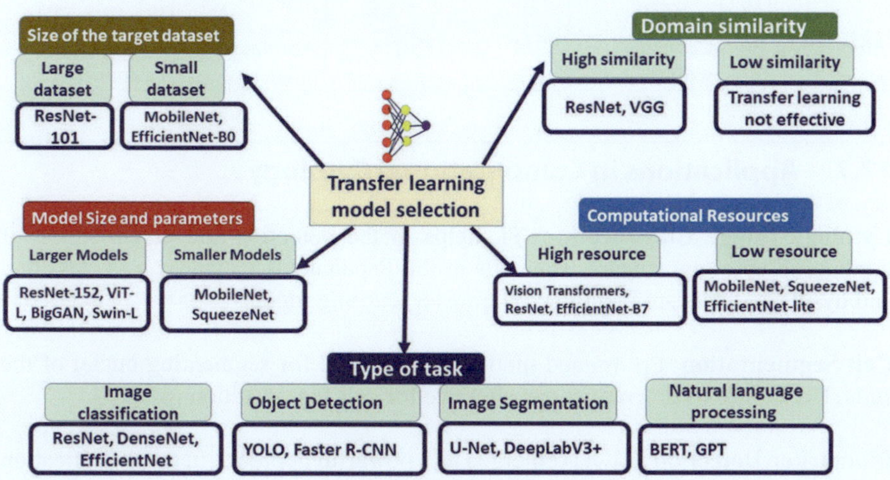

Fig. 17.3 The selection criteria of different transfer learning models

Table 17.2 Comparison of different transfer models

Model	Key Idea	Parameters (Millions)	Inference Speed	Strengths	Limitations
VGG-16	Deep stack of 3×3 convolutions	138M	Slow	Easy to implement	Large size; computationally heavy
ResNet-50	Residual learning	25M	Moderate	Excellent accuracy; No vanishing gradient problem	Slightly slower than MobileNet or EfficientNet
Inception-v3	Multi-scale processing with inception modules	24M	Fast	Efficient, fast inference	Complex structure; harder to modify
Xception	Depthwise separable convolutions	23M	Fast	Efficient, good performance	Needs many training epochs
MobileNetV2	Lightweight CNN	3.4M	Very Fast	Suitable for low memory usage	Slightly lower accuracy compared to heavier models
EfficientNet-B0	Compound scaling	5.3M	Fast	Accurate and efficient	Harder to customize

17.7 Applications in Computational Cytology

Cytology Image Classification TL helps in the detection and classification of tumours in cytology smears. The cells in the Papanicolaou's smear was classified and dysplastic cells are identified by transfer learning models [3–5].

Cell Segmentation Pre-trained models can be used for segmenting nuclei of the cells. U-Net and its derivatives are effective for cell segmentation [6].

Biomarker Detection TL has emerged as a powerful approach in the identification of biomarker expression in tumours. It is particularly helpful when the data is limited and resource is restricted. In histopathology, TL may help in the prediction of HER2, Ki67, or p53 status and microsatellite instability from H&E-stained tissue images [7, 8].

Models used: ResNet-50 or DenseNet pretrained on ImageNet.

17.7.1 Challenges and Limitations

Domain Shift The pre-trained models are often trained in ImageNet which differs in the colour and texture of the tissues. So, the differences in the staining of the slides, resolution and the scanner type may have a significant impact on the performance of the model.

Overfitting There may be a chance of overfitting at the time of fine-tuning of small dataset.

Limited Interpretability and Explainability TL often function as black boxes. So the decision of the model may raise trust in the system.

Negative Transfer Due to the dissimilar task of the source and target domains, TL may harm the model and the model may have worse performance than scratch one.

17.7.2 Conclusions

TL has made a paradigm shift in deep learning and computational cytology. By acquiring knowledge from large-scale dataset and transferring the experience to the base model of a limited dataset, it facilitates the development of a robust tool for diagnosis and management of tumours. The domain shifts, negative transfer and overfitting are the major challenges and limitations of TL. In future, TL will overcome its limitations and will be widely applied in pathology.

References

1. Kim HE, Cosa-Linan A, Santhanam N, et al. Transfer learning for medical image classification: a literature review. BMC Med Imaging. 2022;22:69.
2. Litjens G, Bandi P, Ehteshami Bejnordi B. 1399 H&E-stained sentinel lymph node sections of breast cancer patients: the CAMELYON dataset. Gigascience. 2018;7(6):giy065. https://doi.org/10.1093/gigascience/giy065. PMID: 29860392; PMCID: PMC6007545.
3. Mulmule PV, Kanphade RD. Classification of cervical cytology overlapping cell images with transfer learning architectures. Biomed Pharmacol J. 2022;15:277–84.
4. Zhao S, He Y, Qin J, Wang Z, Urzua U. A semi-supervised deep learning method for cervical cell classification. Anal Cell Pathol. 2022;2022:4376178. https://doi.org/10.1155/2022/4376178.
5. Sellamuthu Palanisamy V, Athiappan RK, Nagalingam T. Pap smear based cervical cancer detection using residual neural networks deep learning architecture. Concurr Comput Pract Exp. 2022;34:e6608. https://doi.org/10.1002/cpe.6608.
6. Durkee MS, Abraham R, Clark MR, Giger ML. Artificial intelligence and cellular segmentation in tissue microscopy images. Am J Pathol. 2021;191(10):1693–701. https://doi.org/10.1016/j.ajpath.2021.05.022. Epub 2021 Jun 12. PMID: 34129842; PMCID: PMC8485056.
7. Kather JN, Pearson AT, Halama N, Jäger D, Krause J, Loosen SH, Marx A, Boor P, Tacke F, Neumann UP, Grabsch HI, Yoshikawa T, Brenner H, Chang-Claude J, Hoffmeister M, Trautwein C, Luedde T. Deep learning can predict microsatellite instability directly from histology in gastrointestinal cancer. Nat Med. 2019;25(7):1054–6. https://doi.org/10.1038/s41591-019-0462-y. Epub 2019 Jun 3. PMID: 31160815; PMCID: PMC7423299.
8. Coudray N, Ocampo PS, Sakellaropoulos T, Narula N, Snuderl M, Fenyö D, Moreira AL, Razavian N, Tsirigos A. Classification and mutation prediction from non-small cell lung cancer histopathology images using deep learning. Nat Med. 2018;24(10):1559–67. https://doi.org/10.1038/s41591-018-0177-5. Epub 2018 Sep 17. PMID: 30224757; PMCID: PMC9847512.

Part V

Hands-On and Practical Applications

18 Software and Tools for Computational Cytology

Abstract

Detailed knowledge of essential software and hardware is necessary to build a deep learning model. Most of the software is freely available on websites and anyone can download the requisite software to work. Python is an open-source programming language which is widely used to build convolutional neural network (CNN) modelling. TensorFlow is an open-source platform for deep learning developed by Google. It is a comprehensive program and gives the facilities to use a vast number of libraries. The various programs can be operated in Jupyter Notebook or Google Colab platforms. This chapter provides the guidance to download and install the essential programs to build a deep learning model.

Keywords

Software · Hardware · Python · TensorFlow · Jupyter Notebook · Google Colab

18.1 Introduction

Detailed knowledge of essential software is necessary to build a deep learning model [1]. In fact, knowledge of the hardware is also needed. Most of the software is freely available on the websites. One can download the requisite software to work.

18.2 Basic Requirements

The basic requirements of the hardware and software are described below:

P. Dey, *Computational Cytology*, https://doi.org/10.1007/978-981-95-3272-8_18

1. *A computer*: A laptop or desktop with good memory and computational power is necessary.
   CPU: Central processing units (CPUs) are enough for pre-processing and running the microscopic images with low space requirements.
   GPUs (Graphics Processing Units) are essential for efficient training of CNNs.
   CPU: Recommended is Intel i7 / AMD Ryzen 7 or higher
   GPU: NVIDIA RTX 3060+ or A100 (cloud)
   RAM: 16GB or more
   Storage space: SSD: 256GB or more
2. *Cloud Platforms*:
   (a) *Google Colab notebook*: It is an open and effective platform built by Google [2]. (website : https://colab.research.google.com/)
   (b) *Jupyter Notebook* [3]: It is an essential and effective open platform to build the CNN model. (website: https://jupyter.org/)
   (c) *Anaconda*: Anaconda consists of multiple platforms. It is highly recommended to install Anaconda along with the latest Python model. Subsequently, you can install other programming languages through Anaconda.
   All these programs are freely available on the webpages. (Website: https://www.anaconda.com/)
   (d) *Programming Language*
   Python [4]: It is the basic language of deep learning. It helps in the image processing and convolutional neural network (CNN) modelling (Box 18.1). It is also useful for the evaluation of the CNN model. It is an open-source language. (website: https://www.python.org/)
   • Recommended version: *Python 3.8+*
   (e) *Deep Learning Frameworks*
   TensorFlow [5]: TensorFlow is an open-source platform for deep learning. The program is developed by Google (Box 18.2). It is a comprehensive program that gives the facilities to use a vast number of libraries.
   Advantages:
   • *Comprehensive Ecosystem*: It supplies a huge number of tools and libraries. TensorFlow helps for developing, implementing and maintaining the CNN model.
   • *Scalability*: TensorFlow is a highly scalable program and it promotes training simple to highly complex CNN models. It can work on large datasets and in different hardwires. TensorFlow can work efficiently in including multiple GPUs and distributed systems. This is crucial for large-scale image analysis tasks, such as those involving microscopic images.
   • *Research and Production Readiness*: TensorFlow is a useful platform to perform research activities along with the real-world applications. It is a very robust platform to do versatile works.
   #Installation
   In python: pip install tensorflow
   Keras: Keras is a very good Application Programming Interface (API). It runs with TensorFlow. It is a highly recommended software to build,

train and deploy CNN model. It is essential for designing multimodal dataset models.

#Install: pip install keras

#Verify Installation:

import keras

print(keras.__version__)

PyTorch: PyTorch is a popular open-source platform. PyTorch provides dynamic computational graphs that can help in debugging. It is recommended for research flexibility.

Install:

pip install torch torchvision torchaudio

(f) Image Processing Libraries

The various image processing libraries are available for loading, manipulating and augmenting image data.

A. *QuPath*

It is a powerful open source application for analysing images particularly tailored for whole slide image (WSI) (Fig. 18.1).

Website: https://qupath.github.io/

Key advantages:

- WSI: It can analyse WSI.
- Interactive annotation: It has interactive annotation tools by which the region of interest can be marked or drawn.
- Cell Detection Algorithms: It has Cell Detection Algorithms that can detect the nuclei or cell.
- Batch processing: It has batch processing facility that can analyse multiple slides with same pipeline.
- Extension Framework: It can connect to external model via python.

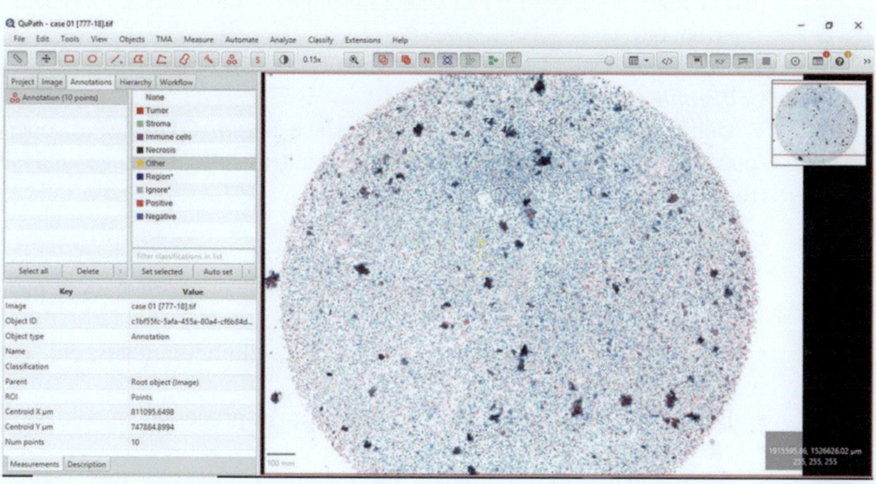

Fig. 18.1 Whole slide image annotation can be done on QuPath system

Applications in cytology:

- *To detect cells of interest*: The cells of interest in effusion, urine cytology smear or cervical smear can be annotated.
- *To generate training data for CNN*: After annotation of the cells, the images can be exported to CNN model.
- *To integrate the data with python for CNN model*

B. *Open Source Computer Vision Library (OpenCV)*: OpenCV is a powerful open source software library which works with interface in Python.

Website: https://opencv.org/

Key functions

- Image Preprocessing: Denoising slides, enhancing contrast, etc.
- Thresholding and Segmentation: Extract cell or nuclei boundaries, detection of overlapping nuclei, etc.
- Object Detection and Measurement: Measurement of nuclear size, analysis of cell shape, etc.
- Feature Engineering: Morphometric and textural analysis.

Limitations

- It does not have any GUI or annotation tool
- Manual training needed

C. Scikit-image: It is purely focused on image analysis and is unrelated to machine learning. Scikit-image algorithms can work on *NumPy*, *SciPy*, and *matplotlib*.

Key features of Scikit-image

(a) Reading/writing: It can read images in different formats and can save after manipulation.
(b) Image filtering: It filters the image by Gaussian, median, Sobel, etc.
(c) Segmentation: It helps in image segmentation.
(d) Morphology: It does erosion, dilatation opening/closing, etc.
(e) Feature extraction: It can detect the edges of the images, blob detection, etc.
(f) Measurements: Label analysis and object counting

D. *CellProfiler*

CellProfiler is a graphical user interface based (GUI-based), open-source software used for automated quantitative cellular image analysis (Fig. 18.2).

Website: https://cellprofiler.org/

Advantages:

- Modular Pipeline: It has an in-built workflow as segmentation, measurement and export.
- Segmentation: The nuclei of the cells, subcellular elements, etc., can be segmented
- Batch Processing: Hundreds of images can be processed immediately.
- No coding is needed.
- Feature extraction: more than 100 features (cell shape, size, texture, etc.) can be extracted.

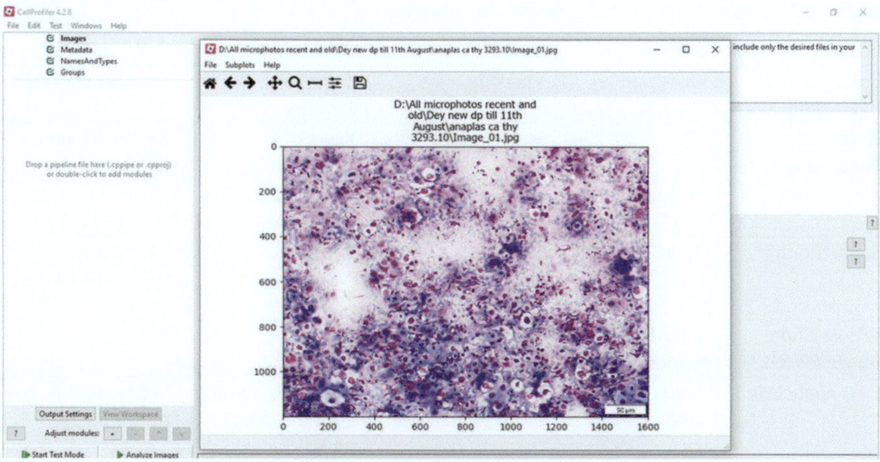

Fig. 18.2 CellProfiler can quantitate cellular parameters

Applications in Cytology:

- Nuclear segmentation in cytology smears
- Morphometric quantifications

Limitations:

- Unfit for WSI
- Not possible in real-time AI
- Table 18.1 shows the comparison of image processing libraries.

E. *Digital Pathology Viewers:* These are tools that help to open, view and annotate the WSI. The WSI images are in different formats and they may be opened only on the company's machine.

The main tools for WSI viewer are:

(a) *Automated Slide Analysis Platform (ASAP):* It is an open source platform that can ran into window.

Main features:

- WSI images of different formats can be opened (.svs, .ndpi, .tiff, .mrxs, .scn)
- Annotations can be done
- Image export facility is present
- Fast and lightweight
- Annotated images can exported
- Deep Learning Integration is possible

(b) SlideRunner: It is a licenced software program that can be operated in window.

Main features:

- Annotations can be done
- Deep Learning Integration is possible
- Image export facility is present

Table 18.1 Comparison of image processing libraries

Feature	QuPath	OpenCV	CellProfiler	Scikit-image
Feature Extraction	Moderate	Via code	Extensive features	Custom via code
Batch Processing	Yes	Yes	Yes	Yes by Python loops
Annotation	Manual	Manual by code	No manual annotation	Manual possible via masks
Segmentation	Good	Excellent	Excellent	Excellent (watershed, edge, etc.)
Whole Slide Image (WSI)	In built support	Needs pre-processing	No	No
Best application	WSIs, annotations, IHC	Pre-processing and segmentation	Feature extraction from the cell/ nuclei	Segmentation and morphology

F. *Data Augmentation*

Keras ImageDataGenerator: It helps in real-time data augmentation, and data pre-processing, particularly helpful in medical images when the datasets are small. It helps in

- *Image rotation*: In different degrees.
- *Image rescaling*: Rescale the size such as: rescale=1./255.
- *Zoom range*: Zoom in and out
- *Efficient image loading* in batches from disk
- *Validation split:* Split training data for validation
- *Code*

```
pip install keras
from keras.preprocessing.image import ImageDataGenerator
from tensorflow.keras.preprocessing.image import ImageDataGenerator
datagen = ImageDataGenerator(
 rescale=1./255,
 rotation_range=40,
 zoom_range=0.2,
 horizontal_flip=True
)
```

Albumentations (advanced): It is a fast, flexible and powerful image augmentation library that helps in the augmentation of medical images.
Strength of Albumentations

- Wide variety of augmentations
- Works with NumPy & OpenCV directly
- Faster than ImageDataGenerator

Basic Setup

```
Install: pip install albumentations
# Import
import albumentations as A
from albumentations.pytorch import ToTensorV2
import cv2
```

G. *Model Evaluation and Metrics*: The model evaluation is essential to assess the performance of the model. We need "scikit-learn": to demonstrate confusion matrix and ROC-AUC. "matplotlib" is used to demonstrate plot loss, accuracy of the curves and confusion matrix and ROC-AUC. For Heatmaps and data visualization, we use "seaborn".
   Install: pip install scikit-learn matplotlib seaborn
   This command can be given to Jupyter Notebook
H. *Model Saving & Deployment*: The saving of the present model is extremely important. The model can be saved by:
   (a) tensorflow.keras.models.save_model()
   (b) joblib, pickle
   (c) Flask, FastAPI
I. *Graphics Processing Units (GPU) Acceleration Support*: GPU Acceleration Support means the ability of software and hardware to speed up the intensive task of computation. Unlike the CPU, the GPU is made of large number of smaller, specialized cores in a parallel architecture. This huge number of parallel cores performs the large number of similar tasks simultaneously to make the work fast.

GPU Acceleration Support in Hardware

GPU: To have the proper GPU support, we need NVIDIA (with its CUDA platform) and AMD (with its ROCm open platform).

Memory: The computer should have sufficient memory to implement the work.

To train faster in a large image dataset, we need NVIDIA CUDA toolkit.

Interconnects: High-speed interconnection between CPU and GPU is needed for efficient data transfer.

GPU Acceleration Support in Software

NVIDIA CUDA: This parallel computing platform contains various toolkit libraries that helps in programming.

AMD ROCm: AMD ROCm is an open-source platform that allows programming by providing libraries, compilers, and development tools.

Box 18.1: Programming Language: Python

- Open source
- Flexible
- Standard language for deep learning
- Simple
- Vast
- Extensive support
- Recommended version: Python 3.8+

Box 18.2: TensorFlow: Overview

- Open source platform for deep learning
- It gives the facilities to use vast number of libraries
- Provides Comprehensive Ecosystem
- Highly scalable
- Ideal for researchers and also fit for real world application

Installation: In python: pip install tensorflow

18.3 Conclusion

The proper computer hardware and various software programs are important to have a successful deep learning model. Currently, most of the important software is freely available on the website. The programs are usually operated either in Jupyter Notebook or in Google colab.

References

1. McGenity C, Clarke EL, Jennings C, et al. Artificial intelligence in digital pathology: a systematic review and meta-analysis of diagnostic test accuracy. NPJ Digit Med. 2024;7:114. https://doi.org/10.1038/s41746-024-01106-8.
2. Meyer TA, Ramirez C, Tamasi MJ, Gormley AJ. A user's guide to machine learning for polymeric biomaterials. ACS Polym Au. 2022;3(2):141–57.
3. Perkel JM. Why Jupyter is data scientists' computational notebook of choice. Nature. 2018;563(7729):145–6.
4. Perkel JM. Programming: pick up Python. Nature. 2015;518(7537):125–6.
5. Vogelsang DC, Erickson BJ. Magician's Corner: 6. TensorFlow and TensorBoard. Radiol Artif Intell. 2020;2(3):e200012.

Practical Examples to Build the Deep Learning Models

19

Abstract

The convolutional neural network (CNN) is the most important type of deep learning model. The practical knowledge of CNN is essential to building a successful model. The codes of the CNN model are usually written in Python language which are operated in Jupyter or Google Colab platform. The current chapter discusses the data collection, labelling, data splitting and the building of different CNN models to detect malignancy.

Keywords

Convolutional neural network · Deep learning · Data labelling · Data splitting · Model building codes · Python · Jupyter · Google Colab

19.1 Introduction

The practical knowledge on a convolutional neural network (CNN) is essential to build a successful model. It is essential to have knowledge of running the code in Jupyter or Google Colab. The data pre-processing, data splitting and data running along with the evaluation of the CNN's performance are important [1]. In this chapter, the practical applications of the CNN code and its implementation are highlighted.

There are certain essential steps to build a successful deep learning model. We commonly use a convolutional neural network (CNN) model for images.

1. *Aims and Objectives*: In any project, you need specific aims and objectives and according to that your code will be built up.
2. *Code running*: Where to run your code: The code given here can be run in Jupyter notebook and alternatively, you can run it in Google Colab.

P. Dey, *Computational Cytology*, https://doi.org/10.1007/978-981-95-3272-8_19

You should download Anaconda (with Anaconda Navigator) to work in the Jupyter notebook.

3. *Data Collection and Labelling*:

   Data collection followed by labelling is the fundamental step in building a CNN model [2]. The microscopic images should be collected in .jpg/ .jpeg or . png format.

JPEG JPEG is a widely used format that occupies relatively less space, making it suitable for large datasets where space and speed are considerations.

PNG (.png) PNG file size is larger than JPEG. However, it retains all the data of the original image.

19.2 Split the Data

Label At first, the data should be labelled properly such as:

Malignant: img001, img002, img003, img004, etc
Benign: img005, img006 etc.
Keep all the malignant images in one folder and the benign images in another folder.

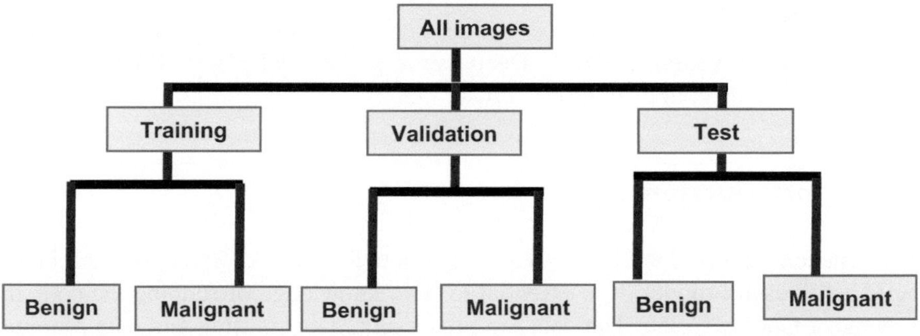

Please make three separate folders for training, validation and test set with two sub-folders named as benign and malignant.

Common Ratios to Split the Folders

- Training set: 70%
- Validation set: 15%
- Test set: 15%

The way to split the cases and keep in the subfolders

19.3 Code to Split Cases

Installation
pip install split-folders

Code

```
import splitfolders
import os
# Original dataset directory structure (e.g., by class)
# input_folder/
# ├── class1/
# │   ├── img_a.jpg
# │   └── img_b.jpg
# └── class2/
# ├── img_c.jpg
# └── img_d.jpg

input_folder = 'path/to/your/image/dataset' # Replace with your dataset path
output_folder = 'path/to/save/splitted_dataset' # Where the new train/val/test
folders will be created

# Split with a ratio: (train, val, test)
# For example, 70% train, 15% validation, 15% test
splitfolders.ratio(input_folder, output=output_folder, seed=42,
ratio=(0.7, 0.15, 0.15), group_prefix=None)

# The output_folder will now have:
```

Train:

- Class1
- Class2

Val

- Class1
- Class2

Test

- Class1
- Class2

```
print(f"Images split into {output_folder}/train, {output_folder}/val, and {output_
folder}/test directories.")
```

4. *Selection and Designing of Model Architecture*

Choice of CNN Architecture Various already pre-trained architectures are available such as ResNet, Inception, EfficientNet, DenseNet, etc. These architectures already have known performance on a large set of images [3]. Alternatively, one can make an individual CNN network and can adopt the pre-trained architectures for fine-tuning.

- *Feature Extraction*: The feature extraction includes the detection of edges, texture, etc.
- *Pooling Layers*: It reduces the dimension of the image.
- *Fully Connected Layers*: It flattens the pixel values of the image to make the final neural network for the regression task [4].

5. *Training and Optimization*

Training from scratch: It indicates building a completely new model and training it from its initial point, where the weights and biases are used randomly. The success of this CNN model depends on the large data set and optimizing the algorithms.

Transfer learning: It is a common and effective approach. Here, a pre-trained architecture on a large dataset is used. The previous knowledge on the large dataset helps to fine-tune the custom model.

- *Loss Function*: Proper selection of the loss function is needed. The primary aim of the loss function is to give a numerical signal to adjust the model's internal parameters such as weight and bias during training. The classification problem cross cross-entropy is used and mean squared error (MSE) is used for regression analysis.
- *Optimizer*: Optimizers help to reduce the loss function.
- *Batch Size:* It means the number of images that are processed in each training iteration.
- *Regularization:* It means techniques to prevent overfitting and make the model more general for use. The main cause of overfitting is limited data. Dropout, data augmentation and early stopping are used to prevent overfitting.
- *Addressing Data Imbalance:* The pathologists must be careful in the selection of biased data inclusion such as too many normal cases.
- *Hardware Requirements:* Running of WSI data requires an extremely powerful computer.

6. *Evaluation and Validation*
   Metrics: The commonly used metrics are accuracy, sensitivity, specificity and Area Under the Curve (AUC) of ROC.
   Cross-validation: k-fold cross-validation is used to ensure the model's robustness.
   Independent Test Set: The model should be evaluated in a completely unknown external dataset which helps to prove its performance in a real world setting.
7. *Integration with Clinical Workflow*: The model should be integrated with the existing digital workflow [5].

19.4 Code to Detect Malignant Cells in Effusion Cytology Smear

#Loading and Pre-processing the Data

```
import os
import numpy as np
import matplotlib.pyplot as plt
from sklearn.metrics import confusion_matrix, classification_report, roc_auc_score, roc_curve

import tensorflow as tf
from tensorflow.keras.models import Model
from tensorflow.keras.layers import Dense, GlobalAveragePooling2D, Dropout
from tensorflow.keras.preprocessing.image import ImageDataGenerator
from tensorflow.keras.applications import ResNet50
from tensorflow.keras.applications.resnet50 import preprocess_input
```

 # Set Paths

```
base_path = "/path/to/effusion_cytology_split" # Replace this by your own path
train_dir = os.path.join(base_path, "train")
val_dir = os.path.join(base_path, "val")
test_dir = os.path.join(base_path, "test")
```

 # Parameters

```
img_size = (224, 224)
batch_size = 32
epochs = 15
```

 # Image Generators

```
train_datagen = ImageDataGenerator(preprocessing_function=preprocess_input)
val_test_datagen = ImageDataGenerator(preprocessing_function=preprocess_input)
```

```
train_gen = train_datagen.flow_from_directory(
 train_dir, target_size=img_size, batch_size=batch_size,
 class_mode='binary', shuffle=True
)

val_gen = val_test_datagen.flow_from_directory(
 val_dir, target_size=img_size, batch_size=batch_size,
 class_mode='binary', shuffle=False
)

test_gen = val_test_datagen.flow_from_directory(
 test_dir, target_size=img_size, batch_size=batch_size,
 class_mode='binary', shuffle=False
)
```

 # Building the CNN Model

```
model = Sequential([
 Conv2D(32, (3, 3), activation='relu', input_shape=(*img_size, 3)),
 MaxPooling2D(2, 2),

 Conv2D(64, (3, 3), activation='relu'),
 MaxPooling2D(2, 2),

 Conv2D(128, (3, 3), activation='relu'),
 MaxPooling2D(2, 2),

 Flatten(),
 Dropout(0.5),
 Dense(128, activation='relu'),
 Dense(1, activation='sigmoid')
])

model.compile(optimizer='adam', loss='binary_crossentropy', metrics=['accuracy'])
model.summary()
```

 # Train the Model

```
history = model.fit(
 train_gen,
 validation_data=val_gen,
 epochs=epochs,
 callbacks=[tf.keras.callbacks.EarlyStopping(patience=3, restore_best_weights=True)]
)
```

#Save the Model

```
model.save("cytology_malignancy_cnn_model.h5")
```

 # Plot Accuracy and Loss

```
plt.figure(figsize=(12, 5))
```

 # Accuracy

```
plt.subplot(1, 2, 1)
plt.plot(history.history['accuracy'], label="Train Acc")
plt.plot(history.history['val_accuracy'], label="Val Acc")
plt.title("Training and Validation Accuracy")
plt.xlabel("Epoch")
plt.ylabel("Accuracy")
plt.legend()
plt.grid(True)
```

 # Loss

```
plt.subplot(1, 2, 2)
plt.plot(history.history['loss'], label="Train Loss")
plt.plot(history.history['val_loss'], label="Val Loss")
plt.title("Training and Validation Loss")
plt.xlabel("Epoch")
plt.ylabel("Loss")
plt.legend()
plt.grid(True)

plt.tight_layout()
plt.show()
```

 # Test Evaluation

```
test_gen.reset()
y_prob = model.predict(test_gen)
y_pred = (y_prob > 0.5).astype(int).flatten()
y_true = test_gen.classes
```

 # Confusion Matrix & Classification Report

```
print("\n--- Classification Report ---")
print(classification_report(y_true, y_pred, target_names=["Benign", "Malignant"]))

print("\n--- Confusion Matrix ---")
print(confusion_matrix(y_true, y_pred))
```

 # ROC Curve & AUC

```
roc_auc = roc_auc_score(y_true, y_prob)
fpr, tpr, _ = roc_curve(y_true, y_prob)

plt.figure(figsize=(6, 6))
plt.plot(fpr, tpr, label=f"AUC = {roc_auc:.4f}")
plt.plot([0, 1], [0, 1], 'k--')
plt.title("ROC Curve on Test Set")
plt.xlabel("False Positive Rate")
plt.ylabel("True Positive Rate")
plt.legend()
plt.grid(True)
plt.show()

print(f"\nTest ROC-AUC Score: {roc_auc:.4f}")
```

Note Please replace the path of basepath (including all your images), train path, validation path and test path according to your local data. (Right-click on the subfolder will show you the path. Please make a forward slash "'/")

19.5 Transfer Learning with ResNet50 in Effusion Cytology

Transfer learning can improve the model's efficiency several times. Here, a previously trained similar type of model ResNet 50 as a base model with an added layer is used to increase the model's efficiency.

ResNet50 Transfer Code

```
import os
import numpy as np
import matplotlib.pyplot as plt
from sklearn.metrics import confusion_matrix, classification_report, roc_auc_score, roc_curve
import tensorflow as tf
from tensorflow.keras.models import Model
from tensorflow.keras.layers import Dense, GlobalAveragePooling2D, Dropout
from tensorflow.keras.preprocessing.image import ImageDataGenerator
from tensorflow.keras.applications import ResNet50
from tensorflow.keras.applications.resnet50 import
preprocess_input
```

 # Set Paths

```
base_path = "/path/to/effusion_cytology_split" # Replace this
train_dir = os.path.join(base_path, "train")
```

```
val_dir = os.path.join(base_path, "val")
test_dir = os.path.join(base_path, "test")
```

Parameters

```
img_size = (224, 224)
batch_size = 32
epochs = 15
```

Image Generators

```
train_datagen = ImageDataGenerator(preprocessing_function=preprocess_input)
val_test_datagen = ImageDataGenerator(preprocessing_function=preprocess_input)

train_gen = train_datagen.flow_from_directory(
 train_dir, target_size=img_size, batch_size=batch_size,
 class_mode='binary', shuffle=True
)

val_gen = val_test_datagen.flow_from_directory(
 val_dir, target_size=img_size, batch_size=batch_size,
 class_mode='binary', shuffle=False
)

test_gen = val_test_datagen.flow_from_directory(
 test_dir, target_size=img_size, batch_size=batch_size,
 class_mode='binary', shuffle=False
)
```

Build Transfer Learning Model

```
base_model = ResNet50(weights='imagenet', include_top=False, input_shape=(*img_size, 3))
base_model.trainable = False # Freeze base layers
```

Add Custom Classification Layers

```
x = base_model.output
x = GlobalAveragePooling2D()(x)
x = Dropout(0.5)(x)
x = Dense(128, activation='relu')(x)
x = Dropout(0.3)(x)
output = Dense(1, activation='sigmoid')(x)

model = Model(inputs=base_model.input, outputs=output)

model.compile(optimizer='adam', loss='binary_crossentropy', metrics=['accuracy'])
model.summary()
```

```
# Train the Model
history = model.fit(
 train_gen,
 validation_data=val_gen,
 epochs=epochs,
 callbacks=[tf.keras.callbacks.EarlyStopping(patience=3, restore_best_weights=True)]
)

# Save the Model
model.save("resnet50_cytology_malignancy_model.h5")

# Plot Training Curves
plt.figure(figsize=(12, 5))

plt.subplot(1, 2, 1)
plt.plot(history.history['accuracy'], label="Train Acc")
plt.plot(history.history['val_accuracy'], label="Val Acc")
plt.title("Accuracy")
plt.xlabel("Epoch")
plt.ylabel("Accuracy")
plt.legend()
plt.grid(True)

plt.subplot(1, 2, 2)
plt.plot(history.history['loss'], label="Train Loss")
plt.plot(history.history['val_loss'], label="Val Loss")
plt.title("Loss")
plt.xlabel("Epoch")
plt.ylabel("Loss")
plt.legend()
plt.grid(True)

plt.tight_layout()
plt.show()

# Test Evaluation
test_gen.reset()
y_prob = model.predict(test_gen)
y_pred = (y_prob > 0.5).astype(int).flatten()
y_true = test_gen.classes

# Confusion Matrix & Report
print("\n--- Classification Report ---")
print(classification_report(y_true, y_pred, target_names=["Benign", "Malignant"]))
```

```
print("\n--- Confusion Matrix ---")
print(confusion_matrix(y_true, y_pred))
```

#ROC & AUC

```
roc_auc = roc_auc_score(y_true, y_prob)
fpr, tpr, _ = roc_curve(y_true, y_prob)

plt.figure(figsize=(6, 6))
plt.plot(fpr, tpr, label=f"AUC = {roc_auc:.4f}")
plt.plot([0, 1], [0, 1], 'k--')
plt.title("ROC Curve")
plt.xlabel("False Positive Rate")
plt.ylabel("True Positive Rate")
plt.legend()
plt.grid(True)
plt.show()

print(f"\nTest ROC-AUC Score: {roc_auc:.4f}")
```

19.6 Urine Cytology Code for Basic CNN Model

#CODE

```
import os
import tensorflow as tf
from tensorflow.keras.preprocessing.image import
ImageDataGenerator
from tensorflow.keras.models import Sequential
from tensorflow.keras.layers import Conv2D, MaxPooling2D, Flatten, Dense, Dropout,
BatchNormalization
from tensorflow.keras.optimizers import Adam
from tensorflow.keras.callbacks import EarlyStopping,
ModelCheckpoint
import matplotlib.pyplot as plt
```

 # Set Parameters

```
IMAGE_SIZE = (224, 224)
BATCH_SIZE = 32

train_dir = 'data/train'
val_dir = 'data/val'
test_dir = 'data/test'
```

 # Image Augmentation for Training

```
train_datagen = ImageDataGenerator(
 rescale=1./255,
```

```
    rotation_range=20,
    zoom_range=0.2,
    shear_range=0.2,
    horizontal_flip=True
)

val_test_datagen = ImageDataGenerator(rescale=1./255)

train_generator = train_datagen.flow_from_directory(
    train_dir,
    target_size=IMAGE_SIZE,
    batch_size=BATCH_SIZE,
    class_mode='binary'
)

val_generator = val_test_datagen.flow_from_directory(
    val_dir,
    target_size=IMAGE_SIZE,
    batch_size=BATCH_SIZE,
    class_mode='binary'
)

test_generator = val_test_datagen.flow_from_directory(
    test_dir,
    target_size=IMAGE_SIZE,
    batch_size=BATCH_SIZE,
    class_mode='binary',
    shuffle=False
)
```

#CNN Model Architecture

```
model = Sequential([
    Conv2D(32, (3, 3), activation='relu', input_shape=(224, 224, 3)),
    BatchNormalization(),
    MaxPooling2D(2, 2),

    Conv2D(64, (3, 3), activation='relu'),
    BatchNormalization(),
    MaxPooling2D(2, 2),

    Conv2D(128, (3, 3), activation='relu'),
    BatchNormalization(),
    MaxPooling2D(2, 2),
```

```
 Flatten(),
 Dense(128, activation='relu'),
 Dropout(0.5),
 Dense(1, activation='sigmoid')
])

model.compile(
 optimizer=Adam(learning_rate=0.0001),
 loss='binary_crossentropy',
 metrics=['accuracy']
)
model.summary()
# Model Training
callbacks = [
 EarlyStopping(patience=5, restore_best_weights=True),
 ModelCheckpoint('best_model.h5', save_best_only=True)
]

history = model.fit(
 train_generator,
 validation_data=val_generator,
 epochs=30,
 callbacks=callbacks
)
```

#Plotting Accuracy & Loss

```
plt.figure(figsize=(12, 5))
plt.subplot(1, 2, 1)
plt.plot(history.history['accuracy'], label='Train Acc')
plt.plot(history.history['val_accuracy'], label='Val Acc')
plt.title('Accuracy')
plt.legend()

plt.subplot(1, 2, 2)
plt.plot(history.history['loss'], label='Train Loss')
plt.plot(history.history['val_loss'], label='Val Loss')
plt.title('Loss')
plt.legend()
plt.show()
```

#Model Evaluation

```
test_loss, test_acc = model.evaluate(test_generator)
print(f"Test Accuracy: {test_acc:.2f}")
# Optional: Confusion Matrix
import numpy as np
```

```
from sklearn.metrics import classification_report, confusion_matrix
import seaborn as sns
```

 # Predictions

```
pred_probs = model.predict(test_generator)
pred_labels = (pred_probs > 0.5).astype(int).flatten()
true_labels = test_generator.classes
```

 # Confusion Matrix

```
cm = confusion_matrix(true_labels, pred_labels)
sns.heatmap(cm, annot=True, fmt='d', cmap='Blues', xticklabels=['Benign',
'Malignant'], yticklabels=['Benign', 'Malignant'])
plt.xlabel('Predicted')
plt.ylabel('True')
plt.title('Confusion Matrix')
plt.show()
```

 # Classification Report

```
print(classification_report(true_labels, pred_labels, target_names=['Benign', 'Malignant']))
#Save Model
model.save('malignant_cell_detector_cnn.h5')
```

19.7 Urine by Transfer Learning (ResNet18) Model

```
# pip install torch torchvision scikit-learn matplotlib
```

#Code

```
import os
import torch
import torch.nn as nn
import torch.optim as optim
from torchvision import models, transforms, datasets
from torch.utils.data import DataLoader
from sklearn.metrics import confusion_matrix, roc_curve, auc
import matplotlib.pyplot as plt
import numpy as np
import seaborn as sns
```

 # Set Device

```
device = torch.device("cuda" if torch.cuda.is_available() else "cpu")
```

Paths
```
data_dir = "urine_cytology_dataset" # Structure: data_dir/train/class_x, /val/
class_y, /test/class_z
train_dir = os.path.join(data_dir, 'train')
val_dir = os.path.join(data_dir, 'val')
test_dir = os.path.join(data_dir, 'test')
```

Data Transforms
```
transform = transforms.Compose([
 transforms.Resize((224, 224)),
 transforms.ToTensor(),
 transforms.Normalize([0.485, 0.456, 0.406],
 [0.229, 0.224, 0.225])
])
```

Datasets
```
train_data = datasets.ImageFolder(train_dir, transform=transform)
val_data = datasets.ImageFolder(val_dir, transform=transform)
test_data = datasets.ImageFolder(test_dir, transform=transform)
```

Dataloaders
```
train_loader = DataLoader(train_data, batch_size=32, shuffle=True)
val_loader = DataLoader(val_data, batch_size=32, shuffle=False)
test_loader = DataLoader(test_data, batch_size=32, shuffle=False)
```

Load Pretrained ResNet18
```
model = models.resnet18(pretrained=True)
```

Modify the Classifier
```
num_ftrs = model.fc.in_features
model.fc = nn.Linear(num_ftrs, 2) # Binary classification: malignant vs benign
model = model.to(device)
```

Loss and Optimizer
```
criterion = nn.CrossEntropyLoss()
optimizer = optim.Adam(model.parameters(), lr=1e-4)
```

Training Loop
```
num_epochs = 10
for epoch in range(num_epochs):
 model.train()
 running_loss = 0.0
 correct = 0
 total = 0
```

```
for inputs, labels in train_loader:
inputs, labels = inputs.to(device), labels.to(device)

optimizer.zero_grad()
outputs = model(inputs)
loss = criterion(outputs, labels)
loss.backward()
optimizer.step()

running_loss += loss.item()
_, predicted = torch.max(outputs, 1)
total += labels.size(0)
correct += (predicted == labels).sum().item()

val_acc = 0
model.eval()
with torch.no_grad():
correct_val = 0
total_val = 0
for inputs, labels in val_loader:
inputs, labels = inputs.to(device), labels.to(device)
outputs = model(inputs)
_, predicted = torch.max(outputs, 1)
total_val += labels.size(0)
correct_val += (predicted == labels).sum().item()
val_acc = correct_val / total_val

print(f"Epoch {epoch+1}/{num_epochs}, Loss: {running_loss/len(train_
loader):.4f}, Train Acc: {correct/total:.4f}, Val Acc: {val_acc:.4f}")
```

Evaluation on Test Set

```
model.eval()
all_preds = []
all_labels = []
all_probs = []

with torch.no_grad():
for inputs, labels in test_loader:
inputs = inputs.to(device)
outputs = model(inputs)
probs = torch.softmax(outputs, dim=1)[:, 1].cpu().numpy()
_, preds = torch.max(outputs, 1)
```

```
 all_preds.extend(preds.cpu().numpy())
 all_labels.extend(labels.numpy())
 all_probs.extend(probs)
```

 # Confusion Matrix

```
cm = confusion_matrix(all_labels, all_preds)
sns.heatmap(cm, annot=True, fmt="d", cmap="Blues", xticklabels=train_data.classes,
yticklabels=train_data.classes)
plt.title("Confusion Matrix")
plt.xlabel("Predicted")
plt.ylabel("Actual")
plt.show()
```

 # ROC Curve

```
fpr, tpr, _ = roc_curve(all_labels, all_probs)
roc_auc = auc(fpr, tpr)

plt.figure()
plt.plot(fpr, tpr, label=f"AUC = {roc_auc:.2f}")
plt.plot([0, 1], [0, 1], linestyle="--")
plt.xlabel("False Positive Rate")
plt.ylabel("True Positive Rate")
plt.title("ROC Curve")
plt.legend(loc="lower right")
plt.show()
```

19.8 Breast Carcinomas for Benign and Malignant Cells

```
pip install tensorflow scikit-learn matplotlib seaborn
```

Code

```
import os
import numpy as np
import matplotlib.pyplot as plt
import seaborn as sns
from sklearn.metrics import classification_report, confusion_matrix, roc_curve, auc
from tensorflow.keras.preprocessing.image import ImageDataGenerator
from tensorflow.keras.applications import EfficientNetB0
from tensorflow.keras.models import Model
from tensorflow.keras.layers import Dense, GlobalAveragePooling2D
from tensorflow.keras.optimizers import Adam
from tensorflow.keras.callbacks import EarlyStopping
```

 # 1. Path Setup

```
IMG_SIZE = 224
BATCH_SIZE = 32
EPOCHS = 10

DATA_DIR = '/path/to/data/' # <- Update this to your actual path
TRAIN_DIR = os.path.join(DATA_DIR, 'train')
VAL_DIR = os.path.join(DATA_DIR, 'val')
TEST_DIR = os.path.join(DATA_DIR, 'test')
```

 # 2. Data Generators

```
datagen = ImageDataGenerator(rescale=1./255)

train_gen = datagen.flow_from_directory(
 TRAIN_DIR,
 target_size=(IMG_SIZE, IMG_SIZE),
 batch_size=BATCH_SIZE,
 class_mode='binary'
)

val_gen = datagen.flow_from_directory(
 VAL_DIR,
 target_size=(IMG_SIZE, IMG_SIZE),
 batch_size=BATCH_SIZE,
 class_mode='binary'
)

test_gen = datagen.flow_from_directory(
 TEST_DIR,
 target_size=(IMG_SIZE, IMG_SIZE),
 batch_size=BATCH_SIZE,
 class_mode='binary',
 shuffle=False # Keep order for evaluation
)
```

 # 3. Transfer Learning Model

```
base_model = EfficientNetB0(weights='imagenet', include_top=False, input_shape=(IMG_
SIZE, IMG_SIZE, 3))
base_model.trainable = False

x = GlobalAveragePooling2D()(base_model.output)
x = Dense(128, activation='relu')(x)
output = Dense(1, activation='sigmoid')(x)
```

```
model = Model(inputs=base_model.input, outputs=output)
model.compile(optimizer=Adam(1e-4), loss='binary_crossentropy', metrics=['accuracy'])
```

4. Training

```
early_stop = EarlyStopping(monitor='val_loss', patience=3, restore_best_weights=True)

history = model.fit(
 train_gen,
 epochs=EPOCHS,
 validation_data=val_gen,
 callbacks=[early_stop]
)
```

#5. Evaluation on Test Set

```
test_gen.reset()
y_true = test_gen.classes
y_pred_probs = model.predict(test_gen).ravel()
y_pred = (y_pred_probs > 0.5).astype(int)
```

Confusion Matrix

```
cm = confusion_matrix(y_true, y_pred)
sns.heatmap(cm, annot=True, fmt="d", cmap="Blues", xticklabels=test_gen.class_
indices.keys(), yticklabels=test_gen.class_indices.keys())
plt.xlabel('Predicted')
plt.ylabel('True')
plt.title('Confusion Matrix')
plt.show()
```

Classification Report

```
print("\nClassification Report:\n")
print(classification_report(y_true, y_pred, target_names=list(test_gen.class_indices.keys())))
```

ROC Curve

```
fpr, tpr, _ = roc_curve(y_true, y_pred_probs)
roc_auc = auc(fpr, tpr)

plt.figure()
plt.plot(fpr, tpr, label=f"ROC Curve (AUC = {roc_auc:.2f})", color='blue')
plt.plot([0, 1], [0, 1], 'k--')
plt.xlabel("False Positive Rate")
```

```
plt.ylabel("True Positive Rate")
plt.title("ROC Curve")
plt.legend(loc="lower right")
plt.grid(True)
plt.show()
```

19.9 CNN Model on Cervical Smears to Detect Normal, Atypical and Dysplastic Cells

19.9.1 Code

#Please Install

```
pip install tensorflow scikit-learn matplotlib
```

#Code

```
import numpy as np
import matplotlib.pyplot as plt
import itertools
from sklearn.metrics import confusion_matrix, roc_curve, auc
from sklearn.preprocessing import label_binarize
import tensorflow as tf
from tensorflow.keras.preprocessing.image import ImageDataGenerator
from tensorflow.keras.models import Sequential
from tensorflow.keras.layers import Conv2D, MaxPooling2D, Flatten, Dense, Dropout
from tensorflow.keras.optimizers import Adam
```

 # Set Parameters

```
img_height, img_width = 128, 128
batch_size = 32
epochs = 15
num_classes = 3
class_names = ['normal', 'atypical', 'dysplasia']
```

 # Paths to Your Data

```
train_dir = 'dataset/train'
val_dir = 'dataset/val'
test_dir = 'dataset/test'
```

 # Image Data Generators

```
train_datagen = ImageDataGenerator(rescale=1./255)
val_datagen = ImageDataGenerator(rescale=1./255)
test_datagen = ImageDataGenerator(rescale=1./255)
```

 # Load Datasets

```
train_gen = train_datagen.flow_from_directory(
 train_dir, target_size=(img_height, img_width),
 batch_size=batch_size, class_mode='categorical'
)

val_gen = val_datagen.flow_from_directory(
 val_dir, target_size=(img_height, img_width),
 batch_size=batch_size, class_mode='categorical'
)

test_gen = test_datagen.flow_from_directory(
 test_dir, target_size=(img_height, img_width),
 batch_size=1, class_mode='categorical', shuffle=False
)
```

 # Define CNN Model

```
model = Sequential([
Conv2D(32, (3, 3), activation='relu', input_shape=(img_height, img_width, 3)),
 MaxPooling2D(2, 2),
 Conv2D(64, (3, 3), activation='relu'),
 MaxPooling2D(2, 2),
 Conv2D(128, (3, 3), activation='relu'),
 MaxPooling2D(2, 2),
 Flatten(),
 Dense(128, activation='relu'),
 Dropout(0.5),
 Dense(num_classes, activation='softmax')
])

model.compile(optimizer=Adam(1e-4), loss='categorical_crossentropy',
metrics=['accuracy'])

model.summary()
```

 # Train Model

```
history = model.fit(
 train_gen,
 validation_data=val_gen,
 epochs=epochs
)
```

 # Evaluate Model on Test Data

```
Y_pred = model.predict(test_gen)
y_pred = np.argmax(Y_pred, axis=1)
y_true = test_gen.classes
```

 # Confusion Matrix

```
def plot_confusion_matrix(cm, classes, normalize=False, title='Confusion Matrix'):
  plt.figure(figsize=(6,6))
  plt.imshow(cm, interpolation='nearest', cmap=plt.cm.Blues)
  plt.title(title)
  plt.colorbar()
  tick_marks = np.arange(len(classes))
  plt.xticks(tick_marks, classes, rotation=45)
  plt.yticks(tick_marks, classes)

  fmt = '.2f' if normalize else 'd'
  thresh = cm.max() / 2.

 for i, j in itertools.product(range(cm.shape[0]), range(cm.shape[1])):
  plt.text(j, i, format(cm[i, j], fmt),
  horizontalalignment="center",
  color="white" if cm[i, j] > thresh else "black")

  plt.ylabel('True label')
  plt.xlabel('Predicted label')
  plt.tight_layout()

 cm = confusion_matrix(y_true, y_pred)
plot_confusion_matrix(cm, classes=class_names, title='Confusion Matrix')
 plt.show()
```

 # Confusion Matrix Plot

```
cm = confusion_matrix(y_true, y_pred)
plot_confusion_matrix(cm, class_names, title='Confusion Matrix')
```

 # Save it as PNG

```
plt.savefig('confusion_matrix.png', dpi=300, bbox_inches='tight')
plt.close()
```

 # ROC Curves

```
y_true_bin = label_binarize(y_true, classes=[0, 1, 2])
fpr, tpr, roc_auc = {}, {}, {}

for i in range(num_classes):
 fpr[i], tpr[i], _ = roc_curve(y_true_bin[:, i], Y_pred[:, i])
 roc_auc[i] = auc(fpr[i], tpr[i])
```

 # Plot ROC

```
plt.figure()
colors = ['blue', 'orange', 'red']
for i in range(num_classes):
 plt.plot(fpr[i], tpr[i], color=colors[i],
label=f'ROC curve for {class_names[i]} (area = {roc_auc[i]:.2f})')

plt.plot([0, 1], [0, 1], 'k--')
plt.xlim([0.0, 1.0])
plt.ylim([0.0, 1.05])
plt.xlabel('False Positive Rate')
plt.ylabel('True Positive Rate')
plt.title('Multi-class ROC Curve')
plt.legend(loc="lower right")
plt.show()
```

 # ROC Curve Plot

```
fpr, tpr, _ = roc_curve(y_true, y_prob)
roc_auc = auc(fpr, tpr)

plt.figure()
plt.plot(fpr, tpr, color='darkorange', lw=2, label=f'ROC curve (area = {roc_auc:.2f})')
plt.plot([0, 1], [0, 1], color='gray', linestyle='--')
plt.xlim([0.0, 1.0])
plt.ylim([0.0, 1.05])
plt.xlabel('False Positive Rate')
plt.ylabel('True Positive Rate')
plt.title('ROC Curve - Normal vs Abnormal')
plt.legend(loc="lower right")
```

 # Save ROC curve

```
plt.savefig('roc_curve.png', dpi=300, bbox_inches='tight')
plt.close()
```

19.10 Transfer Learning in Three Classes with ROC Saving

Code

```
Full Transfer Learning Code (Multiclass with ROC + CM Save)
import numpy as np
import matplotlib.pyplot as plt
import itertools
import os
from sklearn.metrics import confusion_matrix, roc_curve, auc
from sklearn.preprocessing import label_binarize
from tensorflow.keras.preprocessing.image import ImageDataGenerator
from tensorflow.keras.applications import MobileNetV2
from tensorflow.keras.models import Model
from tensorflow.keras.layers import Dense, GlobalAveragePooling2D, Dropout
from tensorflow.keras.optimizers import Adam
```

Parameters

```
img_height, img_width = 224, 224
batch_size = 32
epochs = 10
class_names = ['normal', 'atypical', 'dysplasia']
num_classes = len(class_names)
```

PATHS

```
train_dir = 'dataset/train'
val_dir = 'dataset/val'
test_dir = 'dataset/test'
```

Data Loaders

```
train_datagen = ImageDataGenerator(rescale=1./255)
val_test_datagen = ImageDataGenerator(rescale=1./255)

train_gen = train_datagen.flow_from_directory(
 train_dir, target_size=(img_height, img_width),
 batch_size=batch_size, class_mode='categorical'
)

val_gen = val_test_datagen.flow_from_directory(
 val_dir, target_size=(img_height, img_width),
 batch_size=batch_size, class_mode='categorical'
)

test_gen = val_test_datagen.flow_from_directory(
```

```
 test_dir, target_size=(img_height, img_width),
 batch_size=1, class_mode='categorical', shuffle=False
)
```

#Transfer Learning Model

```
base_model = MobileNetV2(weights='imagenet', include_top=False, input_shape=(img_
height, img_width, 3))
base_model.trainable = False

x = base_model.output
x = GlobalAveragePooling2D()(x)
x = Dropout(0.3)(x)
x = Dense(128, activation='relu')(x)
x = Dropout(0.3)(x)
predictions = Dense(num_classes, activation='softmax')(x)

model = Model(inputs=base_model.input, outputs=predictions)
model.compile(optimizer=Adam(1e-4), loss='categorical_crossentropy',
metrics=['accuracy'])
model.summary()
```

 # Training

```
history = model.fit(train_gen, validation_data=val_gen, epochs=epochs)
```

 # prediction on Test Set

```
Y_prob = model.predict(test_gen)
y_pred = np.argmax(Y_prob, axis=1)
y_true = test_gen.classes
```

 # Confusion Matrix

```
def plot_confusion_matrix(cm, classes, save_path=None):
 plt.figure(figsize=(6,6))
 plt.imshow(cm, interpolation='nearest', cmap=plt.cm.Blues)
 plt.title("Confusion Matrix")
 plt.colorbar()
 tick_marks = np.arange(len(classes))
 plt.xticks(tick_marks, classes, rotation=45)
 plt.yticks(tick_marks, classes)

 fmt = 'd'
 thresh = cm.max() / 2.

 for i, j in itertools.product(range(cm.shape[0]), range(cm.shape[1])):
```

```
 plt.text(j, i, format(cm[i, j], fmt),
 horizontalalignment="center",
 color="white" if cm[i, j] > thresh else "black")

 plt.ylabel('True label')
 plt.xlabel('Predicted label')
 plt.tight_layout()

 if save_path:
 plt.savefig(save_path, dpi=300, bbox_inches='tight')
 plt.close()

cm = confusion_matrix(y_true, y_pred)
plot_confusion_matrix(cm, class_names, save_path='confusion_matrix.png')
```

 # MULTICLASS ROC Curve

```
y_true_bin = label_binarize(y_true, classes=[0, 1, 2])
fpr, tpr, roc_auc = {}, {}, {}

for i in range(num_classes):
 fpr[i], tpr[i], _ = roc_curve(y_true_bin[:, i], Y_prob[:, i])
 roc_auc[i] = auc(fpr[i], tpr[i])
```

 # Plot ROC Curve

```
plt.figure()
colors = ['blue', 'orange', 'green']
for i in range(num_classes):
 plt.plot(fpr[i], tpr[i], color=colors[i], lw=2,
 label=f'ROC curve ({class_names[i]}) - AUC = {roc_auc[i]:.2f}')

plt.plot([0, 1], [0, 1], 'k--')
plt.xlim([0.0, 1.0])
plt.ylim([0.0, 1.05])
plt.xlabel('False Positive Rate')
plt.ylabel('True Positive Rate')
plt.title('Multi-class ROC Curve')
plt.legend(loc="lower right")

plt.savefig('roc_curve.png', dpi=300, bbox_inches='tight')
plt.close()
```

References

1. Greener JG, Kandathil SM, Moffat L, Jones DT. A guide to machine learning for biologists. Nat Rev Mol Cell Biol. 2022;23(1):40–55. https://doi.org/10.1038/s41580-021-00407-0. Epub 2021 Sep 13. PMID: 34518686.
2. Huang Q, Zhao T. Data collection and labeling techniques for machine learning. arXiv:2407.12793.
3. Salehi AW, Khan S, Gupta G, Alabduallah BI, Almjally A, Alsolai H, Siddiqui T, Mellit A. A study of CNN and transfer learning in medical imaging: advantages, challenges, future scope. Sustainability. 2023;15(7):5930.
4. Dey P. The emerging role of deep learning in cytology. Cytopathology. 2021;32(2):154–60.
5. Dey P, Bansal B, Saini T. An emerging era of computational cytology. Diagn Cytopathol. 2023;51(4):270–5.

Part VI

Challenges and Future Directions

Data Storage, Transfer, Security and Ethical Issues in Computational Cytology

20

Abstract

The data is the fundamental component in the implementation of artificial intelligence (AI) in cytology. It provides the basic information and all the raw materials to build up the mansion of AI. So after successful data collection and preprocessing, data storage and sharing are needed. Data can be stored in a local computer or in cloud storage. To have a complete worldwide network, the data sharing is important. The data sharing can be done by direct transferring the data, cloud-based transfer, physical transfer, federated learning, and edge computing. At the time of data sharing, the security of the data component is equally important. Sharing of the stored data is always vulnerable to ethical issues. In fact, the implementation of AI in the medical field is intimately related to various ethical issues. In this chapter, the data storage, data sharing, data security and ethical issues are discussed.

Keywords

Data storage · Data sharing · Data security · Data ethics · Cloud-based transfer · Physical transfer · Federated learning · Edge computing

20.1 Introduction

The data is the fundamental component in the implementation of artificial intelligence (AI) in cytology. It provides the basic information and all the raw materials to build up the mansion of AI. So after successful data collection and preprocessing, data storage and sharing are needed. To have a complete worldwide network the data sharing is important. At the time of data sharing, the security of the data component is equally important. Sharing of the stored data is always vulnerable to ethical issues. In fact, the implementation of AI in the medical field is intimately related

P. Dey, *Computational Cytology*, https://doi.org/10.1007/978-981-95-3272-8_20

to various ethical issues [1–6]. In this chapter, the data storage, data sharing, a security and ethical issues are discussed.

20.2 Data Storage

The data in cytology (pathology) laboratories is stored both as whole slide imaging (WSI) and as metadata. Metadata refers annotations, labels, etc. At times, we need to store clinical data and other relevant laboratory investigations.

20.2.1 Types of Data to Store

1. WSI of microscopic images: WSI is usually saved in formats like .svs, .tiff, .ndpi, etc. WSI images are usually in gigapixels.
2. Tiles or small patches: These are the small images extracted from WSI.
3. Annotations: These are the regions of interest or cancer labels. These images are stored as JSON, XML, etc.
4. Metadata: It consists of various information related to patient identification, type of stain, etc.
5. Labels: The diagnosis of the cases.

20.2.2 Storage Formats

- *WSI*: WSI is usually saved as formats like .svs, .tiff, .ndpi, etc. After preprocessing the image, WSI can be stored as jpg or png format.
- *Metadata*: The metadata and labels are stored as CSV or Parquet.
- *Annotations*: The files are stored as JSON or XML.
- Large dataset: TFRecord (TensorFlow)/LMDB (PyTorch) can be used for storing a large dataset.

20.2.3 Data Storage Spaces

1. *Local Storage*: Files can be stored locally for small to mid-sized datasets (<1TB). The files/folders can be stored in SSD or NVME drive.

Limitations

- Not scalable
- It needs proper backup
- Difficult to collaborate with remote laboratories

Table 20.1 Comparison of different storage systems

Feature	Local SSD	Google Cloud Storage (GCS)	Amazon S3	Azure Blob Storage
Storage Capacity	Usually few TBs	Virtually unlimited	Virtually unlimited	Virtually unlimited
Speed	Very high	High	High	High
Remote Accessibility	No. only local use	Remote via internet	Remote via internet	Remote via internet
Scalability	Not scalable	Auto-scalable	Auto-scalable	Auto-scalable
Cost	One-time hardware cost	Payment depends on storage space and time	Payment depends on storage space and time	Payment depends on storage space and time
Durability	Depends on backup	99.99% durability	99.99% durability	99.99% durability

2. *Cloud Storage*: In case of a huge dataset, the cloud storage is a better option. Moreover, cloud storage has added advantages of scalability and remote access facilities.

The commonly used cloud spaces are:

(a) *Google cloud space (GCS)*: GCS integrates well with the commonly used AI platforms TensorFlow and PyTorch.
(b) *Amazon S3*: Amazon S3 is also popular as it is scalable and works well with Python.
(c) *Azure Blob Storage*: It is compatible with azure-storage-blob SDK
- Used by many institutions with Microsoft infrastructure
- Compatible with azure-storage-blob SDK

Table 20.1 compares different storage systems.

20.3 Data Transfer

The successful and fast transfer of data are important pre-requisites for building an artificial intelligence system.

The data is transferred in following ways:

20.3.1 Direct Data Transfer (Centralized Data Transfer)

Direct transfer of data is a centralized approach where the pathology data from different local sites is sent to the central server. The central server receives the data comprised of WSIs, annotations, and metadata. The data is processed for building AI models.

Advantages

- The central data server provides uniform pre-processing and training of data
- Easily manageable and debuggable AI model.

Disadvantages

- Slow transfer due to the large data volume of WSI
- High risk of breach of data and accidental exposure
- Problems of data privacy or legal issues
- It needs high-bandwidth infrastructure

20.3.2 Cloud-Based Transfer & Collaboration Platforms

In Cloud-Based Transfer, the data is uploaded and stored in a cloud environment. The cloud-based secure environment may be Google Cloud, AWS, Aiforia, PathAI or SlideScore.

Advantages

- Remote sharing: The data is shared across the globe.
- Scalability: Cloud-based transfer can store and compute on huge datasets.
- Readymade tools: It has built-in tools for annotation and training.

Disadvantages

- *Cost*: Overall, costly as there is a recurrent cost
- *Variable regulatory law*: The data transfer may be across the country and so may violate the laws.
- *Trust*: The service providers should be trustful.

20.3.3 Physical Transfer

In case of physical transfer, the data is stored in the Hard Drives or SSDs and then shipped to the other party.

Advantages

- The transfer of a large dataset is relatively fast.
- Simple for the laboratories that work offline.
- No need for high-bandwidth internet service.

Disadvantages

- Damage: Risk of damage to the hard disc or theft
- Data privacy: It may come under data privacy laws
- Time: Time-consuming

20.3.4 Federated Learning (Model-to-Data)

Federated Learning can be said simply as a model to data. Here, the laboratories keep data on-site and AI models are trained in the local site. Instead of the raw data, only weights of the models are shared with the central server to make a global model [7] (Fig. 20.1).

Advantages
- Data privacy: Very high, as there is no option to share raw data.
- Legal restriction: It follows legal and ethical issues.
- Collaboration: No question of data ownership

Disadvantages
- Complexity: It is technically intricate
- Debug: Difficult
- Consistency: It needs a consistent model architecture

20.3.5 Edge Computing (Remote Execution)

In the case of edge computing, the code is sent to the laboratory and the data is executed locally. No raw data transfer is needed in edge computing [8]. So, it is also known as remote execution.

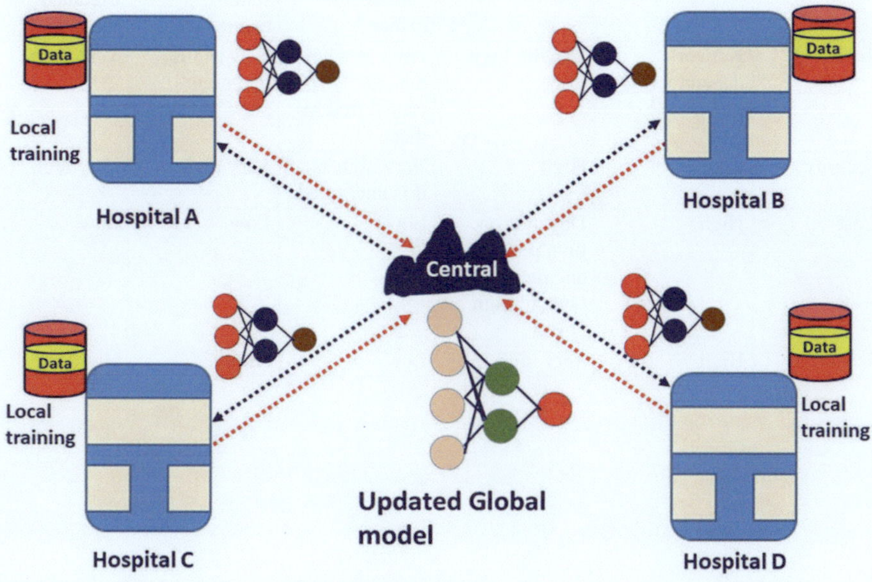

Fig. 20.1 Federated learning transfer of data

Advantages
- Data Transfer: No need to transfer raw data
- Data security: Totally secure

Disadvantages
- Information technology: It is dependent on firewalls, permissions, etc.
- Local resource: Limited due to lack of resource by local computational power
- Update: Complex procedure to update

Table 20.2 compares the different modes of data transfer.

Figure 20.2 shows the schematic diagram of various modes of data transfer.

Table 20.2 Comparison of the different modes of data transfer

Features	Centralized Transfer	Cloud-Based	Physical Media	Federated Learning	Edge Computing
Description	Pathology data from different local sites is sent to the central server	The data is uploaded and stored in a cloud environment	The data is manually transferred to the other party	Instead of the raw data, only weights of the models are shared to the central server	Data is processed locally at the source by the code given by central server
Data Transfer Location	It is located in the central server	Located in the cloud server	Data is transferred in the remote centercentre offline	Updated weights of the model sent to central server	No raw data transfer. Data is executed locally
Speed	Network dependent	Usually high	High as whole data is transferred by disc.	Low as the update is slow process	Very high
Security	Low	High	Very high as it is encrypted	Very high	Very high
Cost	High	Depends on time period and data load. Overall high cost	Low	Low	Low
Scalability	High	Very high	Low	High	High

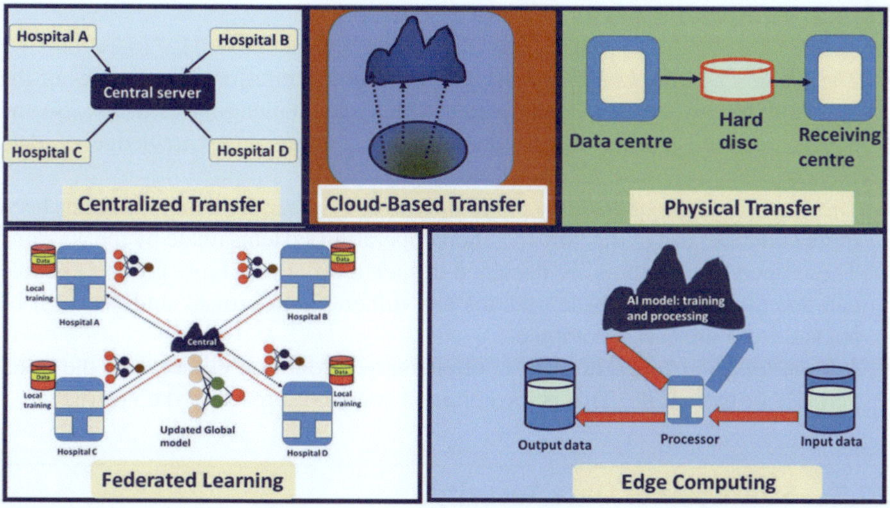

Fig. 20.2 The schematic diagram of various modes of data transfer

20.4 Data Security

Data security means protecting data at the time of collection, processing, storing and training of the AI model. The data is protected from unauthorized access, corruption, modification or leakage [3].

20.4.1 The Key Challenging Areas of Data Security

Data Privacy Data privacy is the most serious concern in AI. However, the term "privacy" is to some extent vague. Overall, data privacy means the personal information should not be disclosed and should be kept as confidential. It is the right of the individual to decide when and how their information will be accessed and shared.

Data Integrity The data should be cleaned and free from manipulation. The wilful insertion of malicious data may affect the entire AI model.

Model Theft The attackers may hack the AI model which is a valuable asset as it contains many sensitive information.

Inference Attacks There may be leakage of information through inference.

20.4.2 Vulnerable Areas of Data Security

- *The Increasing attacks by hackers*: There are now increasing occurrences of the cyber-attacks by evasive technologies which are challenging to detect. So the hackers can do extensive data damage even before any knowledge of data breach [4].
- *The Increasing use of "off-the-shelf" operating systems*: Recently, there has been more and more use of the "off-the-shelf" operating systems made by the vendors. These operating systems are designed in such a way that a large group of people can use the systems. These systems are vulnerable to viruses and data can be hacked from the user's computer.
- *Information Sharing*: The data is often shared from one clinician to the other verbally or by mobile. This is the common source of breach of data privacy.

20.5 Strategies of Data Security

There are certain strategies to Enhance Data Security [5].

The strategies are described below:

20.5.1 Basic Strategies

1. *Data Classification and Inventory:*
   - *Understand priority*: At the time of collection of data, one should identify the location and the importance of sensitive data. The *sensitive data should be prioritized.*
   - *Data Management*: Standardization of processing of data, storing and deletion are important for the health of the data system.
2. *Assessment of vulnerable data:*
   - *Identification of Vulnerabilities*: It is important to identify the potential areas of vulnerability to theft. Those areas should be under vigilance.
   - *Continuous Monitoring*: The system should be monitored in real time. The network infrastructure should be evaluated intermittently.
   - *Data Protection Policies*: There should be well-defined and comprehensive written instructions of data protection policies.

20.5.2 Technical Controls

1. *Data Anonymization*: Highly sensitive information can be masked and it can be used only for training as training dataset.
2. *Encryption*: Data encryption is another novel way to block unauthorized access [6].

(i) *At rest*: The sensitive data can be encrypted at the time of storage.
(ii) *Data transfer*: At the time of data transfer, the strict encryption protocols (e.g., HTTPS, TLS) should be used to protect data.
(iii) *Key Management*: The encryption key should be changed at regular intervals and the key should be strong enough to protect the data.

3. *Access Control*:
   (i) *Principle of Least Privilege*: The access to data should be limited and minimal to perform the specific jobs.
   (ii) *Role-Based Access Control*: The access should be assigned based on the role of the users within the laboratories.
   (iii) *Multi-Factor Authentication*: There should be multiple levels of authentication such as password, biometry, etc.
   (iv) *Regular Access Reviews*: There should be periodic audits of the access of the data by the users.
4. *Network Security*:
   (i) *Firewalls*: The firewalls should be configured properly to create a barrier of data monitoring and network access. The malicious traffic should be blocked.
   (ii) *Network Segmentation*: The network should be segregated into zones for the sensitive data.
   (iii) *Intrusion Detection/Prevention Systems (IDS/IPS)*: The implementation of IDS/ IPS may help to prevent unauthorized access.
5. *Endpoint Security*:
   (i) *Antivirus and Anti-malware*: Installation of proper antivirus and anti-malware software is needed. The software should be regularly updated.
   (ii) *Patch Management*: All the operating systems, software and security system should be regularly updated. It may help to detect an unnoticed data breach.
6. *Federated Learning*:

   As discussed before, Federated Learning helps to prevent raw data transfer. It only deals with the model's internal parameters.

20.5.3 Proactive and Adaptive Measures

1. *Vendor Risk Management*: The assessment of third-party vendors is essential as they have access to the data and may be a potential source of beach of data security.
2. *Threat Intelligence*: One should always be updated regarding the emerging threats and newer techniques of the data-attack.

Figure 20.3 shows the various technical aspects of data security.

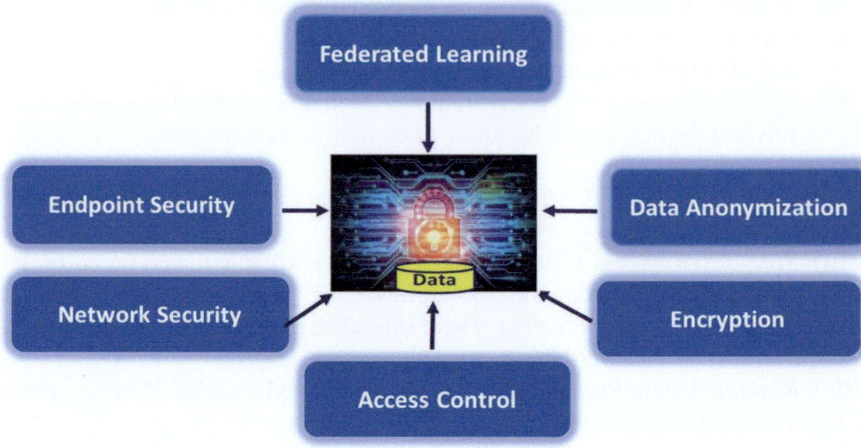

Fig. 20.3 The various technical strategies of data security

20.6 Ethical Issues Related to Data

The data handling in AI is deeply related to various ethical issues, particularly data transparency, bias and privacy. The key ethical issues are discussed here.

20.6.1 Privacy and Consent

(a) *Massive Data Collection and Surveillance*:
- *Issues*: AI system needs a huge amount of data that is collected from various sources and includes sensitive personal data.
- *Ethical question*: The unlimited data collection raises questions about the limit of data collection. How much data should be collected, even if it is anonymous?

(b) *Lack of Informed Consent:*
- *Issue*: The user often agrees to permit the data collection unknowingly. They do not read the lengthy terms and conditions.
- *Ethical Question*: The question is whether the consent is really informed or not? Most of the time, the individuals do not know how the data will be collected and how it will be used.

(c) *Re-identification Risks*:
- *Issue*: The "anonymized" information may not be totally anonymous and the person can be re-identified with the help of advanced AI techniques.
- *Ethical Question*: Is there any guarantee to make the data totally anonymous? What responsibility do we have if the re-identification is done?

20.6.2 Bias and Fairness

- *Concern*: AI model learns from the collected data. If the training data reflects the biases (such as racial, ethnic, etc., gender), then the AI model may wrongly perpetuate the bias.
- *Ethical Issue*: The biased AI model based on skewed data may make wrong decisions and injustice may occur.

20.6.3 Data Ownership and Control

- *Concern*: It is often unclear who owns the data: the individual or organizer or AI developers?
- *Ethical Issues*: As there is no control (or limited control) over the individual's own data so there is enough confusion about the right to profit from this data.

20.6.4 Transparency and Accountability

- *Concern*: The decision taken by AI is made by hidden layers. It is also known as "black box. We do not have any control over the black box. So most of the decisions taken by AI are often opaque, especially when managed by private entities.
- *Ethical Issue*: How can we make AI accountable when we do not know even how it has reached a certain decision.

20.6.5 Data Security

- *Concern*: AI uses a vast amount of data that is vulnerable to cyber-attacks. The hackers may expose the sensitive data.
- *Ethical Issue*: The question of moral obligations of organizers and AI developers to protect the data arises as a serious ethical issue.

20.7 Conclusions

We are in the era of data hacking and other moral issues like illegal data sharing and limited security to the confidentiality of the data. It is extremely important to take adequate measures during data sharing, as the data can be misused in the central cloud-based storage or direct data transfer. Federated learning transfer can prevent data misuse by third parties. Regarding the confidentiality of the data, we need to have data anonymization and strong data encryption facilities. For the successful implementation of AI, we need well-drafted medical ethics and laws.

References

1. Smallman M. Multi scale ethics-why we need to consider the ethics of AI in healthcare at different scales. Sci Eng Ethics. 2022;28(6):63. https://doi.org/10.1007/s11948-022-00396-z. PMID: 36441282; PMCID: PMC9705474.
2. McLennan S, Fiske A, Tigard D, Müller R, Haddadin S, Buyx A. Embedded ethics: a proposal for integrating ethics into the development of medical AI. BMC Med Ethics. 2022;23(1):6. https://doi.org/10.1186/s12910-022-00746-3. PMID: 35081955; PMCID: PMC8793193.
3. Elliott D, Soifer E. AI technologies, privacy, and security. Front Artif Intell. 2022;5:826737.
4. Liu V, Musen MA, Chou T. Data breaches of protected health information in the United States. JAMA. 2015;313(14):1471–3. https://doi.org/10.1001/jama.2015.2252. Erratum in: JAMA. 2015 Jun 23–30;313(24):2497.
5. Basil NN, Ambe S, Ekhator C, Fonkem E. Health records database and inherent security concerns: a review of the literature. Cureus. 2022;14(10):e30168. https://doi.org/10.7759/cureus.30168. PMID: 36397924; PMCID: PMC9647912.
6. Chenthara S, Ahmed K, Wang H, Whittaker F, Chen Z. Healthchain: a novel framework on privacy preservation of electronic health records using blockchain technology. PLoS One. 2020;15(12):e0243043.
7. Bao G, Guo P. Federated learning in cloud-edge collaborative architecture: key technologies, applications and challenges. J Cloud Comput (Heidelb). 2022;11(1):94. https://doi.org/10.1186/s13677-022-00377-4. Epub 2022 Dec 15. PMID: 36536803; PMCID: PMC9753079.
8. Gawande S, Gorde S. Edge computing in the cloud: enabling real-time data processing and analytics. J Emerg Technol Innov Res. 2014;11:206–9.

Future of Artificial Intelligence in Computational Cytology

21

Abstract

Artificial intelligence (AI) has made a paradigm shift in various fields of medical science. It has the full potential to help in the diagnosis, classification, interpretation of immunocytochemistry and molecular biology. AI can give a holistic approach to the disease to the pathologists and the clinicians. There are certain challenges and limitations in the implementation of AI in cytology laboratories such as good-quality data acquisition, ethical issues, black box problems and recognition from the regulatory authorities. It is expected that these limitations will be overcome in the future. The pathologist's effort leveraging AI will bring more effective care to the patients.

The present chapter explores the future pathway of AI in cytology in terms of the opportunities and challenges.

Keywords

Artificial intelligence · Cytology · Data acquisition · Ethical issues · Black box · Federated learning · Edge computing · Digital twin technology

21.1 Introduction

Artificial intelligence (AI) has made a paradigm shift in various fields of medical science [1–3]. The digital cytology, particularly whole slide images (WSI), along with AI can help in diagnosis, management and prognosis prediction [4]. Deep learning (DL) is now equipped with several advanced techniques that help in the generation of synthetic images, working with a small dataset and enhancing the efficiency of the model. The present chapter explores the future pathway of AI in cytology in terms of the opportunities and challenges.

P. Dey, *Computational Cytology*, https://doi.org/10.1007/978-981-95-3272-8_21

21.2 The Turning Points: Advanced Technologies in AI

The DL network (particularly the convolutional neural network, CNN) has made a grand success in the field of cytology in cancer screening, tumour classification and predicting prognosis [5, 6].

Generative Adversarial Networks (GAN) GAN is a newer entity in deep learning networks with the unique power of data creation. The large number of synthetic images generated by GANs help to train the neural network. Moreover, GAN can make high-quality quality realistic images and can be used for different purposes [7].

Multimodal Foundation Models (MFM) MFMs are pre-trained models and can do a wider range of tasks such as generating the data content from one modality to another modality, e.g., text to image and vice versa. MFM has the power to reason the diagram and chart [8].

Self-Supervised Learning (SSL) SSL technique learns by unsupervised learning from the unlabelled data that conventionally needs supervised learning. It can handle a huge amount of raw data and is beneficial to use the unlabelled dataset. So this will be helpful to make a deep learning model in cytology from the large set of unlabelled data [9].

Multimodal Data Fusion Currently, there is an explosion of data from diverse modalities, e.g., WSI, clinical, biochemical, radiological and molecular fields. The extraction of the salient features from these multimodal datasets may be extremely helpful. Multimodal data fusion is the process that integrates the data acquired from different modalities to improve the diagnostic accuracy, management, and to implement personalized medicine. The multimodal data fusion will give a new dimension in cytology [10].

Federated Learning and Edge Computing Techniques The successful and fast transfer of data are important pre-requisites for building an artificial intelligence system. The data safety is intimately related to data transfer. Federated Learning is a new, safer addition of data transfer technology. Instead of raw data sharing, here only the weights of the neural network model are shared to build a global model [11]. Therefore, it bypasses the problems of data secrecy (as no raw data is shared), data ownership and legal restriction.

In Edge Computing techniques, the code is sent to the laboratory and the data is executed locally. So, no transfer of raw data is needed in edge computing and it enhances data security [12].

Digital Twin Technology The digital twin technology is the virtual replica of a physical system. The virtual replica changes in real time with the alteration of the physical system [13]. The key features of digital twin technology are real-time synchronization and simulation.

Example In cytology, the digital twin of papillary carcinoma of the thyroid will integrate:

- Cytology and histopathology image data
- Immunocytochemistry
- Molecular data
- Management of the tumour

The digital twin will now provide the virtual replica of the papillary carcinoma and simulate the therapeutic response.

21.3 Clinical Application: What Is on the Horizon?

Early Cancer Detection and Screening: AI will take a major role in cancer detection and screening.

Cervical Cancer Screening AI can successfully detect dysplastic cells and malignant cells in papanicolaou's stained cervical smear. It is expected that in the near future, the AI system will automatically screen the cervical smear (Figs. 21.1 and 21.2). The cytopathologists may have to screen only the positive smears. This will reduce the workload and improve the efficiency of screening [14–17].

Urine The multiple studies showed the higher specificity and variable sensitivity in the detection of malignant cell in urinary cytology [18–20].
AI system may be useful in supervised screening of urinary cytology (Figs. 21.3 and 21.4).

Effusion Cytology The CNN model is useful in the detection of malignant cells in effusion cytology smears. The studies showed very high sensitivity (95%) and spec-

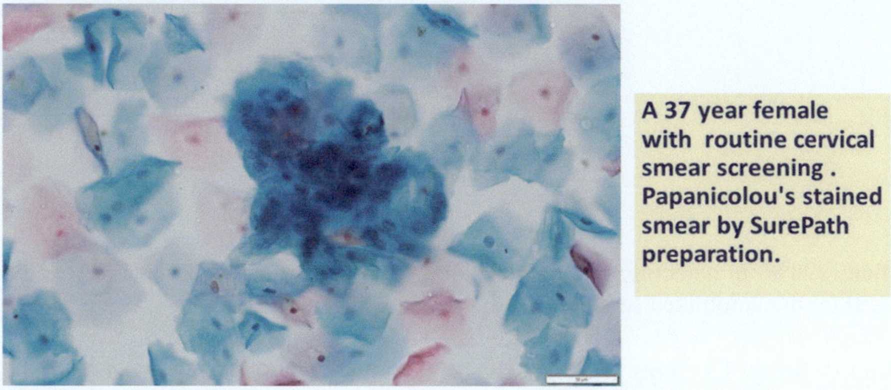

Fig. 21.1 Cervical Papanicolaou's smear for interpretation by AI

Bethesda System Interpretation

1. Specimen Type: Liquid-based cytology (SurePath)

2. Specimen Adequacy: Satisfactory for evaluation

3. General Categorization: Epithelial cell abnormality – Low-grade squamous intraepithelial lesion (LSIL)

4. Interpretation/Result:
LSIL (Low-grade Squamous Intraepithelial Lesion)The smear reveals:
- **Enlarged nuclei with irregular nuclear contours**
- **Perinuclear halos suggestive of HPV effect (koilocytosis)**
- **Background of superficial/intermediate squamous cells**

Recommendation (Based on ASCCP 2019 Guidelines)For a 37-year-old woman with LSIL:
- **If HPV testing is available: Reflex HPV genotyping (preferred):If HPV 16/18 positive → Immediate colposcopy**
- **If other high-risk HPV → Repeat in 1 year or colposcopy depending on algorithm**
- **If HPV testing not available: Proceed to colposcopic evaluation directly**
- **If HPV negative in past 5 years: Still consider colposcopy due to LSIL**

Fig. 21.2 AI-generated report of the cervical smear. Note the complete report is generated by AI

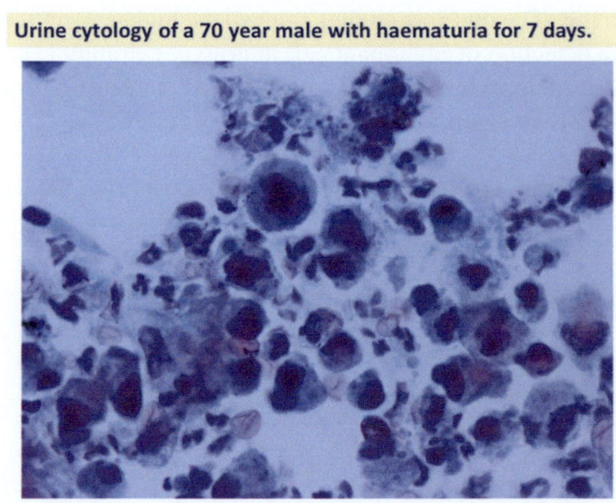

Fig. 21.3 Urine cytology smear for interpretation

ificity (98%) in detecting malignant cells in cytology smear. CNN in WSI can be used for the automated screening of malignant cells [21–23].

Liquid-Based Cytology (LBC) LBC helps to make a monolayer smear from the fluid. There are commercially available partial or totally automated LBC machines and the smears are also stained automatically by the LBC system [24]. In the future,

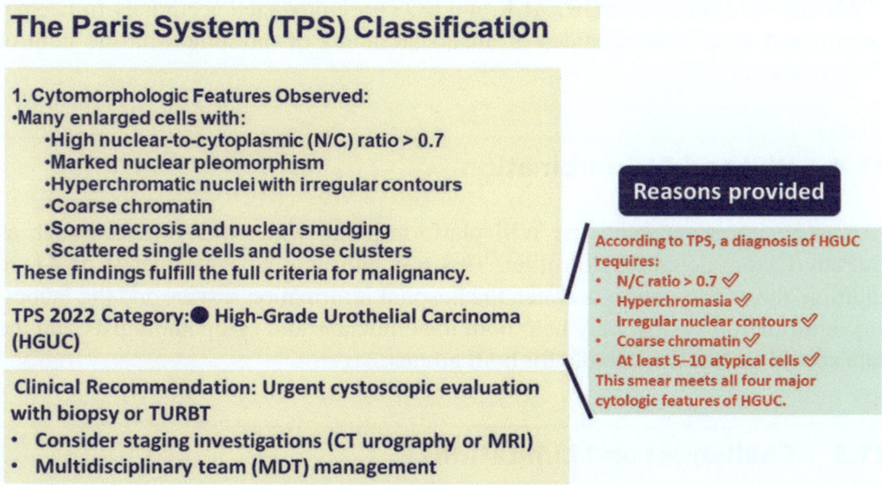

Fig. 21.4 Interpretation of urine cytology smear by AI (unaltered)

the processed and stained cytology smear prepared by the LBC system can go directly for WSI scanning.

21.3.1 Real-Time Diagnostic Assistance

On Screening Diagnosis The AI-based platform may help in on-screen immediate diagnosis of the various cytology smears including fine-needle aspiration cytology. There may be an integrated decision-support system that combines the clinical history, site of the sample and WSI imaging for the diagnosis.

Disease Classification Bethesda reporting of cervical smear, Paris classification of the urine cytology and other international classifications of different samples can be stratified by AI-integrated system.

21.3.2 Biomarker and Molecular Prediction

The AI model can detect the sub-visual changes and can accurately predict the mutational changes of various biomarkers. This prediction is very important for targeted therapy. So, an AI model can bypass the costly and time-consuming tests to detect mutational changes. Cytology smear is used for prediction of the biomarker expression [25].

Wang C-W et al. successfully predicted the BRAF (V600E) mutational changes in Papanicolaou's stained cytology smear of papillary thyroid carcinoma with an accuracy of 87%, a precision of 94%, a sensitivity of 91% and a specificity of 71%.

Mutational status of EFGR, ALK and ROS1 are predicted accurately in haematoxylin and eosin-stained slides of adenocarcinoma of the lung with the help of CNN mode [26–28].

21.4 WSI and AI Combination

AI can be integrated with the WSI platform along with other modules such as QuPath, Cytomine and CellProfiler. This will enhance the performance of AI. In addition, the collaboration between the hospital information service and the laboratory information system may help both the clinicians and cytopathologists and the data should be freely available for both groups.

21.5 Challenges and Limitations

There is little doubt about the potential impact of AI in cytopathology. However, we cannot ignore the challenges and limitations in this field.

Huge Amount of Good Quality Data To make a successful CNN model, we need well-distributed good quality data. In the real world, the quality of WSI is widely variable due to staining defect, bad smear preparation or bad quality section with artefact. WSI may also suffer from the resolution or Z-axis scanning. WSI must be in huge volume to provide a good source of training data for the CNN model. It should be collected from different sources with a clinically equal distribution of age and sex and other factors.

Approval from the Regulatory Organization The data collection, storage, transfer and utilization should be under strict regulation. There should be proper written instruction and it should be approved by the law of the country. Without appropriate rules and regulation, AI may face tremendous setbacks in the near future.

21.6 Ethical Issues: Are We Right?

Many serious ethical issues are related to AI. These issues are: (1) Lack of proper consent, (2) doubtful anonymous information, (3) risk of skewed data producing biased decision, (4) data ownership, (5) transparency and accountability of AI due to black box, (6) data security. These issues have been discussed in the previous chapter (Chap. 20).

21.7 The Role of the Cytopathologists in the New Era: Goodbye to Cytopathologists?

Many cytopathologists are sceptical about their future role in the era of AI. There is a possibility that a deep learning-based advanced model may successfully screen the WSI of the cytology smears and can accurately diagnose and classify according to the international classification. The multimodal data fusion may provide an accurate diagnosis, classification, prediction of mutation and guide for precision medicine. AI may detect the sub-visual changes in the cytology smear that are impossible for the pathologists to detect. Even immunocytochemistry scoring can be done accurately by AI. Then what is the need to hire a cytologist in the laboratory? The cytologist/ pathologist should not be afraid of losing their job. In future, only their role in the laboratory will change. They will be needed to interpret complex cases, set the goals of the AI model, validate the model in a clinical context, change the model for better tuning and give foresight to the medical system. Therefore, the cytologist/pathologist should know basics of AI and continuously learn the newer areas for the better application of AI in cytology/pathology.

21.8 Vision: A Day in the Cytology Laboratory in 2030

Imagine

The cytologist enters in the cytology laboratory. In front of him, there is a large screen and as he presses the key one by one, the whole slide image appears along with the diagnosis.

The case was a fine needle aspiration cytology smear of the thyroid.

Age: 64 year
Sex: Female
Site of FNAC: Midline neck swelling
Size: 1.2 cm diameter
Mode of FNAC: USG-guided FNAC

Microscopy: Fig. 21.5a, b
AI diagnosis: Bethesda classification: Type VI: Malignancy (not classified)

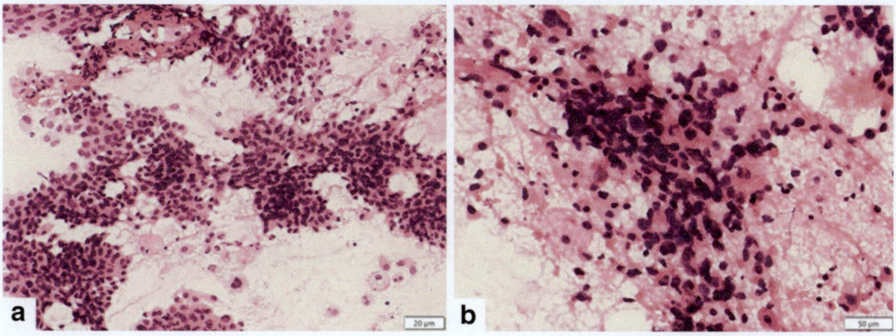

Fig. 21.5 (**a**) Multiple clusters and discrete cells with foamy macrophages in the background. (**b**) The higher magnification showed moderately pleomorphic cells with enlarged hyperchromatic nuclei (Haematoxylin and Eosin stain)

Supportive history: AI system already searched the patient's history and informs that the patient has history of carcinoma of right breast 15 days back
Ancillary tests ordered by AI: It has already ordered immunocytochemistry in cell block section for GATA3, Mammaglobin, HER2 and ER/PR
Duty of cytopathologist: The Cytopathologist approves the initial diagnosis
Next day: Immuncocytochemistry was ready (Fig. 21.6)

AI report: Metastatic carcinoma of the breast in the thyroid.
AI scoring: ER/PR and HER-2 immunostaining.
AI supplies information: All the relevant literature review and the microscopic picture for comparison.
AI Advise: Specific treatment of breast carcinoma.
Duty of cytopathologist: The Cytopathologist approves the final diagnosis. The report is written by AI and is validated by the pathologist.

Report entered in the laboratory information system.

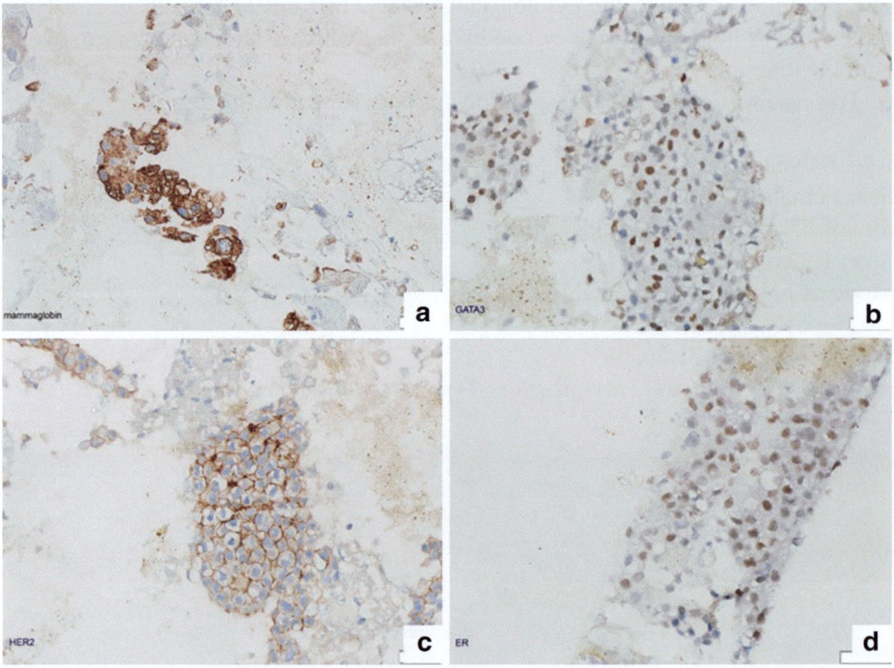

Fig. 21.6 Immunocytochemistry from the cell block section. (**a**) Mammaglobin, (**b**) GATA3, (**c**) HER2, (**d**) ER. All the stains are positive

21.9 Conclusions

AI is a new addition to the pathology laboratory. It has the full potential to help in the diagnosis, classification, interpretation of immunocytochemistry and molecular biology. It can give a holistic approach of the disease to the pathologists and the clinicians. There are certain challenges and limitations in the implementation of AI in cytology laboratories such as data acquisition, ethical issues, black box problems and recognition from the regulatory authorities. It is expected that these limitations will be overcome in the future. There is a need to have a collaboration between the pathologist, clinicians, and software engineers to unlock the new horizon. We should remember that the future of AI in pathology is not "pathologist versus AI", but rather than it is "pathologist with AI". In the future, the pathologist's effort leveraged by AI will bring more effective care to the patients.

References

1. Dey P. Artificial neural network in diagnostic cytology. Cytojournal. 2022;19:27. https://doi.org/10.25259/Cytojournal_33_2021. PMID: 35510103; PMCID: PMC9063555
2. Abiodun OI, Jantan A, Omolara AE, Dada KV, Mohamed NA, Arshad H. State-of-the-art in artificial neural network applications: a survey. Heliyon. 2018;4(11):e00938. https://doi.org/10.1016/j.heliyon.2018.e00938.
3. Hamet P, Tremblay J. Artificial intelligence in medicine. Metabolism. 2017;69S:S36–40. https://doi.org/10.1016/j.metabol.2017.01.011. Epub 2017 Jan 11. PMID: 28126242
4. Saini T, Bansal B, Dey P. Digital cytology: current status and future prospects. Diagn Cytopathol. 2023;51(3):211–8. https://doi.org/10.1002/dc.25099. Epub 2023 Jan 3. PMID: 36594526
5. Dey P. The emerging role of deep learning in cytology. Cytopathology. 2021;32(2):154–60. https://doi.org/10.1111/cyt.12942. Epub 2020 Dec 17. PMID: 33222315
6. McAlpine ED, Pantanowitz L, Michelow PM. Challenges developing deep learning algorithms in cytology. Acta Cytol. 2021;65(4):301–9. https://doi.org/10.1159/000510991. Epub 2020 Nov 2. PMID: 33137806
7. Goodfellow IJ, Pouget-Abadie J, Mirza M, et al. Generative adversarial networks. arXiv:1406.2661v1.
8. Bommasani R, Hudson DA, Adeli E, Altman R, Arora S, von Arx S, Bernstein MS, Bohg J, Bosselut A, Brunskill E, et al. On the opportunities and risks of foundation models. arXiv preprint arXiv:2108.07258; 2021.
9. Raj A, Dutta S. A review on self-supervised learning. Int J New Technol Res. 2023;9(1):6–10.
10. D'Souza NS, Wang H, Giovannini A, Foncubierta-Rodriguez A, Beck KL, Boyko O, Syeda-Mahmood TF. Fusing modalities by multiplexed graph neural networks for outcome prediction from medical data and beyond. Med Image Anal. 2024;93:103064. https://doi.org/10.1016/j.media.2023.103064. Epub 2023 Dec 27. PMID: 38219500
11. Bao G, Guo P. Federated learning in cloud-edge collaborative architecture: key technologies, applications and challenges. J Cloud Comput (Heidelb). 2022;11(1):94. https://doi.org/10.1186/s13677-022-00377-4. Epub 2022 Dec 15. PMID: 36536803; PMCID: PMC9753079
12. Gawande S, Gorde S. Edge computing in the cloud: enabling real-time data processing and analytics. J Emerg Technol Innov Res. 2014;11:206–9.
13. Shen S, Qi W, Liu X, Zeng J, Li S, Zhu X, Dong C, Wang B, Shi Y, Yao J, Wang B, Jing L, Cao S, Liang G. From virtual to reality: innovative practices of digital twins in tumor therapy. J

Transl Med. 2025;23(1):348. https://doi.org/10.1186/s12967-025-06371-z. PMID: 40108714; PMCID: PMC11921680
14. Rahaman MM, Li C, Yao Y, Kulwa F, Wu X, Li X, Wang Q. DeepCervix: a deep learning-based framework for the classification of cervical cells using hybrid deep feature fusion techniques. Comput Biol Med. 2021;136:104649.
15. Wang CW, Liou YA, Lin YJ, Chang CC, Chu PH, Lee YC, Wang CH, Chao TK. Artificial intelligence-assisted fast screening cervical high grade squamous intraepithelial lesion and squamous cell carcinoma diagnosis and treatment planning. Sci Rep. 2021;11(1):16244.
16. Holmström O, Linder N, Kaingu H, Mbuuko N, Mbete J, Kinyua F, Törnquist S, Muinde M, Krogerus L, Lundin M, Diwan V, Lundin J. Point-of-care digital cytology with artificial intelligence for cervical cancer screening in a resource-limited setting. JAMA Netw Open. 2021;4(3):e211740.
17. Hussain E, Mahanta LB, Das CR, Talukdar RK. A comprehensive study on the multi-class cervical cancer diagnostic prediction on pap smear images using a fusion-based decision from ensemble deep convolutional neural network. Tissue Cell. 2020;65:101347. https://doi.org/10.1016/j.tice.2020.101347.
18. Lebret T, Paoletti X, Pignot G, et al. Artificial intelligence to improve cytology performance in urothelial carcinoma diagnosis: results from validation phase of the French, multicenter, prospective VISIOCYT1 trial. World J Urol. 2023;41(9):2381–8.
19. Zhang Z, Fu X, Liu J, Huang Z, Liu N, Fang F, Rao J. Developing a machine learning algorithm for identifying abnormal urothelial cells: a feasibility study. Acta Cytol. 2021;65(4):335–41. https://doi.org/10.1159/000510474. Epub 2020 Oct 6. PMID: 33022673
20. Sanghvi AB, Allen EZ, Callenberg KM, Pantanowitz L. Performance of an artificial intelligence algorithm for reporting urine cytopathology. Cancer Cytopathol. 2019;127(10):658–66. https://doi.org/10.1002/cncy.22176. Epub 2019 Aug 14. PMID: 31412169
21. Park HS, Chong Y, Lee Y, Yim K, Seo KJ, Hwang G, Kim D, Gong G, Cho NH, Yoo CW, Choi HJ. Deep learning-based computational Cytopathologic diagnosis of metastatic breast carcinoma in pleural fluid. Cells. 2023;12(14):1847. https://doi.org/10.3390/cells12141847. PMID: 37508511; PMCID: PMC10377793
22. Sanyal P, Dey P. Using a deep learning neural network for the identification of malignant cells in effusion cytology material. Cytopathology. 2023;34(5):466–71. https://doi.org/10.1111/cyt.13260. Epub 2023 Jun 23. PMID: 37350108
23. Xie X, Fu CC, Lv L, Ye Q, Yu Y, Fang Q, Zhang L, Hou L, Wu C. Deep convolutional neural network-based classification of cancer cells on cytological pleural effusion images. Mod Pathol. 2022;35(5):609–14. https://doi.org/10.1038/s41379-021-00987-4. Epub 2022 Jan 10. PMID: 35013527; PMCID: PMC9042694
24. Dey P. Chapter 2: sample collection, liquid based cytology and automated screening. In: Handbook on cervical cytology: special emphasis on liquid based cytology. 2nd ed. Jaypee Brothers Medical Publishers; 2023.
25. Wang C-W, Muzakky H, Lee Y-C, Lin Y-J, Chao T-K. Annotation-free deep learning-based prediction of thyroid molecular cancer biomarker BRAF (V600E) from cytological slides. Int J Mol Sci. 2023;24(3):2521. https://doi.org/10.3390/ijms24032521.
26. Pao JJ, Biggs M, Duncan D, Lin DI, Davis R, Huang RSP, Ferguson D, Janovitz T, Hiemenz MC, Eddy NR, et al. Predicting EGFR mutational status from pathology images using a real-world dataset. Sci Rep. 2023;13:4404. https://doi.org/10.1038/s41598-023-31284-6.
27. Mayer C, Ofek E, Fridrich DE, Molchanov Y, Yacobi R, Gazy I, Hayun I, Zalach J, Paz-Yaacov N, Barshack I. Direct identification of ALK and ROS1 fusions in non-small cell lung cancer from hematoxylin and eosin-stained slides using deep learning algorithms. Mod Pathol. 2022;35:1882–7. https://doi.org/10.1038/s41379-022-01141-4.
28. Tomita N, Tafe LJ, Suriawinata AA, Tsongalis GJ, Nasir-Moin M, Dragnev K, Hassanpour S. Predicting oncogene mutations of lung Cacer using deep learning and histopathologic features on whole-slide images. Transl Oncol. 2022;24:101494.

MIX
Papier aus verantwortungsvollen Quellen
Paper from responsible sources
FSC® C105338

If you have any concerns about our products,
you can contact us on
ProductSafety@springernature.com

In case Publisher is established outside the EU,
the EU authorized representative is:
Springer Nature Customer Service Center GmbH
Europaplatz 3, 69115 Heidelberg, Germany

Printed by Libri Plureos GmbH
in Hamburg, Germany